METHODS IN MOLECULAR BIOLOGY

Series Editor
John M. Walker
School of Life and Medical Sciences
University of Hertfordshire
Hatfield, Hertfordshire, AL10 9AB, UK

For further volumes:
http://www.springer.com/series/7651

High-Throughput RNAi Screening

Methods and Protocols

Editors

David O. Azorsa

Institute of Molecular Medicine, Phoenix Children's Hospital, Phoenix, Arizona, USA

Shilpi Arora

Constellation Pharmaceuticals, Cambridge, Massachusetts, USA

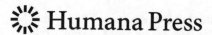 Humana Press

Editors
David O. Azorsa
Institute of Molecular Medicine
Phoenix Children's Hospital
Phoenix, Arizona
USA

Shilpi Arora
Constellation Pharmaceuticals
Cambridge, Massachusetts
USA

ISSN 1064-3745   ISSN 1940-6029   (electronic)
Methods in Molecular Biology
ISBN 978-1-4939-8168-7   ISBN 978-1-4939-6337-9   (eBook)
DOI 10.1007/978-1-4939-6337-9

Printed on acid-free paper

This Humana Press imprint is published by Springer Nature
The registered company is Springer Science+Business Media LLC New York

Preface

Ever since the discovery of small interfering RNA-mediated transcriptional inhibition by Craig Mello and Andrew Fire, there have been great advances in manipulating this cellular mechanism to achieve targeted gene silencing. Short interfering RNA (siRNA) and short hairpin RNA (shRNA) are commonly used for gene silencing and validation of gene function. Both can be implemented using standard techniques of transferring nucleic acids into cells. With the completion of the human genome project and other advances in genomics, nucleic acid sequences that target specific gene transcripts have become available. In addition, both commercial and academic institutions have made advances in chemical synthesis of double-stranded RNA and the development of large shRNA libraries. Through the use of these libraries and high-throughput methodologies, it has become possible to advance RNAi research from observing the phenotypic/cellular response after silencing a few genes to silencing hundreds or thousands of genes in a single experiment. This type of high-throughput RNAi (HT-RNAi) or loss-of-function screening has become a powerful tool in the field of functional genomics.

The power of HT-RNAi screening is in its ability to provide large amounts of functional data for a particular biological assay. These large data sets can provide valuable insight into the role of specific genes or groups of genes in a biological process. Many research groups working with various cell models and organisms from different species have recognized the potential of HT-RNAi assays. Studies have been done in whole organisms like *C. elegans* and *drosophila* as well as plant and mammalian cell systems, including established cell lines and primary cells. HT-RNAi screening in mammalian cells has routinely been applied to identify genes that modulate specific biological responses or result in a particular phenotype. Although there are many advantages in using HT-RNAi, there are also some potential downsides, particularly in mammalian cell HT-RNAi screening. These include the cost of large genome-wide libraries, the infrastructure and equipment needed to perform the assays, and the analysis and management of large data sets.

In this volume, we cover the various aspects and methodologies for performing HT-RNAi screens, including the use of various RNAi platforms and delivery methods in mammalian cells, as well as various applications such as drug sensitizer identification. We also cover methods for HT-RNAi screening in non-mammalian, whole organism and cell models including *C. elegans, drosophila, S. cerevisiae, S. frugiperda, P. patens* and zebrafish. Finally, we examined the latest advancements in the fields of assay development, library screening, data analysis, and hit selection. The goal of this volume is to provide a comprehensive source of protocols and other necessary information to make robust and successful assays possible for all who wish to use HT-RNAi in their research.

Phoenix, AZ   *David O. Azorsa*
Cambridge, MA   *Shilpi Arora*

Contents

Contributors

ANUPRIYA AGARWAL • *Division of Hematology and Medical Oncology, Department of Molecular and Medical Genetics, Oregon Health and Science University, Portland, OR, USA; Knight Cancer Institute, Oregon Health and Science University, Portland, OR, USA*

SHILPI ARORA • *Constellation Pharmaceuticals, Lexington, MA, USA*

DAVID O. AZORSA • *Institute of Molecular Medicine, Phoenix Children's Hospital, Phoenix, AZ, USA; Department of Child Health, University of Arizona College of Medicine—Phoenix, Phoenix, AZ, USA*

GEOFFREY A. BARTHOLOMEUSZ • *Division of Cancer Medicine, Department of Experimental Therapeutics, The University of Texas M.D. Anderson Cancer Center, Houston, TX, USA*

RODERICK L. BEIJERSBERGEN • *Division of Molecular Carcinogenesis and NKI Robotics and Screening Center, The Netherlands Cancer Institute, Amsterdam, The Netherlands*

MARIANA G. BEXIGA • *School of Biology and Environmental Science & UCD Conway Institute of Biomolecular and Biomedical Research, University College Dublin, Dublin, Ireland*

RAJ K. BHATNAGAR • *Insect Resistance Group, International Centre for Genetic Engineering and Biotechnology, New Delhi, India*

MICHAEL BOUTROS • *Division of Signaling and Functional Genomics, German Cancer Research Center (DKFZ), Heidelberg, Germany; Department of Cell and Molecular Biology, Medical Faculty Mannheim, Heidelberg University, Heidelberg, Germany*

ALESSANDRO CERONI • *Adaptimmune Ltd, Oxford, UK*

DANIEL V. EBNER • *Target Discovery Institute, Nuffield Department of Medicine, University of Oxford, Oxford, UK*

BASTIAAN EVERS • *Division of Molecular Carcinogenesis and NKI Robotics and Screening Center, The Netherlands Cancer Institute, Amsterdam, The Netherlands*

SUBHANITA GHOSH • *Insect Resistance Group, International Centre for Genetic Engineering and Biotechnology, New Delhi, India*

DANIEL F. GILBERT • *Institute of Medical Biotechnology and Erlangen Graduate School in Advanced Optical Technologies (SAOT), Friedrich-Alexander Universität Erlangen-Nürnberg, Erlangen, Germany; Division of Signaling and Functional Genomics, German Cancer Research Center (DKFZ), Heidelberg, Germany; Department of Cell and Molecular Biology, Medical Faculty Mannheim, Heidelberg University, Heidelberg, Germany*

GOHTA GOSHIMA • *Division of Biological Science, Graduate School of Science, Nagoya University, Nagoya, Japan*

GEOFF S. HIGGINS • *Department of Oncology, University of Oxford—Old Road Campus, Oxford, UK*

LAKESLA R. ILES • *Division of Cancer Medicine, Department of Experimental Therapeutics, The University of Texas M.D. Anderson Cancer Center, Houston, TX, USA*

KATARZYNA JASTRZEBSKI • *Division of Molecular Carcinogenesis and NKI Robotics and Screening Center, The Netherlands Cancer Institute, Amsterdam, The Netherlands*

YUN-JIN JIANG • *Institute of Molecular and Genomic Medicine, National Health Research Institutes, Miaoli, Taiwan*

MICHELLE KASSNER • *Cancer and Cell Biology Division (CCB), Translational Genomics Research Institute (TGen), Phoenix, AZ, USA*

RYAN R. KNOERDEL • *Department of Pediatrics and Cell Biology, University of Pittsburgh School of Medicine, Pittsburgh, PA, USA; Children's Hospital of Pittsburgh, Magee-Women's Hospital Research Institute, University of Pittsburgh Medical Center, Pittsburgh, PA, USA*

AJIT KUMAR • *Centre for Bioinformatics, M.D. University, Rohtak, India*

JUAN LI • *Suzhou Genoarray Biotech Co. Ltd., Suzhou, China*

PAWAN MALHOTRA • *Malaria Group, International Centre for Genetic Engineering and Biotechnology, New Delhi, India*

TOMOHIRO MIKI • *Division of Biological Science, Graduate School of Science, Nagoya University, Nagoya, Japan*

JUSTIN J. MONTOYA • *Department of Child Health, University of Arizona College of Medicine—Phoenix, Phoenix, AZ, USA; Institute of Molecular Medicine at Phoenix Children's Hospital, Phoenix, AZ, USA*

SUNIL K. MUKHERJEE • *Department of Genetics, University of Delhi South Campus, New Delhi, India*

YUKI NAKAOKA • *Division of Biological Science, Graduate School of Science, Nagoya University, Nagoya, Japan*

LINDA P. O'REILLY • *Departments of Pediatrics and Cell Biology, University of Pittsburgh School of Medicine, Pittsburgh, PA, USA; Children's Hospital of Pittsburgh, Magee-Women's Hospital Research Institute, University of Pittsburgh Medical Center, Pittsburgh, PA, USA*

STEPHEN C. PAK • *Departments of Pediatrics and Cell Biology, University of Pittsburgh School of Medicine, Pittsburgh, PA, USA; Children's Hospital of Pittsburgh, Magee-Women's Hospital Research Institute, University of Pittsburgh Medical Center, Pittsburgh, PA, USA*

ROBBIE RAE • *School of Natural Sciences and Psychology, Liverpool John Moores University, Liverpool, UK*

JANI SAARELA • *Institute for Molecular Medicine Finland (FIMM), University of Helsinki, Helsinki, Finland*

BINDIYA SACHDEV • *Insect Resistance Group, International Centre for Genetic Engineering and Biotechnology, New Delhi, India*

CARINA VON SCHANTZ-FANT • *Institute for Molecular Medicine Finland (FIMM), University of Helsinki, Helsinki, Finland*

CHRIS SEREDUK • *Cancer and Cell Biology Division (CCB), Translational Genomics Research Institute (TGen), Phoenix, AZ, USA*

TONG SI • *Carl R. Woese Institute for Genomic Biology, University of Illinois at Urbana-Champaign, Urbana, IL, USA*

GARY A. SILVERMAN • *Department of Pediatrics and Cell Biology, University of Pittsburgh School of Medicine, Pittsburgh, PA, USA; Children's Hospital of Pittsburgh, Magee-Women's Hospital Research Institute, University of Pittsburgh Medical Center, Pittsburgh, PA, USA*

JEREMY C. SIMPSON • *School of Biology and Environmental Science & UCD Conway Institute of Biomolecular and Biomedical Research, University College Dublin, Dublin, Ireland*

GATIKRUSHNA SINGH • *Insect Resistance Group, International Centre for Genetic Engineering and Biotechnology, New Delhi, India; College of Veterinary Medicine, Columbus, OH, USA*

AMIT SINHA • *University of Massachusetts Medical School, Worcester, MA, USA*

NANYUN TANG • *Cancer and Cell Biology Division (CCB), Translational Genomics Research Institute (TGen), Phoenix, AZ, USA*

CHIH-HAO TANG • *Institute of Molecular and Genomic Medicine, National Health Research Institutes, Miaoli, Taiwan*

CHAO TONG • *Life Sciences Institute and Innovation Center for Cell Signaling Network, Zhejiang University, Hangzhou, China*

LI-CHUAN TSENG • *Institute of Molecular and Genomic Medicine, National Health Research Institutes, Miaoli, Taiwan*

MEGAN A. TURNIDGE • *Department of Child Health, University of Arizona College of Medicine—Phoenix, Phoenix, AZ, USA; School of Life Sciences, Arizona State University, Tempe, AZ, USA*

JEFFREY W. TYNER • *Knight Cancer Institute, Oregon Health & Science University, Portland, OR, USA; Department of Cell, Developmental & Cancer Biology, Oregon Health & Science University, Portland, OR, USA*

HONGWEI YIN • *Cancer and Cell Biology Division (CCB), Translational Genomics Research Institute (TGen), Phoenix, AZ, USA*

HANSHUO ZHANG • *Biomedical Engineering Department, College of Engineering, Peking University, Beijing, China*

HUIMIN ZHAO • *Carl R Woese Institute for Genomic Biology, University of Illinois at Urbana-Champaign, Urbana, IL, USA; Department of Chemical and Biomolecular Engineering, University of Illinois at Urbana-Champaign, Urbana, IL, USA; Departments of Chemistry, Biochemistry, and Bioengineering, University of Illinois at Urbana-Champaign, Urbana, IL, USA*

JIA ZHOU • *Life Sciences Institute and Innovation Center for Cell Signaling Network, Zhejiang University, Hangzhou, China*

Chapter 1

Establishing an Infrastructure for High-Throughput Short-Interfering RNA Screening

Hongwei Yin, Chris Sereduk, and Nanyun Tang

Abstract

RNA interference (RNAi) is a readily available research tool that can be used to accelerate the identification and functional validation of a multitude of new candidate drug targets by experimentally perturbing gene expression and function. High-throughput RNAi technology using libraries of short-interfering RNA (siRNA) makes it possible to rapidly identify genes and biomarkers associated with biological processes such as diseases or a cellular response to therapy. Thus, RNAi-based screening is an extremely powerful technology that can provide tremendous insights into the mechanisms of action and contexts of vulnerability of a particular drug treatment. This chapter describes the infrastructure requirements needed to successfully perform HT-RNAi screening. Information on the methodology, instrumentation, experimental design, and workflow aspects is provided, as well as insights on how to successfully implement a high-throughput RNAi screen.

Key words High-throughput, RNA interference, RNAi, siRNA, Functional genomics, Screening workflow, HTS equipment

1 Introduction

High-throughput RNAi (HT-RNAi) screening has been widely applied in drug discovery and drug development for targeting diseases, such as viral infection and cancer. The application of large-scale and genome-wide RNAi has become an integral functional genomics tool for drug target identification and validation, pathway analysis, and drug discovery [1, 2]. Potential targets for anti-cancer therapies can be identified and validated with RNAi lethality screening. This type of screen can target individual oncogenes to reduce their expression, which can lead to a loss of anchorage-independent growth or a decrease in tumorigenic capacity of different tumor types [3–5]. Additionally, RNAi-based drug modifier screens called synthetic lethality screens can be used to identify enhancers or suppressors of a specific chemical compound or specific loss-of-function mutation. These screens have been shown to successfully identify important molecules that mediate drug response and

David O. Azorsa, Shilpi Arora (eds.), *High-Throughput RNAi Screening: Methods and Protocols*, Methods in Molecular Biology, vol. 1470, DOI 10.1007/978-1-4939-6337-9_1, © Springer Science+Business Media New York 2016

resistance [6–12]. A number of discoveries utilizing RNAi chemical synthetic lethality screens in different cancer types have pinpointed genes, pathways, and cellular processes that are involved in the mechanism of action of particular drugs [13]. Such studies not only provide important clues into the mechanism of action of a drug, but they also help to identify the potential rational combination strategies and functional candidates to serve as biomarkers for drug response and patient stratification. To empower such studies, this chapter will specify the steps necessary to set up the screening workflow and provide detailed materials and methods on how to prepare for HT-RNAi screening using siRNA libraries.

1.1 HT-RNAi Screening Design

It is recommended to invest the necessary time and effort into planning and customizing an HT-RNAi screen to fit the specific goals of each experiment. This would ensure a more successful screen and a greater payoff in results. One should also gather input from the discovery biology team and clinical development teams (if applicable) that are responsible for the development and study of the drug of interest. Their insight will help reveal the best questions to ask and help focus the study on specific goals and outcomes that are most relevant and useful for the development needs of that particular drug. The choice of cell lines, siRNA library, and measurement endpoints are critical factors (*see* Table 1) that these groups may be able to assist with.

Table 1
Guidelines on high-throughput RNAi synthetic lethality studies to determine genetic determinants of drug response in vitro

Parameter	Recommendation
Cell line	Limit to 2 (based on compound sensitivity, genetic context or tumor type)
Library	Smaller library (Focused pathway collection (e.g., PI3K pathway), gene family cassettes (e.g., GPCRs or kinases), disease-specific library (e.g., cancer))[a]
Assay readout	Simple homogeneous plate reader assay (e.g., Cell titer Glo) over high-content assays[b]
Drug concentration(s)*	DDR format: 7 non-zero concentration points, 1 dose per plate, with at least 2 replicate runs over single dose with replicates[c]
Controls	Pre-tested sensitizer, positive and negative controls; control plates to be included in the screen

[a]We recommend using siRNA libraries with multiple siRNAs per target (e.g., our Qiagen libraries contain four siRNAs per gene of interest)
[b]In our experience, the multiparametric nature of high-content assays poses significant challenges in data generation, quality and interpretation without robust assay development upfront. Therefore, we recommend high-content assays as a final step to gain deeper insights into biological mechanism of select targets/hits (50 max)
[c]For drug sensitizer screens, our past experience indicates that the drug dose response (DDR) format that was developed provides a powerful means for detecting shifts in drug sensitivity. Future screens would benefit from using the DDR format, but also incorporating additional replicates (2–3 per siRNA). For large-scale screens, if a choice needs to be made between number of replicates and concentration points, we recommend using more concentration points
*single concentration or multiple concentrations can be applied here.

1.1.1 Cell Line Selection

Experimental system/cell line models, such as commercial cell lines, patient-derived cell lines, patient-derived xenografts (PDX) cell lines, and iPSC cell lines, need to be chosen based on either practical or scientific grounds. Many siRNA screens will benefit from the incorporation of more than one cell line. In some instances, cell lines of the same or different genetic background or indication should be selected. In other instances, selecting cell lines with confirmed differential sensitivity toward the drug/compound of interest would be more useful. For some screens, diversity in genetic backgrounds or alternative indications may be important. A point to note for assay development (Subheading 1.2) is that time spent in assay optimization increases with the number of cell lines used. While there is likely to be a tolerable "loss" of information from fewer primary screens, subsequent post-screening follow-up analysis can incorporate diversity in terms of sensitivity, indication, genetic backgrounds, or pharmacology. For example, four cell lines with various genetic backgrounds may be selected for initial assay optimization that will test for drug sensitivity and robust and reproducible results. Based on the results of this optimization and analysis, only one cell line will be selected for primary RNAi screening. The remaining cell lines can be used during the hits validation step (Subheading 1.4).

1.1.2 Choice of the Library

As with cell line selection, the goal of each experiment should be taken into consideration when choosing a siRNA library for screening. For mechanistic and exploratory investigations, a genome-wide screen maybe helpful, but for quick results and rapid clinical transition, we recommend working with smaller focus libraries. Furthermore, running smaller initial screens over a more diverse set of cell lines may have a greater impact when studying a specific process. While large collections, such as druggable genome library, provide numerous novel hits, often times a clear application is not obvious (e.g., an unknown or lesser known gene as a combination therapy target). While smaller collections, such as those that focus on a disease of interest, gene families of interest, or a pathway of relevance, offer fewer choices, they can be rationally followed up. A point to note is that due to automation and parallel throughput, unless a library is significantly smaller, there maybe payoffs in terms of time but not cost. Whichever the choice, we recommend siRNA-based libraries and multiple siRNAs per target for the primary screen (≥ 3) and secondary validation step (≥ 4) [14]. For genome-wide screens, it maybe of economic interest to use siRNA pools. However, this may introduce pooling artifacts that can make deconvolution and follow-up challenging and time consuming.

1.1.3 Endpoint Preference

Plate-reader-based chemiluminescence assays provide cell viability endpoints and have consistently produced high quality, reproducible data in HT-RNAi screens. These endpoint assays have high sensitivity allowing for a large dynamic range and thus are commonly used in many published RNAi screens. As such, we recommend this type of readout as one of the most reliable endpoints for primary screens. An important point to note is that other assays that produce robust endpoints can be used for the primary screening, though the cost of the screen can be increased significantly. For instance, cell proliferation assays using BrdU, apoptotic assay using Caspase Glo (Promega), or cytotoxicity assays using CellTox Green (Promega) are all reliable alternatives. We also strongly recommend using the same endpoint for the hits confirmation step while exploring different secondary assays/endpoints for the hits validation step.

In addition to plate-based assays, many commercial high-content or image-based assays are also available. High-content assays have the benefit of being tightly linked with the biological question addressed. They are also more amenable to perform with time lapse and high-resolution image analysis [15]. Unfortunately, while high-content assays can be used for high-throughput screening, the flood of data obtained from the screening can be overwhelming and it may require a significantly longer time for data processing as well as data analysis [16]. However, these assays are very informative when analyzed using appropriate data analysis tools. High-content assays can also be very powerful tools for the hits validation step when following up a handful of genes or for screening of a focused library set, and they are often more manageable in these lower-throughput applications.

1.1.4 Assay Controls

It is very important to select various and suitable controls during assay development in order to properly evaluate the robustness of the assay and the upcoming screens. Analysis of all available information about the drug target, pathway of focus, disease of interest, or drug/compound of interest can be very helpful in choosing the appropriate controls. Spending some time in searching for informative assay development controls is necessary. Selecting a few genes to serve as controls based on prior knowledge and testing their ability to serve as robust controls will contribute significantly to the success of the screen. Once controls for the screens are confirmed and validated, it is important to test them against a panel of cell lines as an in vitro surrogate for expected clinical applications. This test will allow for bioinformatic analyses to be carried out, in particular, analyses of correlating genomic data with chemosensitivity profiles and retrospectively integrating sensitizer hits from a screen [17].

1.2 Assay Development and Optimization

Assay development and optimization, which involves the establishment of optimal parameters, is a critical determinant of screening success. A list of parameters to be optimized during assay development and optimization has been previously described [13]. Application of extensive assay development by our group has contributed to the generation of robust HT-RNAi data [13, 17–19].

1.3 High-Throughput Primary Screening

After taking the factors discussed above into consideration, the recommendations for each aspect of the screen are outlined in Table 1. The procedure of such a HT-RNAi primary screens is detailed in subsequent chapters.

1.4 Confirmation and Validation

The successful outcome of an HT-RNAi screen, with robust and reproducible data, requires stringent quality control as well as a multi-step confirmation and validation plan. Once hits are selected from a primary screen, they are advanced to a hit confirmation assay. This assay involves performing a small-scale screen with appropriate controls and conditions similar to those used in the primary screen. Based on our experience, we recommend confirming the top (~5–10%) hits, under conditions identical to those employed in the primary screen, to weed out false positives. In the subsequent steps, based on how large the screens are and the nature of the investigation, we recommend:

1. *Knockdown verification* of target gene expression by qPCR and/or by Western blotting/ELISA/immunocytochemistry (not always possible but recommend for high confidence hits) assays to confirm RNAi-mediated effect in ascribing phenotypic observations to target gene suppression.

2. *Testing additional siRNAs* for the target of interest. We recommend testing ≥4 siRNAs per target in secondary validation runs.

3. *Testing additional cell lines* either in isogenic cell line pairs to identify specific hits, or testing activity against in cell lines with diverse genetic backgrounds or having alternative indications.

4. *Secondary validation assays* are recommended to characterize target biology in more detail. The exact nature of the assay may differ as a function of the target pathway, biological process, or disease biology. Validated high-content assays (i.e., Acumen, Cellomics, GE InCell Analyzer) may be particularly informative in this regard. It is also important to remember that the widespread relevance of a few hits can be complicated by the genetic dependence of some cells on abnormally expressed proteins (e.g., p53 aberrations) and drug mediated pharmacodynamic effects (e.g., a marker that is over expressed upon treatment). These factors need to be evaluated in follow up studies.

1.5 Analysis

Guidelines for quality control (QC) and normalization methods for RNAi screening experiments are covered in Chapter 19. When analyzing drug sensitizer screen hit selection, we suggest excluding hits that result in high cytotoxicity due to siRNA treatment alone (without drug) since siRNA toxicity could make it difficult to ascertain any potentiation affects of drug activity. As an example, we have often excluded hits that cause >50% loss of viability from the further analysis. Other threshold values for siRNA toxicity can be obtained by using population-based methods suggested by statisticians (such as 2 or 3 standard deviations from the mean). For drug sensitizer hits, we also recommend using a multiple concentration drug dose response (DDR) format. All valid (filtering spurious point and transfection artifacts) sigmoidal drug response curves (±siRNA) should be compared in order to pick hits that demonstrate a significant shift of dose response curves with the addition of siRNA. Statistical tests like t-test (comparing IC_{50}/EC_{50} estimates), F test (curve fittings comparison), and information criteria are useful for testing significance between the two sets of data. In general, we recommend hits that show at least a three-fold EC_{50} shift with respect to the negative control. In both lethality and synthetic lethal (drug sensitizer) screens, we highly recommend applying the probability-based redundant siRNA activity (RSA) method or other similar method, which takes into account the behavior of all siRNA sequences of the same target, thus reducing the siRNA off-target effect [14].

2   Materials

2.1   Equipment

1. Biomek® FX Laboratory Automation Workstation (Fig. 1a) (Beckman-Coulter) (*see* **Note 1**).

2. Biomek® NX Laboratory Automation Workstation (Fig. 1b) (Beckman-Coulter) (*see* **Note 2**).

3. Biomek P20 96-well and P30 384-well tips (Beckman-Coulter).

4. XL20® Tube Handler (Fig. 1c) (BioMicroLab).

5. ALPS-300® thermal plate sealer (Fig. 1d) (Thermo/Abgene).

6. Allegra® 25R Plate centrifuge (Fig. 1e) (Beckman-Coulter).

7. Micronic Automatic De-capper (Fig. 1f) (Micronic).

2.2   Library Preparation and Screening

1. Lyophilized whole human genome siRNA library pre-arrayed in 96-well microplate format (Source plates): (Qiagen).

2. 96-well, round-bottom, polypropylene plates (Daughter plates).

3. siRNA buffer: 30 mM HEPES (pH 7.4), 100 mM Potassium Acetate, 2 mM Magnesium Acetate.

4. 384-well black, clear bottom, barcoded microplates (Daughter plates).

5. 384-well white, solid-bottom, barcoded microplates (Assay plates).

6. 0.65 mL Micronic 2D barcoded tubes with racks and lids (Micronic).

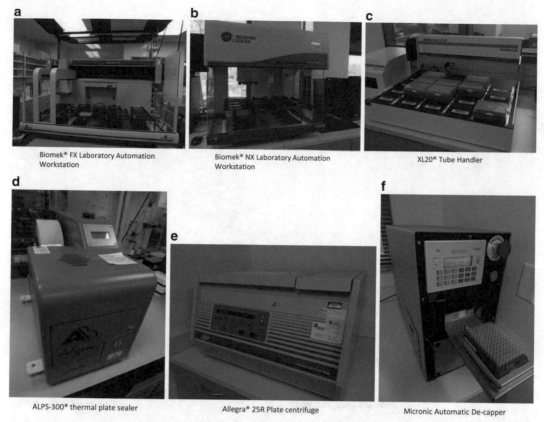

Biomek® FX Laboratory Automation
Workstation

Biomek® NX Laboratory Automation
Workstation

XL20® Tube Handler

ALPS-300® thermal plate sealer

Allegra® 25R Plate centrifuge

Micronic Automatic De-capper

Fig. 1 Equipment used for high-throughput RNAi screening. (**a**) Biomek FX workstation is a liquid handler for library plate printing. (**b**) Biomek NX workstation is a liquid handler for library preparation. (**c**) Micronic XL20 is used for hit picking 2D tubes. (**d**) ALP-300 is to seal the plates with foils. (**e**) Beckman Allegra plate centrifuge to spin down the plates and tubes. (**f**) Micronic automatic de-capper is used to un-cap the 2D tubes

3 Methods

HT-RNAi screening with siRNA begins with access to a large siRNA library. The library we use is a commercially available siRNA library supplied by Qiagen. Several commercial sources have various libraries available that target specific genes, gene families, or pathways. We routinely use a large siRNA library known as the whole human genome library (WHGv1) that contains approximately 15,000 gene targets, which includes the druggable genome library (~7000 genes) as well as the validated kinase library (711 genes). There are generally four siRNA sequences for each target, which are referred to as sequences A, B, C, and D. This library arrives in a lyophilized form contained in 888 96-well polypropylene microplates (222 plates for each of the four sequences). The original stock library is aliquoted into three working sets that will each be used for a different process (Fig. 2): a 384-well microplate set that will be used for full library screens, a 96-well microplate set that will used for replenishing the

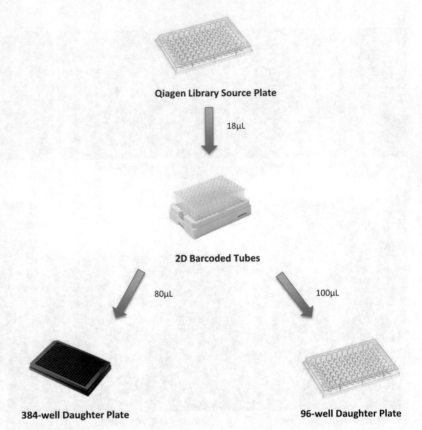

Fig. 2 Library plate preparation flowchart. The original stock library is aliquoted into three working sets: a 384-well microplate set that will be used for full library screens, a 96-well microplate set that will used for replenishing the 384-well library, and a Micronic 2D labeled tube set that will be used later for confirmation and validation

384-well library, and a Micronic 2D labeled tube set that will be used later for confirmation and validation.

3.1 Library Preparation

The following process describes the re-allocation of our stock Qiagen siRNA library into a more diverse and accessible format at a preferred working concentration (Fig. 2). The 2D tube library will provide us with the ability to access specific siRNA sequences by assigning each of them a barcode that can be easily tracked. The 384-well microplates are referred to as daughter plates and will each contain two of the four sequences. This means there will be two sets of daughter plates: an A/B set and a C/D set. The 96-well microplates are also referred to as daughter plates and will be used primarily for replenishing the 384-well daughter plates.

1. Reconstitute and thoroughly mix lyophilized library plates with 50 μL of siRNA buffer to a concentration of 20 μM, using a Biomek FX liquid handler with a 96-well head and Biomek P20 tips (*see* **Note 3**).

2. Manually remove 50 μL from the following wells in Column 12 of the Qiagen library plates and add 50 μL of the corresponding stock controls at a 20 μM concentration (*see* **Note 4**):

(a) C12: Allstar non-silencing negative control siRNA (Qiagen)

(b) D12: Non-silencing negative control siRNA (Qiagen)

(c) E12: UBBs1 positive control siRNA (Qiagen)

(d) F12: ACDC positive control siRNA (Qiagen)

(e) G12: Non-silencing negative control siRNA (already supplied in library plate) (Qiagen)

(f) H12: Qiagen GFP negative control (already supplied in library plate) (Qiagen)

(g) A12 and B12: Qiagen siRNA buffer (already supplied in library plate)

3. Label the 2D tube racks and the 96-well daughter plates (e.g., DGv3_A01_667nM) (*see* **Note 5**).

4. Pre-fill 2D tubes with siRNA buffer.

(a) Remove column 1 from 2D tube racks and column 1 tips from Biomek P20 tip box (see Note 6).

(b) Dispense 522 μL of siRNA buffer into the 2D tube racks using Biomek NX liquid handler with 96-well head and Biomek P20 tips (see Note 7).

5. Pre-fill 384-well daughter plates and 96-well daughter plates with siRNA buffer.

(a) Manually dispense 100 μL of siRNA buffer to each well in column 1 of the 96-well daughter plates using a 96-well multi-channel pipette (see Note 6).

(b) Manually dispense 80 μL of siRNA buffer to each well in columns 1 and 2 of the 384-well daughter plates using a 384-well multi-channel pipette (*see* **Note 6**).

6. Perform transfer method on Biomek FX.

(a) Remove tips from column 1 of Biomek P20 tip box to account for the manually added buffer columns.

(b) Transfer 18 μL from the Qiagen library source plate to the corresponding pre-labeled and pre-filled 2D tube rack and mix using Biomek FX with 96-well head and Biomek P20 tips and mix thoroughly (see Note 8).

(c) Transfer 100 μL from the 2D tube rack to corresponding pre-labeled 96-well daughter plate using the same Biomek P20 tips (*see* **Note 8**).

(d) Transfer 80 μL from the 2D tube rack to 384-well daughter plate using the same Biomek P20 tips. Four different

2D tube racks make up one 384-well daughter plate (1 quadrant per tube rack) (*see* **Note 8**).

7. Seal the 96-well daughter plates, the 384-well daughter plates, and the 96-well Qiagen library plates using an Abgene microplate heat sealer and store the plates at –20 °C (*see* **Note 9**).

8. Cap the 2D tube racks using a manual capper and 2D tube caps, and record gene sequences and their corresponding 2D barcodes in the database (*see* **Note 10**).

9. The library now consists of:

    (a) Original Qiagen library plates (888 total)—32 μL [20 μM]

    (b) 96-well daughter plates (888 total)—100 μL [667 nM]

    (c) 384-well daughter plates (222 total)—80 μL [667 nM]

    (d) 2D tube racks (888 total)—360 μL [667 nM]

3.2 Preparation of Screening Plates

Assay plates for screening are prepared in advance.

1. Remove the 384-well daughter plates from –20 °C to thaw at room temperature for 1 h.

2. Centrifuge daughter plates for 1 min. at $200 \times g$ in the Beckman plate centrifuge.

3. Transfer 1 μL from each well of the 384-well daughter plates to the corresponding wells of pre-barcoded 384-well assay plates using a Biomek FX with a 384-well head and Biomek P30 tips (*see* **Note 11**).

4. Seal the daughter plates and the assay plates using a microplate heat sealer (*see* **Note 9**).

5. Return the daughter plates to –20 °C. Store the assay plates at –80 °C until needed for screening (*see* **Note 12**).

3.3 Hitpicking for Assay Validation/ Confirmation

Hitpicking involves choosing a specific set of sequences from the 2D tube library by utilizing the database of siRNA sequences and their corresponding barcodes.

1. Generate a hitpick list from the database based on the genes/sequences of interest. This list will be formatted for the BioXL software and will indicate which of the 2D tubes and racks will be needed (*see* **Note 13**).

2. Remove the necessary 2D tube racks from –20 °C and re-array 2D tubes into an empty 2D tube rack using the BioXL system.

3. Thaw the re-arrayed tube racks at room temperature for 2 h and centrifuge in a plate centrifuge for 20 s at $200 \times g$.

4. De-cap tubes using Micronic de-capper.

5. Transfer the desired volume from the 2D tubes to a 384-well daughter plate using the Biomek FX with 96-well dispense head and tips (*see* **Note 14**)

6. Transfer 1 µL of siRNA from the 384-well daughter plate to 384-well assay plate(s) using the Biomek FX using a 384-well dispense head and Biomek P30 tips.

7. Seal the daughter plates and the assay plates using a microplate heat sealer and store the printed plates at –80 °C until needed for screening.

8. Re-cap 2D tubes using a manual capper.

9. Return the 2D tubes to their original location in the 2D tube rack using a reverse hitpick worklist on the BioXL system.

10. Return the 2D tube racks to storage at –20 °C.

4   Notes

1. An alternate liquid handler may be used, but it will need to accurately dispense a 1 µL volume to a 384-well microplate with CV <5 %.

2. It may be possible to use the same liquid handler to dispense the 384-well assay and daughter plates, 96-well daughter plates, and 96-well 2D tubes. However, this will likely require changing the dispense head. For this reason, we use separate, dedicated instruments.

3. The library can be purchased in different moles/sequence of siRNA. It will contain specifications for reconstitution to a 20 µM concentration, thus the final volume may vary.

4. This step is only to introduce additional positive and/or negative controls. Other controls may be used (e.g., GFP) or this step may be omitted altogether, as Qiagen provides their own positive and negative controls already in the plate.

5. It is important to pre-label as many components as possible. This will help ensure that the library is transferred accurately to the appropriate daughter plates. We prefer a labeling system indicating library_plate #_concentration. However, label according to your own needs.

6. The first column in every plate of the stock library is a buffer-only column. By removing the column at this time and manually filling this column in the corresponding daughter plates eliminates having hundreds of 2D tubes that are filled with only buffer.

7. The final volume will be 540 µL after 18 µL of 20 µM siRNA stock is added, for a final library concentration of 667 nM. This will give us a final assay concentration of 13 nM (when we use a 50 µL-assay), which is a high enough concentration to observe knockdown, but low enough to minimize off-target hits (false positives).

8. **Steps 6b**, **6c** and **6d** are performed using one method (or script) written on the Biomek FX.

9. Plates can be sealed manually using standard foil plate seals if a plate sealer is not available.

10. This is a simple spreadsheet database that associates each siRNA sequence with a specific 2D barcoded tube.

11. This is essentially making exact copies of the 384-well daughter plate. We prefer to make multiple copies of the daughter plate to allow for multiple cell lines or multiple replicates being screened. This also avoids multiple freeze and thaw cycles of the 384-well daughter plate.

12. Because of the extremely low volume of the assay plates and to avoid potential evaporation, we prefer to store the 384-well assay plates at an additionally protective temperature of –80 °C for long-term storage –20 °C is sufficient for short-term storage.

13. This file is generated according to our preferred layout. We can group specific genes together and/or leave blank spaces for additional controls or buffer to be added. It is exported as a text file to be used on the BioXL system.

14. This is a necessary intermediate step due to the low volume that is dispensed to the assay plates in the next step. This volume will vary based on the number of assay plates needed. It is advisable to consider future use of this specific daughter plate and adjust volume accordingly. The minimal working volume for the daughter plates is 5 μL to account for dead volume in the well.

Acknowledgments

We would like to thank TGen for their support and Mr. Donald Chow for providing the images as well as critical discussion.

References

1. Caldwell JS (2007) Cancer cell-based genomic and small molecule screens. Adv Cancer Res 96:145–173

2. Perrimon N, Friedman A, Mathey-Prevot B et al (2007) Drug-target identification in Drosophila cells: combining high-throughout RNAi and small-molecule screens. Drug Discov Today 12:28–33

3. Berns K, Horlings HM, Hennessy BT et al (2007) A functional genetic approach identifies the PI3K pathway as a major determinant of trastuzumab resistance in breast cancer. Cancer Cell 12(4):395–402

4. Giroux V, Iovanna J, Dagorn JC (2006) Probing the human kinome for kinases involved in pancreatic cancer cell survival and gemcitabine resistance. FASEB J 20:1982–1991

5. Schlabach MR, Luo J, Solimini NL et al (2008) Cancer proliferation gene discovery through functional genomics. Science 319:620–624

6. Whitehurst AW, Bodemann BO, Cardenas J et al (2007) Synthetic lethal screen identification of chemosensitizer loci in cancer cells. Nature 446(7137):815–819

7. Iorns E, Lord CJ, Ashworth A (2009) Parallel RNAi and compound screens identify the PDK1 pathway as a target for tamoxifen sensitization. Biochem J 417:361–370

8. MacKeigan JP, Murphy LO, Blenis J (2005) Sensitized RNAi screen of human kinases and phosphatases identifies new regulators of apoptosis and chemoresistance. Nat Cell Biol 7:591–600

9. Bartz SR, Zhang Z, Burchard J et al (2004) A large-scale RNAi screen in human cells identifies new components of the p53 pathway. Nature 428:431–437

10. Brummelkamp TR, Fabius AW, Mullenders J et al (2006) An shRNA barcode screen provides insight into cancer cell vulnerability to MDM2 inhibitors. Nat Chem Biol 2(4):202–206

11. Morgan-Lappe S, Woods KW, Li Q et al (2006) RNAi-based screening of the human kinome identifies Akt-cooperating kinases: a new approach to designing efficacious multi-targeted kinase inhibitors. Oncogene 25(9):1340–1348

12. Turner NC, Lord CJ, Iorns E et al (2008) A synthetic lethal siRNA screen identifying genes mediating sensitivity to a PARP inhibitor. EMBO J 27:1368–1377

13. Yin H, Kiefer J, Kassner M et al (2010) The application of high-throughput RNAi in pancreatic cancer target discovery and drug development. In: Drug discovery in pancreatic cancer. Springer Science + Business Media, LLC, New York, NY, pp 153–170

14. König R, Chiang CY, Tu BP et al (2007) A probability-based approach for the analysis of large-scale RNAi screens. Nat Methods 4(10):847–849

15. Haney SA (2008) High content screening: science, techniques and applications. Wiley-Interscience, New York

16. Gasparri F (2009) An overview of cell phenotypes in HCS: limitations and advantages. Expert Opin Drug Discov 4(6):643–657

17. Kiefer J, Yin HH, Que QQ et al (2009) High-throughput siRNA screening as a method of perturbation of biological systems and identification of targeted pathways coupled with compound screening. Methods Mol Biol 563:275–287

18. Luo Q, Kang Q, Song WX et al (2007) Selection and validation of optimal siRNA target sites for RNAi-mediated gene silencing. Gene 395(1-2):160–169

19. Alabi CA, Love KT, Sahay G et al (2013) Multiparametric approach for the evaluation of lipid nanoparticles for siRNA delivery. Proc Natl Acad Sci U S A 110(32):12881–12886

Chapter 2

Optimization of Transfection Conditions for siRNA Screening

Justin J. Montoya and David O. Azorsa

Abstract

RNAi screening of mammalian cells is often performed using siRNAs and cationic lipids as transfection reagents. Efficiency of transfection depends on growth characteristics of the cells and the cationic lipid used. With a large selection of cationic lipids available, it can often be difficult to select the optimal lipid and lipid:siRNA (vol:wt) ratio. Here, we describe the process of optimizing siRNA transfection conditions for efficient reverse transfection of mammalian cells using specific positive and negative siRNA controls.

Key words siRNA, Cationic lipid, RNAi screening, Assay

1 Introduction

There are multiple methods currently being used for transfecting siRNA into cells including cationic lipid or polymer mediated transfection, electroporation, and viral mediated transduction [1]. Initial protocols for introducing siRNA into eukaryotic cells were similar to those introducing other nucleic acids such as plasmid DNA. These methods primarily involved the use of cationic lipids [2]. Although the use of cationic lipids provided efficient transfection, the complexing of siRNA with the lipid was a step that made it difficult to adapt for high throughput screening. Reverse transfection of nucleic acids, a method originally developed for cell arrays [3], was eventually adapted to plate-based high throughput siRNA screening [4, 5] as a more manageable alternative to forward cationic lipid transfection. The use of reverse transfection has allowed for siRNA screening to be expanded to many more cell types than the easily transfectable HeLa and HEK-293 cells; however, these cell types may have different transfection efficiencies under the same transfection conditions. In order to improve siRNA transfection conditions, many laboratories use a transfection optimization assay that helps select the best transfection reagent and lipid:siRNA (vol:wt)

David O. Azorsa, Shilpi Arora (eds.), *High-Throughput RNAi Screening: Methods and Protocols*, Methods in Molecular Biology, vol. 1470, DOI 10.1007/978-1-4939-6337-9_2, © Springer Science+Business Media New York 2016

ratio for most cell types. We have successfully used this approach to optimize siRNA transfection for many cell types, including ovarian cancer [6], pancreatic cancer [7], Ewing sarcoma [8], AML, and fibroblast cell lines [9]. This simple technique optimizes high throughput siRNA screening using 384-well plates, and utilizes negative control non-silencing siRNAs and positive control lethal siRNAs, both of which are commercially available. Moreover, the assay can test several commercially available transfection reagents at various ratios at once. The resulting conditions from this optimization step can rapidly be applied to siRNA library screening.

2   Materials

Prepare reagents in a BSL2 laboratory safety hood at room temperature (unless indicated otherwise) and use RNase-free water. Maintain a sterile RNase-free environment using proper PPE, tissue culture, and biohazard waste disposal techniques.

2.1   siRNA Plate Printing Components

1. Negative control siRNA: AllStar Negative Control siRNA (Qiagen) or Non-silencing siRNA (Qiagen). Reconstitute the siRNA in RNase-free water at room temperature to make 20 µM stock reagent. Store at –20 °C for long-term use.

2. Positive control siRNA: AllStars Hs Cell Death siRNA (Qiagen). Reconstitute the siRNA in RNase-free water at room temperature to make 20 µM stock reagent. Store at –20 °C for long-term use.

3. White 384-well plates, tissue culture treated (Greiner Bio-One).

4. RPMI-1640 medium.

5. 12-channel pipette. Pipette must be able to effectively dispense 2 µl of liquid.

6. 50 ml reservoirs (Must be of appropriate length to support 12-channel pipette delivery, and preferably one with a ridge for low volumes).

7. Foil adhesive seals for 384-well plates.

2.2   Transfection Reagent Dilution Components

1. Cationic lipid transfection reagents. *See* Table 1 for a list of commercially available transfection reagents.

2. Opti-MEM® reduced serum medium (Thermo Fisher).

3. Sterile, polypropylene 2 ml deep 96-well plate.

4. 8-channel pipette. Pipette must effectively dispense 1000 µl of liquid.

5. 12-channel pipette. Pipette must effectively dispense 20 µl of liquid.

6. Incubator set to 37 °C and 5 % CO_2.

Table 1
Commercially available transfection reagents

siRNA transfection reagent	Supplier	Source
DeliverX	Affymetrix	http://www.affymetrix.com
siLentFect™	Bio-Rad	http://www.bio-rad.com
Xfect	Clontech	http://www.clontech.com
DharmaFECT 1 Transfection Reagent	Dharmacon	http://dharmacon.gelifesciences.com
DharmaFECT 2 Transfection Reagent	Dharmacon	http://dharmacon.gelifesciences.com
DharmaFECT 3 Transfection Reagent	Dharmacon	http://dharmacon.gelifesciences.com
DharmaFECT 4 Transfection Reagent	Dharmacon	http://dharmacon.gelifesciences.com
RiboJuice™ siRNA Transfection Reagent	EMD Millipore	http://www.emdmillipore.com
GeneSilencer® Transfection Reagent	Genlantis	http://www.genlantis.com
Torpedo siRNA Transfection Reagent	ibidi	http://ibidi.com
TransIT-TKO® Reagent	Mirus	https://www.mirusbio.com
TransIT-siQUEST® Reagent	Mirus	https://www.mirusbio.com
siTran	OriGene	http://www.origene.com
Lullaby	OZBiosciences	http://www.ozbiosciences.com
INTERFERin®	Polyplus	http://www.polyplus-transfection.com
HiPerFect Transfection Reagent	Qiagen	https://www.qiagen.com
X-tremeGENE	Roche	https://lifescience.roche.com
GenJet™ siRNA Transfection Reagent	SignaGen® Laboratories	http://signagen.com
siRNA Transfection Reagent	Santa Cruz Biotechnology	http://www.scbt.com
MISSION® siRNA Transfection Reagent	Sigma-Aldrich	http://www.sigmaaldrich.com
Lipofectamine® RNAiMax Transfection Reagent	ThermoFisher Scientific	https://www.thermofisher.com
Lipofectamine® LTX with Plus™ Reagent	ThermoFisher Scientific	https://www.thermofisher.com

2.3 Cell Plating Components

1. Cells to be tested.
2. Trypsin.
3. Phosphate-Buffered Saline (PBS).
4. RPMI 1640 media supplemented with 10% fetal bovine serum and 2 mMl-glutamine (*see* **Note 1**).
5. 15 ml conical tubes.
6. Centrifuge with the capacity to spin 15 ml conical tubes.
7. 12-channel pipette. Pipette must effectively dispense 20–200 µl of liquid.
8. CO_2 Incubator.

2.4 Bioluminescence Assay Components

1. Cell-Titer Glo (CTG; Promega).
2. Orbital plate shaker.
3. Luminescence plate reader.

3 Methods

The following method describes a siRNA reverse transfection assay for optimization of four transfection reagents in human cell lines using a luminescent-based viability assay. Sufficient reagents are prepared to test three assay plates that correspond to three variables, usually different cell lines, cell densities, incubation times, assay plates, etc. We refer to each assay as a Transfection Reagent Test or TRT. Printing of the TRT plates can be done using a variety of control siRNAs, though we routinely use a non-silencing control siRNA and a lethal positive control siRNA. A final plate layout of the printed TRT plate is shown in Fig. 1. Additional control siRNAs can be found in Table 2.

3.1 Transfection Reagent Test Printing

1. In separate reservoirs, dilute 40 µl of stocks (20 µM negative control siRNA and 20 µM positive control siRNA) in 2.5 ml RPMI media (without additives) and mix well (*see* **Note 2**).
2. Remove the lids of ten 384-well plates for printing (*see* **Note 3**).
3. Using a 12-channel pipette, transfer 2 µl of negative control siRNA to all wells in rows C-F of a 384-well assay plate (*see* **Notes 4** and **5**).
4. Transfer 2 µl of positive control siRNA to all wells in rows K-N.
5. Transfer 2 µl of dilution buffer to all wells in rows G-J (*see* **Note 6**)
6. Seal plates with foil plate seal for long-term use.
7. Label plates and store at −80 °C.

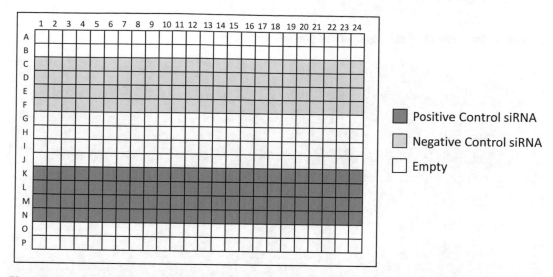

Fig. 1 Plate layout for printing of siRNA onto Transfection Reagent Test (TRT) plate. Desired amount of siRNA is printed onto the plate in a low volume of 1–2 μl using a multichannel pipet. Printed plates can be sealed and stored at −80 °C until needed

3.2 Transfection Reagent Test Set Up

1. Before beginning the TRT assay, remove the selected number of TRT plates from the freezer and thaw to room temperature.

2. In a 2 ml deep 96-well plate, add 1 ml of Opti-MEM to each well of rows A and B.

3. Add 1–5 μl of the first transfection reagent, in 1-μl increments, to wells A2–A6, respectively as indicated in Fig. 2.

4. Add 1–5 μl of the second transfection reagent to wells A7–A11, respectively.

5. Repeat **steps 3** and **4** in row B for the third and fourth transfection reagents (*see* Fig. 2).

6. Mix well by using a multichannel pipette with six tips, changing tips with each set.

7. Using a 12-channel pipette, transfer 20 μl of diluted transfection reagent from Row A of the 96-well plate to the odd numbered columns of an assay plate (*see* **Notes 7** and **8**).

8. Repeat this process for transferring the diluted transfection reagents in Row B of the 96-well plate to the even columns of the assay plate.

9. Check the plate for complete transfer of transfection reagents. The completed pattern should resemble Fig. 3.

10. Allow the transfection reagent and siRNA to complex for 30 min at room temperature.

Table 2
Commercially available siRNA negative and positive controls

Positive control siRNA	Supplier	Source
AccuTarget Control siRNA	Bioneer	http://us.bioneer.com/
ON-TARGETplus Cyclophilin B Control siRNA	Dharmacon	http://dharmacon.gelifesciences.com
Control siRNA Duplex Beta-aactin	Eurogentec	http://www.eurogentec.com
Trilencer-27 siRNA	ORIGENE	http://www.origene.com
AllStars Hs Cell Death Control siRNA	Qiagen	https://www.qiagen.com/
MISSION® Positive Control siRNA	Sigma-Aldrich	http://www.sigmaaldrich.com
Silencer® GAPDH	ThermoFisher Scientific	https://www.thermofisher.com
Negative Control siRNA	Supplier	Source
Negative Control siRNA vector	Abcam	http://www.abcam.com/
AccuTarget Control siRNA	Bioneer	http://us.bioneer.com/
ON-TARGETplus Non-targeting Control siRNAs	Dharmacon	http://dharmacon.gelifesciences.com
Control siRNA Duplex Negative Control	Eurogentec	http://www.eurogentec.com
Trilencer-27 Universal Scramble negative control siRNA	ORIGENE	http://www.origene.com
AllStars Negative Control siRNA	Qiagen	https://www.qiagen.com/
MISSION® siRNA Universal Negative Control #1	Sigma-Aldrich	http://www.sigmaaldrich.com
Silencer® Negative Control No. 1 siRNA	ThermoFisher Scientific	https://www.thermofisher.com

3.3 Cell Plating

While the siRNA and transfection reagents are complexing, the cells can be prepared for plating. This protocol can be used for both adherent cells and cells grown in suspension. Cells should be in logarithmic growth phase and have high viability.

1. Wash the cells in PBS, trypsinize the cells as needed and resuspend them in 5 ml of fresh growth media without antibiotics. Transfer the cell suspension to a 15 ml conical tube.

2. Count the cells and transfer 1.5 million cells to a 50 ml conical tube.

3. Add growth media without antibiotics to bring the volume to 30 ml (*see* **Note 9**) and transfer the cells to a reagent reservoir.

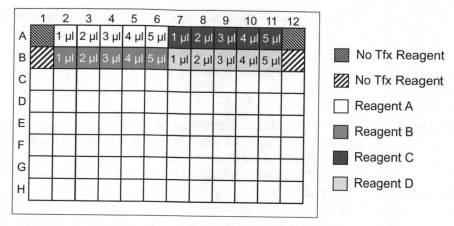

Fig. 2 Plate layout for transfection reagent dilution preparation. In a 2 ml deep 96-well plate containing Opti-MEM, the indicated amount (1–5 µl) of four different transfection reagents is added. The diluted transfection reagents can then be added to the TRT assay plate. One plate preparation can test up to three TRT plates

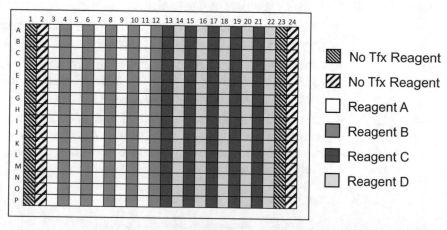

Fig. 3 Plate layout of the distributed transfection reagents on a TRT assay plate. The diluted transfection reagents are added to the TRT assay plates using a 12-channel pipette. Reagents from row A of the 96-well preparation plate are added to the odd numbered columns and reagents from row B are added to the even numbered columns. After allowing the siRNA and transfection reagents to complex for 30 min, cells are added to initiate reverse transfection

4. Using a 12-channel pipette, add 20 µl of cells to all of the wells in the assay plate (*see* **Note 10**).

5. Place the plate in an incubator at 37 °C and 5 % CO_2 for 72–96 h.

3.4 Cell Viability Assay

1. Remove the plates from incubator and allow them to equilibrate to room temperature.

2. Prepare Cell-Titer Glo and equilibrate to room temperature. Transfer to a reagent reservoir.

3. Using a 12-channel pipette, add 25 μl of CTG to all wells in the assay plate (*see* **Note 10**).

4. Place the assay plate on an orbital shaker at 200 rpm for 30 min to complete cell lysis.

5. Read the assay plate using a luminescence reader.

3.5 Data Analysis

Data is analyzed to determine the optimal transfection reagent and ratio for the selected cell line and assay condition. We routinely normalize the data to the "no transfection reagent" and "no siRNA" controls in columns 1–2 and 23–24 and call this "% Control." The most optimal condition(s) will have the lowest cell viability for the positive control (lethal) siRNA and little to no decrease in viability with the negative control siRNA. A decrease in cell viability in conjunction with increasing amounts of cationic lipids in the buffer samples indicates cationic lipid toxicity. An efficient transfection reagent and cationic lipid ratio for a tested cell line can usually be ascertained by this assay.

1. Transfer raw data as a spreadsheet.

2. Normalize data to the average of the "no transfection reagent/ no siRNA" wells (wells G1-J2, G23-J24) (*see* **Note 11**).

3. Calculate the % control of each well by dividing by average of the "no transfection reagent/no siRNA" well as follows: % control well $X = (\mathrm{RLU}\,X / \mathrm{RLU}_{\mathrm{Control}}) \times 100$.

4. Plot the % control values (Fig. 4) and select the transfection reagent and ratio which shows the greatest and least toxicity induced by the positive and negative control siRNAs, respectively (*see* **Note 11**).

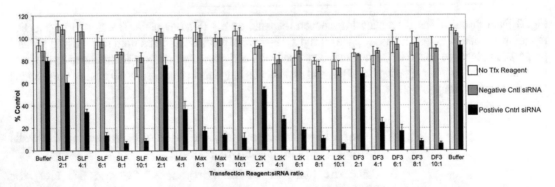

Fig. 4 Representative data from a TRT analysis of MCF-7 breast cancer cells. The raw data from the Cell-Titer Glo assay in RLU is normalized to the average of the "no transfection reagent" well containing only buffer. The normalized average of four wells per complex is plotted showing standard deviation. Transfection reagents analyzed include siLentFect (SLF), RNAiMAX (Max), Lipofectamine 2000 (L2K) and Dharmafect 3 (DF3). The preferred transfection reagent and ratio that showed a high % control without siRNA and with negative control siRNA and low % control with the positive (lethal) control siRNA (i.e., SLF at 2:1 or Max at 4:1)

4 Notes

1. Antibiotics should not be added to the growth medium as they may interfere with transfection efficiency. We routinely use RPMI-1640 media, though this protocol can be adjusted for cells using any growth media.

2. The selection of the 384-well plate is important. We have noticed transfection efficiency difference between plates from different manufacturers. If the high throughput screening demands a specific type of plate, we recommend testing several for transfection efficiency difference.

3. The siRNA can also be diluted in an siRNA dilution buffer for printing. We use RPMI since its color allows for visual confirmation of low volume printing, and comparison of diluents showed no difference in the assay results. Diluting the siRNA in 2.5 ml of media will be sufficient to print ten siRNA test assay plates.

4. Printing of 2 µl of diluted siRNA/well can be achieved by using a programmable 12-channel pipette with a 2–20 µl volume range. Setting the pipette to pick up 16 µl and dispense 8×2 µl will thus print one plate per pick up.

5. Using a printed volume of 2 µl of diluted siRNA and a final well volume of 40 µl results in an assay concentration of 16 nM siRNA. Adjustments can be made in dilution of the control siRNA and diluted cationic lipid to obtain the desired assay concentrations and volumes.

6. If using non-supplemented RPMI media as the siRNA diluent, addition of RPMI media can be omitted.

7. Printing of 20 µl of diluted transfection reagent can be achieved by using a programmable 12-channel pipette with a 20–200 µl volume range. Setting the pipette to pick up 160 µl and dispense 8×20 µl will thus dispense enough diluted transfection reagent to complete dispensing onto half of a plate.

8. When dispensing into wells, angle tips at a 45° angle and make sure they are touching the side half way down the well. The plate can be centrifuged at $100 \times g$ for 30 s to bring liquid to the bottom.

9. For most fast growing adherent cells, we seed 500–1000 cells/well. For slower growing cells or adherent cells a higher cell concentration can be used.

10. Liquid transfers that involve dispensing to all the wells of a 384-well plate can be done using a microplate-based liquid dispenser such as a Multidrop (Thermo) or a Multiflo (BioTek).

11. Although this TRT test should help identify an optimal transfection condition, it should be repeated if one is not found. We usually aim to see at least 70% toxicity by the positive control siRNA and less than 10% toxicity using the negative control siRNA. Follow up TRT assay can include the testing of other transfection reagents.

References

1. Kim TK, Eberwine JH (2010) Mammalian cell transfection: the present and the future. Anal Bioanal Chem 397(8):3173–3178. doi:10.1007/s00216-010-3821-6

2. Brazas RM, Hagstrom JE (2005) Delivery of small interfering RNA to mammalian cells in culture by using cationic lipid/polymer-based transfection reagents. Methods Enzymol 392:112–124. doi:10.1016/S0076-6879(04)92007-1

3. Ziauddin J, Sabatini DM (2001) Microarrays of cells expressing defined cDNAs. Nature 411(6833):107–110. doi:10.1038/35075114

4. Aza-Blanc P, Cooper CL, Wagner K, Batalov S, Deveraux QL, Cooke MP (2003) Identification of modulators of TRAIL-induced apoptosis via RNAi-based phenotypic screening. Mol Cell 12(3):627–637

5. Henderson MC, Azorsa DO (2013) High-throughput RNAi screening for the identification of novel targets. Methods Mol Biol 986:89–95. doi:10.1007/978-1-62703-311-4_6

6. Arora S, Bisanz KM, Peralta LA, Basu GD, Choudhary A, Tibes R, Azorsa DO (2010) RNAi screening of the kinome identifies modulators of cisplatin response in ovarian cancer cells. Gynecol Oncol 118(3):220–227. doi:10.1016/j.ygyno.2010.05.006

7. Azorsa DO, Gonzales IM, Basu GD, Choudhary A, Arora S, Bisanz KM, Kiefer JA, Henderson MC, Trent JM, Von Hoff DD, Mousses S (2009) Synthetic lethal RNAi screening identifies sensitizing targets for gemcitabine therapy in pancreatic cancer. J Transl Med 7:43. doi:10.1186/1479-5876-7-43

8. Arora S, Gonzales IM, Hagelstrom RT, Beaudry C, Choudhary A, Sima C, Tibes R, Mousses S, Azorsa DO (2010) RNAi phenotype profiling of kinases identifies potential therapeutic targets in Ewing's sarcoma. Mol Cancer 9:218. doi:10.1186/1476-4598-9-218

9. Arora S, Beaudry C, Bisanz KM, Sima C, Kiefer JA, Azorsa DO (2010) A high-content RNAi-screening assay to identify modulators of cholesterol accumulation in Niemann-Pick type C cells. Assay Drug Dev Technol 8(3):295–320. doi:10.1089/adt.2009.0240

Chapter 3

High Throughput siRNA Screening Using Reverse Transfection

Carina von Schantz and Jani Saarela

Abstract

RNA interference (RNAi) is a commonly used technique to knockdown gene function. Here, we describe a high throughput screening method for siRNA mediated gene silencing of the breast cancer cell line MDA-MB-231 using reverse transfection. Furthermore, we describe the setup for two separate methods for detecting viable and dead cells using either homogenous assays or image-based analysis.

Key words RNAi, Reverse transfection, Gene silencing, Acoustic droplet ejection, siRNA screening, High throughput screening

1 Introduction

RNA interference (RNAi) mediated gene knockdown [1] is a widely used method to study gene functions. Introduction of a double stranded short interfering RNA (siRNA) into a cell allows formation of an RNA-induced silencing complex (RISC), which degrades the associated messenger RNA. siRNAs are used to link the identity of a gene with a function. Reducing the expression of specific genes one at a time shed light on various intracellular pathways and disease mechanisms. In plate-based reverse transfection of siRNAs, siRNAs are first mixed with the transfection reagent to form complexes within wells of a multiwell plate. Subsequently, cells suspended in medium are added to the wells, allowing the siRNA complexes to enter the cells. Reverse transfection is shown to be a more efficient transfection method than the traditional forward transfection method, where the transfection reagent is added on top of previously plated cells. It also requires smaller amounts of siRNAs and is able to silence larger numbers of cells/well [2, 3]. Reverse transfection is often used in high throughput RNAi screening because it also allows separating the preparation of the assay plates from the actual screening phase. High throughput screening (HTS) provides a practical method to investigate large numbers of

David O. Azorsa, Shilpi Arora (eds.), *High-Throughput RNAi Screening: Methods and Protocols*, Methods in Molecular Biology, vol. 1470, DOI 10.1007/978-1-4939-6337-9_3, © Springer Science+Business Media New York 2016

siRNAs, or siRNA libraries, in miniaturized in vitro assays to identify those capable of modulating the biological target of interest [4]. High throughput siRNA screens are typically performed in 384-well plate format, allowing for screening in low (µl-scale) volumes. HTS involves the usage of automation and large-scale sample processing [5]. Acoustic droplet ejection (ADE) technology provides the means to dispense very low volumes of liquid with high precision in noncontact fashion. The benefits of ADE are many: automated siRNA transfer to assay plates; increased quality due to accurate dispensing; reduced siRNA, plate, and reagent costs; ability to screen at a medium to high throughput; and randomized placement of combinations across plates [6].

In our laboratory, we prepare assay plates by transferring siRNAs from library plates onto assay plates using ADE, and store the assay plates in –20 °C until needed in screening [7]. We use reverse transfection with adherent cell lines and monitor the proliferation and death of cells using homogenous assays, often combined with live cell imaging. Alternatively, cells are fixed and stained with antibodies for microscopic imaging. When the specific assay tolerates usage of assay-ready cells, we use these cells in siRNA experiments to disconnect the workflow of preparing the cells from the screening procedure. This also helps to improve consistency between experiments. We have optimized several different cell lines for the siRNA screening pipeline where we most often use 384-well plates and typically incubate the cells for 3–5 days prior to final readout. As an example, here we describe how siRNA screening for the breast cancer cell line MDA-MB-231 is performed at the FIMM High Throughput Biomedicine unit using a homogenous cell viability readout or imaging (*see* Fig. 1 for an overview of the protocol).

2   Materials

2.1   siRNA Library

1. Purchase the siRNA library from a commercial vendor in tubes or in multiwell plates. If acoustic droplet ejection using Labcyte Echo equipment is used for siRNA transfer, order the siRNA library on Labcyte Echo® Qualified 384-Well Polypropylene Source Microplates (384PP) (*see* **Notes 1** and **2**).

2. To dissolve the siRNAs, add DEPC-treated sterilized Milli-Q water to reach a concentration of 1–10 µM. For 0.1 nmol of siRNA, add 40 µL of water for a 2.5 µM stock concentration. Mix 30 min with gentle shaking at room temperature (RT) and spin down. If the siRNA library is in a multiwell plate, seal the plate with an adhesive plate seal (for example Corning® 384 Well Microplate Aluminum Sealing Tape, Non sterile). Store dissolved siRNA libraries at –20 °C (*see* **Note 3**).

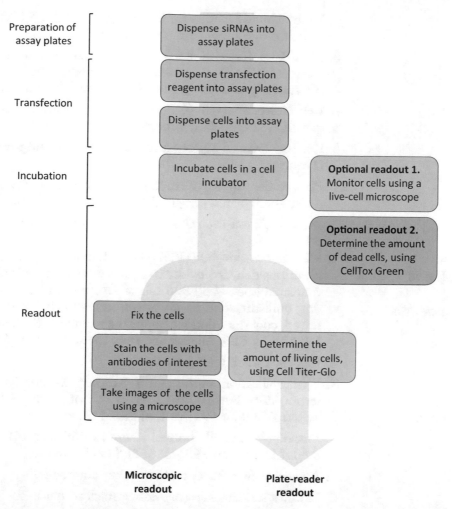

Fig. 1 Workflow for siRNA-mediated gene silencing in plate-based high throughput screening. Using acoustic dispensing, assay plates can be prepared in advance and stored until transfection of cells. The transfected cells can be monitored during incubation using live cell imaging prior to final plate reader based or microscopic readouts

2.2 Reagents and Equipment for Reverse Transfection

1. Lipofectamine® RNAiMAX Transfection Reagent (Thermo Fisher Scientific).

2. 10 mL and 50 mL tubes for liquids (Corning).

3. 384-well assay plates: Corning® 384 Well Flat Clear Bottom White Polystyrene TC-Treated Microplates, Sterile (Product #3707; #3712 for clear bottom black plates).

4. Opti-MEM® I Reduced Serum Medium, without phenol red (Thermo Fisher Scientific).

5. Phosphate-buffered saline (PBS; 1×): 137 mM NaCl, 2.7 mM KCl, 10 mM Na_2HPO_4, 1.8 mM KH_2PO_4, adjust the pH to 7.4 using HCl and then add H_2O to 1 L.

6. 70 % ethanol: 70 % ethanol diluted with sterilized Milli-Q H_2O.

7. Echo® Liquid Handler for Screening and OMICS (Echo 550) or Echo® 525 Liquid Handler (Labcyte).

8. MultiFlo™ FX with RAD module; 5 µL increment single-channel RAD peri cassettes with plastic tips (BioTek). Alternatively, Multidrop Combi dispenser (Thermo Scientific).

9. CellTiter-Glo® Assay (CTG) or CellTiter-Glo® 2.0 Assay for detecting viable cells (Promega).

10. CellTox™ Green Cytotoxicity Assay for detecting dead cells (Promega).

11. Plate reader capable of reading luminescence and fluorescence on 384-well plates, e.g., PHERAstar FS (BMG Labtech).

12. Incucyte Zoom-live cell imager (Essen BioScience).

2.3 Reagents and Equipment for Fixing and Staining Cells

1. 8% paraformaldeyhde (PFA): For 1 L of 8% PFA, add 80 g of paraformaldehyde powder to a glass beaker on a stir plate in a ventilated hood. Add 800 mL of 1× PBS and heat while stirring until the solution clears (do not let it boil). When dissolved, cool the solution. Adjust the volume of the solution to 1 L with 1× PBS. Aliquot and store the solution at –20 °C.

2. PBS (*see* earlier description).

3. Permeabilization buffer: 0.3% Triton™ X-100/5% normal serum/PBS. For 100 mL, add 5 mL of serum, 300 µL of Triton X-100 into 94.7 mL of PBS. Mix well.

4. Blocking buffer: 5% normal serum in PBS. For 100 mL add 5 mL of serum into 95 mL of PBS (*see* **Note 4**).

5. Assay-specific primary and secondary antibodies.

6. Hoechst nuclear stain (or another nuclear stain).

7. Jumbo Mobile filter trolley (Ourex Oy).

8. Multidrop Combi dispenser (Thermo Scientific).

9. 70% ethanol: 70% ethanol diluted with H_2O.

10. Milli-Q H_2O.

11. EL406 plate washer/dispenser (BioTek).

12. Olympus ScanR high content screening system (or equivalent microscope).

3 Methods

Before starting with the actual screen, carefully plan the assay plate layout in advance. Plan how each library or control siRNA and its replicates should be placed within the plate. For transfection controls, negative and positive controls are needed. The positive control should give a phenotype easy to detect, e.g., cell death. A "scrambled" siRNA that doesn't target any gene in the genome is usually used as a negative control. The negative control shouldn't give any aberrant phenotype. It is preferable to include a few wells with only cells as well, to compare this phenotype to the one from the negative control (Fig. 2). If available, specific internal controls can be used to detect the phenotype of interest in that specific assay.

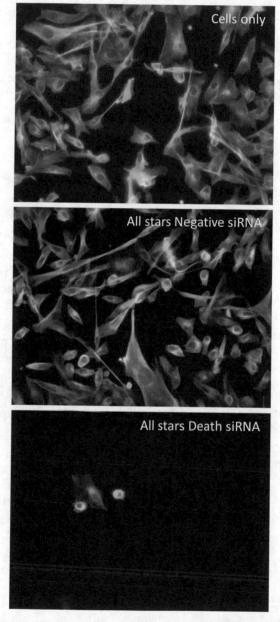

Fig. 2 MDA-MB-231 cells visualized by microscopic readout. MBA-MB-231 cells were transfected with All Stars Negative or All Stars Positive control siRNA. In the *top panel*, non-transfected cells are shown. Nuclei of the cells are stained with Hoechst, while actin is stained with Phalloidin (*red*) and tubulin with a *green-labeled* antibody

Choose assay plate type according to choice of readout. To detect luminescence, choose a white walled plate (e.g., Corning #3707). White walled plates will result in a higher signal for luminescent assays, because they reflect the light maximally. White plates are, however, not the preferred option for microscopic assays, because they tend to result in higher background fluorescence. For staining and imaging cells with fluorescent markers, choose a black walled plate (e.g., Corning #3712).

3.1 Dispensing siRNAs into Assay Plates Using Labcyte Echo® Liquid Handler

The final volume on the assay plates will be 25 µL/well (including transfection reagent, siRNA and cell suspension). The final concentration of siRNAs will be 10 nM. The stock concentration for control siRNAs is 10 µM, whereas the stock concentration for library siRNAs is 2.5 µM.

1. Design the assay plate layout and prepare ECHO transfer files (*see* **Note 1**).

2. Thaw siRNA library plates and equilibrate to RT.

3. Spin down the siRNA library plates for 1 min at $220 \times g$ (*see* **Note 5**).

4. Prepare a source plate for the control siRNAs by pipetting the siRNAs manually on an Echo source plate (*see* **Note 6**).

5. Transfer siRNAs to assay plates using Labcyte Echo 550 or 525. Transfer 25 nL of each control siRNA to the assay plates into at least 16–32 wells per plate. Transfer 100 nL of library siRNAs onto assay plates (*see* **Note 2**).

6. Check visually that transfers were successful. The assay plates can be used right away or used later. Keep (sealed) plates in –20 °C until used (*see* **Note 3**).

3.2 Dispensing Transfection Reagent into Assay Plates Using BioTek MultiFlo FX Dispenser

1. Equilibrate assay plates at RT.

2. Use 10–50 mL tubes for dispensing the wash solutions and the transfection reagent mix.

3. For each transfection well, 50 nL of transfection reagent is mixed with 4.95 µL of Opti-MEM (OM) and the total dispensed volume per well is 5 µL. Multiply these volumes with the amount of transfected wells in order to calculate the total volume of the transfection reagent/OM mix that is needed and an extra 2 mL of total mixture to take into account the dead volume of the BioTek MultiFlo FX with 5 µL single-channel RAD cassette. Mix well (*see* **Note 7**).

3.2.1 Washing the Instrument Before Use

1. Prime the BioTek MultiFlo FX cassette (5 µL increment, single channel) with 3 mL of sterile Milli-Q H_2O.

2. Prime the cassette with 3 mL of 70% EtOH.

3. Prime the cassette with 3 mL of sterile Milli-Q H_2O.

4. Prime the cassette with 2 mL of sterile 1× Opti-MEM and empty the tubing.

3.2.2 Dispensing the Transfection Reagent

1. Check the settings of the BioTek MultiFlo FX (dispense 5 μL/ well into the desired layout).

2. Prime the cassette with the transfection reagent mixture in short pulses until the air bubbles disappear from the tubing and liquid is dispensed from the tip (*see* **Note 8**).

3. Prime very shortly and dispense transfection reagent to assay plates.

4. Move the plates to a plate shaker. Shake the assay plates at 450 rpm for at least 15 min (do not exceed 2 h) at RT before adding the cells.

3.2.3 Washing the Instrument After Use

1. Prime the BioTek MultiFlo FX cassette with 6 mL of sterile Milli-Q H_2O.

2. Prime the cassette with 6 mL of sterile Milli-Q H_2O from a second tube.

3. Prime the cassette with 6 mL of 70% EtOH.

4. Empty the tubing by purging.

3.3 Dispensing of Cells onto Assay Plates Using BioTek MultiFlo FX Dispenser

3.3.1 Washing the Instrument Before Use

1. Prime the BioTek MultiFlo FX cassette with 6 mL of sterile Milli-Q H_2O.

2. Prime the cassette with 6 mL of 70% EtOH.

3. Prime the cassette with 6 mL of sterile Milli-Q H_2O.

4. Prime the cassette with 6 mL of sterile cell culture medium and subsequently empty the tubing.

3.3.2 Dispensing the Cells

Prepare the cell suspension while assay plates are in shaker.

1. Thaw an ampule of assay ready cells and wash the cells with normal culture medium (*see* **Note 9**).

2. Count the cells with a hemocytometer or an automated cell counter.

3. Suspend the cells in normal culture medium: 25,000 cells/mL in a 50 mL conical tube. Prepare enough cell suspension to allow for priming with 6 mL of cell suspension.

4. Check the settings of the BioTek MultiFlo FX (dispense 20 μL/well into the desired layout).

5. Prime the BioTek MultiFlo FX cassette with 6 mL of the cell suspension.

6. Dispense cells into the assay plates (*see* **Note 10**).

7. Place assay plates into a humidified 37 °C cell incubator with 5% CO_2 and incubate the cells for 72–120 h.

8. *Optional*: Image cells using Incucyte ZOOM. IncuCyte ZOOM is a live-cell microscope that resides in a cell incubator. Incucyte is used for kinetic cell monitoring and surveillance. These measurements can be performed label-free without disturbing the cells. This readout can be combined with any other

readout of interest. Some fluorescent markers, e.g., CellTox Green, can be also monitored during incubation.

3.3.3 Washing the Instrument After Use

1. Prime the BioTek MultiFlo FX cassette with 6 mL of sterile PBS.
2. Prime the cassette with 6 mL of sterile Milli-Q H_2O.
3. Prime the cassette with 6 mL of 70 % EtOH.
4. Empty the tubing by purging.

3.4 Determine the Amount of Dead Cells Using CellTox Green (Optional Readout)

CellTox Green is a fluorescent dye that enters dying eukaryotic cells and binds to nuclear DNA. The fluorescent signal correlates with loss of eukaryotic cell viability and can be normalized to positive and negative controls to give a fractional measure of cell death or cell viability [8]. CellTox Green can be used in combination with e.g., CellTiter-Glo.

1. CellTox Green is added to assay plates 24 h after transfection using acoustic dispensing. Transfer 12.5 nL of CellTox Green per well to 384-well plate (final dilution 1:2000). Alternatively, dilute CellTox Green with medium (1:400) and transfer 5 μL per well to 384-well plate using BioTek MultiFlo FX. Put plates back into cell incubator.
2. Prior to CellTiter-Glo measurement, read fluorescence from screening plates using a plate reader (e.g., BMG Labtech Pherastar FS). The data are normalized to negative and positive control wells. Alternatively, imaging can be used to detect living cells and the nuclei of dead cells.

3.5 Determine the Amount of Living Cells Using Cell Titer-Glo (Alternative Readout 1)

CellTiter-Glo (CTG) is a highly sensitive single-step homogeneous assay for the quantification of viable cells. The luminescence produced is proportional to the amount of ATP present, an indicator of cellular metabolic activity [9].

1. After 3–5 day incubation, take out the assay plates from the incubator and let them equilibrate at RT.
2. Let CTG equilibrate at RT.
3. 25 μL of CTG is needed for each transfected well. Multiply this volume with the amount of transfected wells to get the total volume of CTG. Then add an extra 10 mL to allow for priming the Thermo Multidrop Combi dispenser.

3.5.1 Washing the BioTek MultiFlo FX Dispenser Before Use

1. Prime the cassette with 50 mL of sterile Milli-Q H_2O.
2. Prime the cassette with 50 mL of 70 % EtOH.
3. Prime the cassette with 50 mL of sterile Milli-Q H_2O. Leave the tubes empty before priming with CTG.

3.5.2 Dispensing CTG

1. Prime the BioTek MultiFlo FX cassette with 10 mL of CTG (*see* **Note 8**).

2. Check the settings of the BioTek MultiFlo FX (384 standard plate, 25 μL/well) and dispense.

3. Move the assay plates to a plate shaker. Shake the plates at 450 rpm for 5 min.

4. Spin the plates for 5 min ($220 \times g$) in order to remove air bubbles from the wells.

3.5.3 Washing the BioTek MultiFlo FX Dispenser After Use

1. Prime the cassette with $50 + 50$ mL of sterile Milli-Q H_2O.

2. Prime the cassette with 25 mL of 70% EtOH.

3. Empty the tubing by purging.

3.5.4 Detecting Luminescence Using Plate Reader

1. Read luminescence from screening plates using a plate reader (e.g., BMG Labtech Pherastar FS). The data are normalized to negative and positive control wells.

3.6 Fixing and Staining the Cells with Antibodies for Microscopic Imaging (Alternative Readout 2)

Intracellular organelles and biomolecules can be visualized with immunofluorescence [10] using a fluorescence microscope. Fluorescently labeled antibodies bind their antigens and allow visualization of their target molecule in the sample. Several different antibodies can be combined (e.g., several parameters can be measured from the same cell at the same time) as long as they are coupled with different fluorochromes. A nuclear dye, such as Hoechst, is also useful when using high throughput microscopy to focus the microscope based on the cell nucleus and to calculate the number of cells per microscope image based on the amount of nuclei.

3.6.1 Washing the Thermo Multidrop Combi Dispenser Before Use

1. Prime the Multidrop cassette with sterile 50 mL of Milli-Q H_2O (*see* **Note 10**).

2. Prime with 50 mL of 70% PBS. Leave the tubes empty before priming with PFA.

3.6.2 Fixing the Cells with PFA

1. Prime the cassette with 5 mL of 8% PFA (*see* **Notes 8** and **12**).

2. Check the settings of the Multidrop Combi (384 standard plate, 25 μL/well) and dispense. Incubate for 20 min at RT.

3.6.3 Washing the Thermo Multidrop Combi Dispenser After Use

1. Prime the cassette with sterile 50 mL of 1× PBS.

2. Prime the cassette with 50 mL of sterile Milli-Q H_2O.

3. Wipe the tips with a tissue paper.

4. Empty the tubing by purging

3.6.4 Staining the Cells with Antibodies, Using the BioTek EL406 Plate Washer

1. Run the washing programs for the EL406 (washing the manifold and the syringes), while incubating the PFA (*see* **Note 13**).

2. Wash away the PFA with PBS, using the EL406 (in short; 3× (aspirate, then add 50 μL of PBS/well from syringe A)).

3. Add 20 μL of permeabilization buffer/well with the EL406 (in short; aspirate and add 20 μL of buffer/well from syringe B). Incubate at RT for 15 min.

4. Wash away the permeabilization buffer with PBS, using the EL406 (in short; 3× (aspirate, then add 50 μL of PBS/well from syringe A)).

5. Add 20 μL of blocking buffer/well with the EL406 (in short; aspirate and add 20 μL of buffer/well from syringe A). Incubate at RT for 60 min.

6. Wash the peri-pump for the EL406, while incubating the blocking buffer (prime with Milli-Q H_2O, 70 % EtOH, Milli-Q H_2O; 5 mL of each).

7. Dilute the primary antibody of interest in the blocking buffer according to previously optimized concentrations. Make the dilution in a conical tube (15 mL tube for smaller volumes and 50 mL for bigger volumes). Mix well.

8. Add 10 μL of antibody dilution/well with the EL406 (in short; aspirate and add 10 μL antibody/well from peri-pump). Incubate at RT for 60 min (*see* **Note 14 and 15**).

9. Wash the peri-pump for the EL406, while incubating the primary antibodies (by priming with 10 mL of PBS).

10. Wash away the antibody with PBS×3, using the EL406 (in short; 3× (aspirate, then add 50 μL of PBS/well from syringe A)).

11. Dilute the secondary antibody of interest in PBS according to previously optimized concentrations. Make the dilution in a conical tube (15 mL tube for smaller volumes and 50 mL for bigger volumes). Mix well. Cover with a foil to protect the fluorophores from light. Add Hoechst (or another nuclear stain) to the dilution according to previously optimized concentrations.

12. Add 10 μL of secondary antibody dilution/well with the EL406 (in short; aspirate and add 10 μL antibody/well from peri-pump) (*see* **Note 14 and 15**). Incubate at RT for 60 min. Keep the plates covered from light.

13. Wash away the antibody with PBS×3 using the EL406; 3× (aspirate, then add 50 μL of PBS/well from syringe A). The volume of the final addition of PBS is 80 μL/well.

14. Store the plates at 4 °C covered from light.

15. Run the washing programs for the EL406 (washing the manifold and the syringes).

16. Wash the peri-pump of the EL406 (prime with Milli-Q H_2O, 70 % EtOH, Milli-Q H_2O, 5 mL of each).

17. Use a high throughput inverted microscope (e.g., Olympus ScanR) for imaging the plates. Depending on the assay, 10–40× objectives are recommended. Four to nine image fields of view should at least be recorded for each well. If plates have been stored in 4 °C, let them equilibrate at RT before imaging.

4   Notes

1. siRNAs can be purchased also in tubes. In this case, dissolve the siRNAs in the tubes by adding DEPC-treated sterilized Milli-Q water to reach a concentration of 1–10 μM. Then transfer the siRNAs manually by pipetting onto Echo® 384LDV or 384PP plate for transferring onto assay plates with acoustic dispensing. We use barcodes on all of our library and assay plates to track the plates through the pipeline from making the assay plates to analyzing the results.

2. It's recommended to use at least three different siRNA sequences/gene when performing a siRNA screen. In larger screens, such as full genome screens, all three different sequences can be pooled in the same well, in order to reduce cost and time. If pooling, the final siRNA concentration is to remain the same as in single siRNA experiments. If the primary screen is pooled, a secondary screen should be performed where the siRNAs of the hits are screened once more separately.

3. Avoid repeated freeze-thaw cycles of the siRNA stock plates. For short-term storage of the stock plates 4 °C is recommended.

4. When making the blocking buffer, keep in mind that the blocking buffer is also used for the washing steps before the primary antibodies and that the primary antibodies are diluted into it. Therefore make enough buffer for all of these steps.

5. Spin down the source plate before using it to remove air bubbles.

6. Consider how many sets are printed at once, what the total volumes of the controls are (for all the printed assay plates in total), and how much extra control siRNA is needed to use in order to cover for the dead volume. If larger than 8 μL total volume/siRNA are transferred, a Labcyte Echo® 384PP plate is recommended. In cases of smaller volumes, the Echo® LDV plate is preferable. The dead volumes for 384LDV and 384PP plates are; 3 μL and 20 μL, respectively. The working volumes of these plates are: 384LDV 3–12 μL, 384PP 20–50 μL (15–65 μL for Omics 2 calibrations). The remaining liquid can be collected back from the source well after the transfer to be used later.

7. Always pipet Opti-MEM first into the tube and subsequently transfection reagent into the Opti-MEM.

8. Check that the liquid is coming out straight from the dispensing tips and that there are no droplets or bubbles in the dispensing tips; wipe the tips with a tissue paper if needed.

9. Making and using assay ready cells: Prepare freezing medium by mixing 90% FBS and 10% DMSO (e.g., 90 mL FBS and 10 mL DMSO to prepare 100 mL of freezing medium). Use cells that are in an exponential growth phase. Wash cells twice with PBS and detach cells from the culture bottle. Re-suspend

the cells in 10 mL complete medium required for that cell type. Calculate the total number of cells using a hemocytometer. Centrifuge the cell suspension at $100-200 \times g$ for 3 min. Remove the supernatant carefully. Re-suspend the cell pellet in cold freezing medium to get the right cell density/mL medium (we are routinely using 1–2 million cells/mL). Dispense 1 mL aliquots of the cell suspension into cryogenic storage vials. Place the cryovials containing the cells in an isopropanol chamber and store them at −80 °C overnight and subsequently transfer frozen cells to a liquid nitrogen tank. When thawing cells, take a cell vial form the liquid nitrogen and thaw it quickly in a water bath (37 °C). Transfer the cells to a conical tube and add complete medium, mix well, spin down as described previously, and remove the supernatant. Wash the cells twice. Re-suspend the cells in 10 mL complete medium, count cells and finally re-suspend the cells in the complete medium to obtain the right amount of cells/mL needed for assay.

10. While dispensing the cells, it is important to gently mix the cell suspension. This can be done by gently mixing a 50 mL conical tube by hand. If dispensing to a large number of assay plates, a small flat bottom plastic bottle with a small flea can be used and cells can be mixed using a magnetic stirrer.

11. We have a dedicated Multidrop cassette for PFA only. This cassette is only washed with PBS and Milli-Q (before and after use), to avoid fixing the tubing. It is recommended to use only standard size cassette to dispense PFA.

12. All procedures involving paraformaldehyde (PFA) should be carried out under a fume hood to avoid exposure to toxic formaldehyde vapors. We use 8 % PFA for fixing cells. 25 µL of 8 % PFA is added straight on living cells in 25 µL of media in the well resulting in 4 % PFA. This helps to preserve sensitive cells that could otherwise be easily detached by a plate washer. Some pins of the manifold get clogged rather easily. After the manifold wash program is completed, the manifold should be tested using an empty clear bottom plate. First, dispense a small amount of PBS in each well of the plate, then aspirate the PBS, and visually check whether every well is empty. If needed, rerun the wash program until every well is empty after aspiration.

13. PFA should be collected separately as toxic waste. We are using a portable Jumbo mobile filter trolley, which is placed above the EL406 to reduce the PFA fumes from spreading into the lab.

14. We have a dedicated 1 µL peri-pump cassette for antibody staining, from which tubing has been cut as short as possible to reduce the dead volume.

15. When aspirating with the BioTek EL406 plate washer/dispenser, the wells are not aspirated completely dry. When adding antibodies, the concentration should not be diluted by the

excess liquid remaining in the wells. We therefore shortly spin the plate upside-down in a plate centrifuge with a piece of paper placed between the plate and the lid to collect the extra liquid. We also keep the now moist paper in place between the plate and the lid during the 1 h incubation in order to keep the wells humidified and to prevent evaporation of the antibody.

References

1. Fire A, Xu SQ, Montgomery MK, Kostas SA, Driver SE, Mello CC (1998) Potent and specific genetic interference by double-stranded RNA in Caenorhabditis elegans. Nature 391:806–811

2. Amarzguioui M (2004) Improved siRNA-mediated silencing in refractory adherent cell lines by detachment and transfection in suspension. Biotechniques 36:766–770

3. Ovcharenko D, Jarvis R, Hunicke-Smith S, Kelnar K, Brown D (2005) High-throughput RNAi screening in vitro: from cell lines to primary cells. RNA 6:985–993

4. Pereira DA, Williams JA (2007) Origin and evolution of high throughput screening. Br J Pharmacol 152(1):53–61

5. Kiefer J, Yin HH, Que QQ, Mousses S (2009) High-throughput siRNA screening as a method of perturbation of biological systems and identification of targeted pathways coupled with compound screening. Methods Mol Biol 563:275–287

6. Griffith D, Northwood R, Owen P, Simkiss E, Brierley A, Cross K, Slaney A, Davis M, Bath C (2012) Implementation and development of an automated, ultra-high-capacity, acoustic, flexible dispensing platform for assay-ready plate delivery. J Lab Autom 5:348–358

7. Pietiainen V, Saarela J, von Schantz C, Turunen L, Östling P, Wennerberg K (2014) The High Throughput Biomedicine unit at the Institute for Molecular Medicine Finland: high throughput screening meets precision medicine. Comb Chem High Throughput Screen 17:377–386

8. Chiaraviglio L, Kirby JE (2014) Evaluation of impermeant, DNA-binding dye fluorescence as a real-time readout of eukaryotic cell toxicity in a high throughput screening format. Assay Drug Dev Technol 12(4):219–228

9. Hannah R, Beck M (2001) Celltiter-Glo™ luminescent cell viability assay: a sensitive and rapid method for determining cell viability. Promega Cell Notes

10. Fritschy J-M, Härtig W (2001) Immunofluorescence. Encyclopedia of Life Science. doi: 10.1038/npg.els.0001174

Genome-Wide siRNA Screening Using Forward Transfection: Identification of Modulators of Membrane Trafficking in Mammalian Cells

Mariana G. Bexiga and Jeremy C. Simpson

Abstract

RNA interference (RNAi) has become an essential tool for molecular and cellular biologists to dissect cell function. In recent years its application has been extended to genome-wide studies, enabling the systematic identification of new cell regulation mechanisms and drug targets. In this chapter, a protocol for a genome-wide RNAi screen coupled to high-content microscopy is presented. Specifically we describe key features of assay design, plate layout, and a protocol for forward transfection of small interfering RNAs (siRNAs) in a 384-well plate format. As an example of its application in identifying modulators of membrane trafficking, we also provide a protocol to measure the efficacy of intracellular delivery of the B subunit of Shiga-like toxin to the Golgi complex. Finally we show an automated image analysis routine that can be used to extract single cell data from the screen, thereby providing a quantitative ranking of how a large panel of siRNAs affects this biological process.

Key words Genome-wide RNAi screen, High-content microscopy, Image analysis, Membrane trafficking, Mammalian cells

1 Introduction

RNA interference (RNAi) is a conserved biological response to the presence of double-stranded RNA, which mediates resistance to both endogenous parasitic and exogenous pathogenic nucleic acids, and regulates the expression of protein-coding genes [1]. Due to its characteristics, researchers have used RNAi as a tool to selectively study the function of genes, and with the advent of genome-wide libraries of small interfering RNAs (siRNAs) targeting different organisms, its application is now possible in a truly systematic way. RNAi screens, when combined with fluorescence-based imaging readouts, are particularly powerful as they facilitate the study of processes at a genome level, providing a level of phenotypic information that has not been possible using classical genetic approaches. Genome-wide RNAi screens have identified

David O. Azorsa, Shilpi Arora (eds.), *High-Throughput RNAi Screening: Methods and Protocols*, Methods in Molecular Biology, vol. 1470, DOI 10.1007/978-1-4939-6337-9_4, © Springer Science+Business Media New York 2016

new genes, or gene networks, that are involved in a wide variety of biological functions such as cell division [2], apoptosis [3], and protein secretion [4] to name a few. To facilitate the implementation of this technology, several genome-wide RNAi libraries have been developed and are commercially available.

Here we present a protocol to perform genome-wide RNAi screening in cultured mammalian cells using forward transfection. The type and variety of phenotypic outputs from such screens are totally determined by the biological question being addressed, but large-scale RNAi screens are often combined with automated high-content screening microscopy, as this provides large volumes of complex image data that can be interrogated in multiple ways in a quantitative manner. One common readout type is to look for changes in distribution of a fluorescence marker in the presence of a particular siRNA molecule. In the example detailed here, we describe how this technology can be used to study membrane trafficking, specifically of the Shiga-like toxin B subunit (SLTxB) as it moves from the plasma membrane of cells to the Golgi complex [5], and we present an image analysis routine that can be used to quantify this process. This protocol can be easily adapted to study other membrane trafficking events, such as the cellular uptake of nanoparticles, a process relevant to the drug discovery and delivery fields [6]. The protocol we present here for forward transfection uses instruments that are readily available in most laboratories, and does not require any large complex instrumentation, such as liquid handling robots. However, if a higher level of automation is available, solid phase reverse transfection in either plates or in spotted array format [7–9], should be considered, as these methods allows for preparation and storage of transfection-ready plates or arrays, thereby increasing the number of replicates that can be prepared in parallel, in turn improving the reproducibility across screens and reducing the influence of the individual operator.

2 Materials

2.1 Forward Transfection

1. Adherent mammalian cell line (e.g., HeLa cells) (*see* **Note 1**).
2. Genome-wide siRNA library.
3. RNase-free water.
4. Oligofectamine (Life Technologies).
5. Opti-MEM reduced serum medium, no phenol red (Life Technologies).
6. Serum-free medium (for HeLa cells DMEM containing 1 g/L glucose).
7. Medium supplemented with 3× fetal bovine serum (FBS).
8. 384-well (shallow) plate.

9. 384-well (deep storage) plate.

10. 384-well (optical-plastic bottom) Viewplate-384 FTC (PerkinElmer).

11. 384-well plate lids.

12. Handheld automated cell counter for example, Scepter 2.0 (Merck Millipore).

13. Automated cell/liquid dispenser compatible with 384-well plates, for example, Multidrop 384 Reagent Dispenser (Thermo Fisher Scientific).

14. Multichannel pipettes (0.5–10 µl and 30–300 µl).

15. Semi-automated multichannel electronic pipette, ideally with a 96- or 384-well head, for example, VIAFLO (Integra Biosciences).

16. Heated plate sealer.

2.2 Shiga Toxin Assay and Immuno-fluorescence Staining

1. Cy3-labeled SLTxB.

2. Mouse anti-GM130 antibody.

3. Goat anti-mouse antibody conjugated to Alexa 488.

4. Serum-free culture medium.

5. Complete culture medium.

6. Phosphate buffered saline (PBS).

7. 3% Paraformaldehyde (PFA): In a fume hood, add 15 g of paraformaldehyde to 400 ml of PBS preheated to 60–70 °C. Mix well until dissolved and add 50 µl of 1 M $CaCl_2$ and 50 µl of $MgCl_2$. Adjust pH to 7.4 using 1 N NaOH and finally adjust volume to 500 ml. Use immediately or prepare aliquots and store at –20 °C.

8. 0.1% Triton X-100: To 500 ml of PBS, pH 7.4, add 500 µl of Triton X-100. Store at 4 °C.

9. Hoechst 33342 nucleic acid stain.

2.3 Image Acquisition and Analysis

1. Fully automated HCS microscope with appropriate filter sets and objectives, for example, Scan^R (Olympus).

2. High-content analysis software, for example, CellProfiler (Broad Institute) or Columbus Image Data Storage and Analysis System (PerkinElmer).

3 Methods

3.1 Plate Format Design

The key to a successful genome-wide RNAi screen is careful assay design and planning. All individual steps of the screening protocol need to be optimized and typically several pilot experiments should be performed to validate the pipeline. Additionally, since a genome-wide screen normally involves the processing and analysis of numerous samples, it is important to test individual batches of each compound that is going to be used and stock a batch that will be sufficient for the execution of the complete screen. This is of vital importance to ensure reproducibility not only within one plate but also across the entire screen.

Another important aspect to take into consideration during the planning is the correct selection of the positive controls as they will be essential to determine the efficiency of the transfection and of the assay itself. It is also advisable to identify positive controls with different phenotypic strengths, so that weak and strong hits can be calibrated. In our hands, we find it advisable to test at least 20 target genes in order to select the 4–5 most appropriate. In addition to the assay-specific controls, the addition of siRNAs targeting the INCENP mRNA provides for a visual transfection efficiency control. This gene encodes a protein that is involved in cytokinesis and its depletion leads to cells with large multi-lobed nuclei. Negative control siRNAs should also be added to the plate and should give a phenotype similar to that of non-transfected cells. As a guide, 20 wells should be allocated to positive controls and 16 wells should be reserved for negative controls.

Of equal importance is the distribution of the controls throughout the plate, as RNAi screens are particularly susceptible to edge effects or drifting values across a plate. Markedly different readouts from the same controls may indicate that the transfection efficiency was not uniform across the plate. Ideally, all positive and negative controls should be distributed such that they are present at different positions in each plate quadrant. Depending on the plate type and specific assay, in some cases it is preferable not to use the outer wells for the screen and fill these with cell culture medium (*see* **Note 2**).

3.2 Forward Transfection

All procedures involving siRNAs and cells should be performed under aseptic conditions.

1. Centrifuge the lyophilized siRNA plate at $50 \times g$ for 1 min. Resuspend each siRNA (1 nmol) with 33 µl of RNase-free water to prepare a stock plate at 30 µM. Cover the plate with a lid and centrifuge at $50 \times g$ for 1 min.

2. Add 40 µl of RNase-free water to each well of a new 384-well (deep storage) plate and add 10 µl from the stock plate to the corresponding well to prepare a daughter plate at 6 µM. Cover the plate with a lid and centrifuge at $50 \times g$ for 1 min. Seal both the stock and daughter plates using a heat sealer. Both plates can be stored for several months at –20 °C.

3. On the day prior to the transfection, an automated multi-well dispensing system (e.g., MultiDrop 384 Reagent Dispenser) should be used to plate cells in a 384-well optical quality imaging plate such that they are 20 % confluent on the following day. For example, 300 HeLa cells seeded in a volume of 40 µl of complete medium is appropriate for a 72 h transfection and assay (*see* **Note 3**).

4. On the day of transfection, remove the medium from the cells by flicking the plate and blot any remaining liquid on a paper towel. Using a semi-automated pipetting system equipped with a 96- or a 384-head, wash the cells once with 20 μl of serum-free medium. Add 21 μl of serum-free medium and return the plate to the 37 °C incubator (*see* **Note 4**).

5. Add 85 μl of Opti-MEM to each well of a new 384-well (deep storage) plate. Cover the plate with a lid and centrifuge at $50 \times g$ for 1 min.

6. Prepare a master mix of diluted Oligofectamine, containing 0.1 μl of Oligofectamine and 1.4 μl Opti-MEM per well (*see* **Note 5**).

7. Centrifuge the plate containing 6 μM siRNA (daughter plate) at $50 \times g$ for 1 min (*see* **Note 6**).

8. Carefully remove the seal from the siRNA daughter plate and transfer 1.5 μl of siRNA to each well of the 384-well prepared in **step 5**. Place a lid on both plates and centrifuge them at $50 \times g$ for 1 min.

9. Using a multichannel pipette, transfer 1.5 μl of the Oligofectamine master mix to each well of a new 384-well (shallow) plate.

10. Using a multichannel pipette, add 8.5 μl of the diluted siRNA to the plate prepared in **step 9**.

11. Incubate the plate for 20 min at room temperature. During this period, seal the siRNA daughter plate using a heat sealer.

12. Add 7 μl of the transfection mixture prepared in **step 11** to each well of the plate containing the cells (**step 4**). Return the plate to the incubator and incubate for 4 h at 37 °C.

13. Add 14 μl of cell medium containing 3× FBS to each well. Return the plate to the incubator and incubate at 37 °C for a further 68 h.

3.3 Shiga Toxin Assay and Immunofluorescence Staining

As an example, we provide a protocol to detect changes in the accumulation of SLTxB in the Golgi complex after its addition to cells. This protocol can be easily adapted to measure the presence of other molecules in a variety of organelles depending on the biological question. Unless stated otherwise, all procedures are performed at room temperature and all pipetting steps are carried out using a semi-automated pipetting system. Care should be taken in all steps involving fluorophores in order to reduce their exposure to light.

1. Remove the transfection medium from the cells by flicking the plate and wash cells once with 40 μl of ice-cold PBS for 5 min at 4 °C (*see* **Note 7**).

2. Prepare an appropriate dilution of SLTxB-Cy3 (15 μl per well) in cold complete medium (4 °C). Wrap the tube in aluminum foil to protect from light (*see* **Note 8**).

3. Pipette 15 μl of the diluted toxin into each well and incubate at 4 °C for 30 min (*see* **Note 9**).

4. Remove the toxin solution by flicking the plate and wash cells once with 40 μl of ice-cold PBS for 5 min at 4 °C.

5. Remove the PBS by flicking the plate and add 40 μl of pre-warmed complete medium. Incubate the plate for 45 min at 37 °C.

6. Remove the medium and fix the cells by adding 40 μl of 3 % PFA to each well. Incubate for 15 min at room temperature.

7. Remove the PFA and wash once with 40 μl of PBS for 5 min.

8. Permeabilize the cells using 40 μl of 0.1 % Triton X-100 for 5 min.

9. Remove the Triton X-100 and incubate for 5 min with 40 μl of PBS containing 0.2 μg/ml of Hoechst 33342.

10. Prepare an appropriate dilution (for example 1:400) of mouse anti-GM130 antibodies in PBS (15 μl per well) (*see* **Note 10**).

11. Add 15 μl of the anti-GM130 antibody solution to each well and incubate in the dark for 1 h.

12. Discard the antibody solution and wash once with 40 μl PBS for 5 min.

13. Prepare an appropriate dilution (for example 1:400) of goat anti-mouse-Alexa 488 antibody solution in PBS (15 μl per well).

14. Add 15 μl of the antibody solution prepared in **step 13** to each well and incubate for 30 min.

15. Discard the antibody solution and wash the cells once with 40 μl PBS for 5 min.

16. Remove the PBS by flicking the plate and add 40 μl of fresh PBS. Store the plates at 4 °C in the dark until imaging (*see* **Note 11**).

3.4 Image Acquisition and Analysis

In the case of the analysis routine presented here (Fig. 1), the image acquisition will utilize an Olympus Scan^R automated wide-field microscope, equipped with an Olympus 20× LucPlan FLN 0.45NA objective. Acquisition of six fields of view with this objective is sufficient to image typically between 100 and 500 cells per well. For a simple fluorescence intensity measurement this setup is sufficient, however if a more detailed analysis is required, a higher power objective should be used instead. The microscope used here is equipped with a hardware autofocus, which is used at the first sub-position to be imaged in each well. Subsequently, software autofocus will be used to find the appropriate focal plane in the remaining sub-positions.

Fig.1 (continued) prior to analysis. This step removes cells touching the image borders, dividing cells (marked with an *arrow*), and multinucleated cells (marked with an *arrowhead*). In these filtered cells the organelles for measurement (in this case the Golgi complex) are then segmented, and a cell-by-cell measurement of the amount of SLTxB present in this organelle is made. Data are visualized as a mean values per well for each plate across the entire screen. Scale bar represents 10 μm

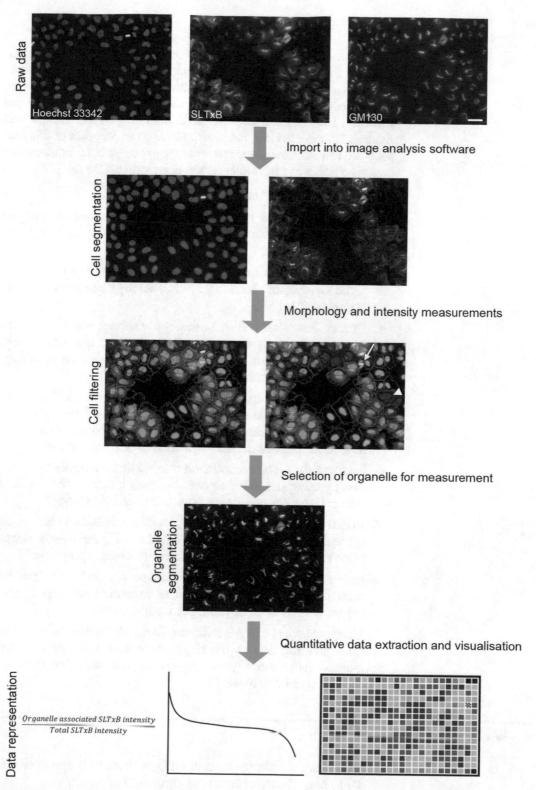

Fig. 1 Example analysis pipeline for quantifying SLTxB accumulation in the Golgi complex. HeLa cells transfected with siRNAs and incubated with Shiga-like toxin B subunit (SLTxB) are fluorescently stained for the nucleus (Hoechst 33342) and Golgi complex (GM130). Images are acquired on an automated screening microscope and then imported into image analysis software. Cells are segmented based on identification of their nuclei and cytoplasm areas, and then morphology and intensity measurements used to filter the population

When the image acquisition is complete, the images should be exported from the microscope and archived safely, preferably in duplicate in two separate locations. Currently several good options exist for image analysis including both open source (e.g., CellProfiler, Broad Institute) and commercial (e.g., Columbus Image Data Storage and Analysis System, PerkinElmer) software. For the purposes of this protocol we will use the Columbus software as an example, but a similar analysis pipeline can be implemented using other software.

1. Import all images into the Columbus system.

2. Using the building block "Find Nuclei", segment the nucleus using the Hoechst 33342 channel, thereby defining the "Nucleus" region.

3. Segment the cells using the Hoechst 33342 channel and the "Find Cytoplasm" building block, thereby defining the "Cell" region (*see* **Note 12**).

4. Extract intensity and morphology measurements on both regions defined in **steps 2** and **3** using the building blocks "Calculate intensity properties" and "Calculate morphology properties", respectively (*see* **Note 13**).

5. Filter cells for analysis using the "Select Population" building block. Here, cells close to the border of the field of view, apoptotic, dividing and abnormal cells will be excluded from analysis and a new "Cell" population will be defined as "Cells for analysis".

6. Segment the Golgi complex on the "Cells for analysis" population by using the "Find Spots" building block on the GM130 channel, thereby creating a population called "Golgi."

7. Extract intensity measurements per cell for the SLTxB channel on the regions defined in **steps 3** and **6** of the "Cells for analysis" population using the building block "Calculate intensity properties".

8. Using the building block "Calculate properties", calculate the ratio between the two intensities measured in **step 7** and export it as an average value per well.

9. Using statistical analysis software (e.g., Microsoft Excel or R), normalize the data to the negative control and plot the normalized values on a graph, removing wells with less than 50 cells analyzed (*see* **Note 14**).

4   Notes

1. We routinely passage our cells and use them only up to passage 10 to keep the experiments as consistent as possible.

2. Based on a library of 22,000 genes, and 36 controls per plate, use of all wells would require the library to be spread across 64 plates, whereas exclusion of the outermost wells would result in 82 plates being needed.

3. We prefer to use an automated cell counter such as the Scepter (EDM Millipore) as this improves reproducibility across the large number of plates required for a genome-wide screen. The number of cells to be plated should be optimized in advance as it will vary with the cell type and transfection time.

4. Alternative techniques, such as aspiration, can be used to change the medium and perform the different washing steps in this protocol, however we find that by flicking and blotting the plate fewer cells are lost.

5. Include extra volume to allow for pipetting errors and void volume. For example, for a 384-well plate we would typically prepare sufficient diluted Oligofectamine for an extra 50 wells, i.e., enough for 434 wells. The volumes would be 43.4 μl of Oligofectamine and 607.6 μl of Opti-MEM.

6. The plate should be fully thawed prior to use, we recommend thawing at room temperature for 45 min to 1 h.

7. To prepare the ice-cold PBS, place the PBS bottle at 4 °C the day prior to the experiment.

8. Care should be taken when choosing the fluorophores for the assay. They should be spectrally compatible, and also be sufficiently bright such that the image acquisition time is reduced to a minimum, thereby reducing the overall acquisition time for each plate.

9. To ensure that the temperature of the cells does not fluctuate during the different manipulation steps, we keep the plate on top of an aluminum block precooled at –20 °C.

10. As an alternative to immunostaining, use of a suitable stably transfected cell line expressing a fluorescently labeled organelle marker may be preferable, as its use will reduce the number of pipetting steps in the protocol, thereby minimizing cell loss.

11. After preparation, the plates should be incubated overnight at 4 °C. This final step promotes a uniform uptake of the nuclear stain by all cells before imaging, thereby aiding the focusing and image analysis.

12. The precision of cell segmentation may be increased if there is a marker present for either the plasma membrane (e.g., CellMask, Life Technologies) or the entire cytoplasm. However, consideration must be given to the spectral properties of that fluorophore, and the additional acquisition time required for this extra channel

13. This step is important for the identification and removal of apoptotic and dividing cells as they will have a brighter nuclear signal and a smaller size. It will also allow removal of cells with an aberrant nucleus or a size larger than normal.

14. Several methods can be used for hit selection, such as definition of a Z-score or the strictly standardized mean difference and are discussed elsewhere [10].

Acknowledgements

Work in the JCS lab is funded by a Principal Investigator (PI) grant (09/IN.1/B2604) from Science Foundation Ireland (SFI). The JCS lab and the UCD Cell Screening Laboratory are supported by a grant from the UCD College of Science.

References

1. Hannon GJ (2002) RNA interference. Nature 418(6894):244–251. doi:10.1038/418244a

2. Neumann B, Walter T, Heriche JK, Bulkescher J, Erfle H, Conrad C, Rogers P, Poser I, Held M, Liebel U, Cetin C, Sieckmann F, Pau G, Kabbe R, Wunsche A, Satagopam V, Schmitz MH, Chapuis C, Gerlich DW, Schneider R, Eils R, Huber W, Peters JM, Hyman AA, Durbin R, Pepperkok R, Ellenberg J (2010) Phenotypic profiling of the human genome by time-lapse microscopy reveals cell division genes. Nature 464(7289):721–727. doi:10.1038/nature08869

3. Aza-Blanc P, Cooper CL, Wagner K, Batalov S, Deveraux QL, Cooke MP (2003) Identification of modulators of TRAIL-induced apoptosis via RNAi-based phenotypic screening. Mol Cell 12(3):627–637

4. Simpson JC, Joggerst B, Laketa V, Verissimo F, Cetin C, Erfle H, Bexiga MG, Singan VR, Heriche JK, Neumann B, Mateos A, Blake J, Bechtel S, Benes V, Wiemann S, Ellenberg J, Pepperkok R (2012) Genome-wide RNAi screening identifies human proteins with a regulatory function in the early secretory pathway. Nat Cell Biol 14(7):764–774. doi:10.1038/ncb2510

5. Johannes L, Romer W (2010) Shiga toxins—from cell biology to biomedical applications. Nat Rev Microbiol 8(2):105–116. doi:10.1038/nrmicro2279

6. Brayden DJ, Cryan SA, Dawson KA, O'Brien PJ, Simpson JC (2015) High-content analysis for drug delivery and nanoparticle applications. Drug Discov Today 20(8):942–957. doi:10.1016/j.drudis.2015.04.001

7. Galea G, Simpson JC (2013) High-content screening and analysis of the Golgi complex. Methods Cell Biol 118:281–295. doi:10.1016/B978-0-12-417164-0.00017-3

8. Erfle H, Neumann B, Liebel U, Rogers P, Held M, Walter T, Ellenberg J, Pepperkok R (2007) Reverse transfection on cell arrays for high content screening microscopy. Nat Protoc 2(2):392–399. doi:10.1038/nprot.2006.483

9. Erfle H, Neumann B, Rogers P, Bulkescher J, Ellenberg J, Pepperkok R (2008) Work flow for multiplexing siRNA assays by solid-phase reverse transfection in multi-well plates. J Biomol Screen 13(7):575–580. doi:10.1177/1087057108320133

10. Birmingham A, Selfors LM, Forster T, Wrobel D, Kennedy CJ, Shanks E, Santoyo-Lopez J, Dunican DJ, Long A, Kelleher D, Smith Q, Beijersbergen RL, Ghazal P, Shamu CE (2009) Statistical methods for analysis of high-throughput RNA interference screens. Nat Methods 6(8):569–575. doi:10.1038/nmeth.1351

Chapter 5

Pooled shRNA Screening in Mammalian Cells as a Functional Genomic Discovery Platform

Katarzyna Jastrzebski, Bastiaan Evers, and Roderick L. Beijersbergen

Abstract

Functional genomic screens using shRNA technology are a great tool in biomedical research. As more labs gain access to the necessary reagents and technology to perform such screens, some may lack in-depth knowledge on the difficulties often encountered. With this protocol, we aim to point out the most important caveats of performing shRNA based screens and provide a streamlined workflow that can be easily adapted to meet the specific needs of any particular screening project.

Key words Functional genetics, RNAi, shRNA, Screens

1 Introduction

Over the last decade, RNA interference has evolved into a powerful method for the analysis of gene function, not only in model organisms such as *C. elegans* and *D. melanogaster*, but also in mammalian cells. Initially, loss-of-function studies in mammalian cells were performed using transient transfection of short interfering RNAs (siRNAs) leading to a robust but transient knockdown [1]. Short hairpin RNA (shRNA) expression technology was developed soon after and viral delivery of these vectors allowed for a more stable gene knockdown as well as use in cell types that are difficult to transfect [2]. After retroviral integration, the shRNA is stably expressed in the cell and processed into a short duplex RNA, which acts similarly to siRNA. Importantly, viral infections can be used to create a large population of cells, each containing a single integration of an shRNA-encoding construct knocking down a specific gene. Such complex pooled populations can be used to simultaneously interrogate large numbers of genes for the identification of key genes involved in diverse cellular processes.

The concept of pooled screening was initially developed in yeast through the construction of a barcoded gene deletion

David O. Azorsa, Shilpi Arora (eds.), *High-Throughput RNAi Screening: Methods and Protocols*, Methods in Molecular Biology, vol. 1470, DOI 10.1007/978-1-4939-6337-9_5, © Springer Science+Business Media New York 2016

collection [3]. This work demonstrated that the presence of an integrated molecular tag, a DNA barcode, linked to loss of expression and the associated phenotype can be used to determine, in a quantitative manner, the selective enrichment or depletion of cells in a heterogeneous population. To this end, barcodes are recovered from the genomic DNA extracted from different populations (selected for the phenotype of interest) by PCR amplification, followed by hybridization to DNA microarrays with the complementary barcode sequences or, more recently, high throughput sequencing. Subsequently, the relative abundance of each barcode under the specific conditions compared to controls can be used to identify the genes of interest. This strategy has been used to profile, in parallel, large numbers of yeast genes for their role in cell survival, drug response, or specific biological processes such as ER biogenesis and DNA damage signaling [4–6]. In contrast to the yeast knockout collections with extrinsic barcodes, in pooled screening approaches using shRNA vectors in mammalian cells, the sequence of the encoded hairpin itself can serve as a tag for quantifying the amount of cells knocked down for any particular gene. The feasibility of this approach was shown in a screen for bypass of a TP53 induced cell cycle arrest, utilizing the first large-scale shRNA collection [7]. Pooled shRNA screening has subsequently been explored by many groups in diverse screening models including the identification of essential genes in tumor cell lines [8–11], synthetic lethal genes [12], drug resistance screens [13], drug enhancer screens [14, 15], in vivo screens [16–19] as well as screens for genes involved in proliferation of tumor associated T-cells [20]. The ability to identify individual perturbing agents by virtue of their specific and unique sequences can be more broadly applied, for example to cDNA sequences in ORF libraries or to sgRNA sequences in the various CRISPR/Cas9 systems, including CRISPRi and CRISPRa. Recently, several other pooled screening systems have been developed mainly as a result of the rapid development of high throughput sequencing. Examples include insertional mutagenesis screens in haploid cells [21] and the analysis of chromatin position effects through the measurement of both the integrated barcode location as well as the corresponding gene expression levels [22].

Pooled shRNA screening is based on the selective enrichment (positive selection) or depletion (negative selection) of tags in one population of cells versus another. These populations can differ in time after infection (to query for straight lethal genes), genotype (to search for synthetic lethal or rescuing genes), treatment (to find genes that either enhance or diminish the activity of a drug, radiation or other perturbing agent) or any phenotype of interest. FACS sorting followed by high throughput sequencing provides a versatile approach to determining differential enrichment or depletion based on phenotypes such as the expression of a cell surface marker, the activity of an integrated reporter driving expression of a fluorescent protein, antibody staining of fixed cells using intracellular (phospho-)epitopes or gene-specific mRNA expression using mFISH [23]. Other selectable phenotypes include anchorage independent growth, migration, and adhesion. Indeed, many examples of positive- and negative-selection pooled screens have been described and with the increasingly easy access to high-throughput screening reagents and deep sequencing pipelines, this number is likely to expand significantly in the coming years.

Despite their well-established status, carrying out pooled shRNA screens is not a trivial endeavor. They are technically complicated, and numerous factors directly or indirectly affect the efficiency and accuracy of the screening results. Important parameters are the complexity and composition of the pooled shRNA library, the viral titer used, and the type of selection (positive and/or negative) screened for, as together these determine the number of cells required for any screen to result in accurate and reproducible data.

High fold representation of each shRNA in a library, that is multiple independent genomic integrations of each shRNA in a cell population, averages out inherent noise in the screen resulting from sampling errors, position effects of viral integration and intrinsic heterogeneity of cell proliferation rates, ensuring high reproducibility between replicates. In addition, the phenotypic penetrance of any shRNA vector is usually not absolute, which limits the resolution in any negative selection screen, whereas in a positive selection screen, overgrowth of positively selected cells will eventually occur, making hit detection easier. Thus, as a rule of thumb, experimental setups for positive selection screens typically require 50- to 100-fold representation of the library, whereas for negative selection screens, 500 to 1000 cells carrying the same shRNA vector are required. Whenever the shRNAs that make up the library are equally distributed, the cell number required for infection is simply a product of the library size and fold representation, but large deviations from this equal distribution may require even higher cell numbers.

It is also important to ensure that cells only express a single unique shRNA. Otherwise, an shRNA with a desired phenotype will alter the relative frequency of other shRNA(s) present in the same cell, which likely do not lead to the phenotype of interest, confounding findings of the screen. This can be achieved by transducing with a relatively low MOI, resulting in ~20% to 30% transduction efficiency. Assuming that viral infections follow a Poisson distribution, it can be calculated that with such transduction efficiencies >80% of cells will carry a single integration (*see* Fig. 1).

Although the design rules for active shRNAs have been improved and alternative systems for the expression of shRNAs have been developed, such as miRNA-embedded shRNAs [24, 25], it remains necessary to include multiple different shRNAs for

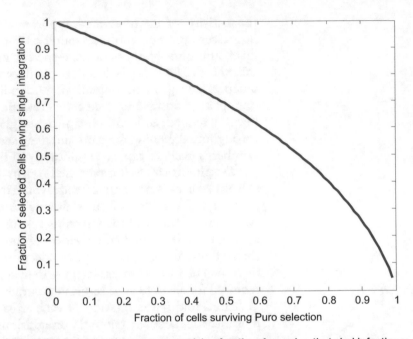

Fig. 1 Single integrations versus surviving fraction. Assuming that viral infections follow a Poisson distribution, it can be derived that the relation between the surviving fraction of cells after puromycin selection (φ) and the fraction of those surviving cells having only a single integration (α) is: $\alpha\left(\varphi\right) = \left(1 - \dfrac{1}{\varphi}\right) \cdot \ln\left(1 - \varphi\right)$.

each gene in a screening collection. The presence of multiple shR-NAs for each gene not only increases the ability to identify multiple active shRNAs for any given gene but also serves to rule out potential off-target effects associated with specific shRNAs. All these parameters together imply that high cell numbers are needed when large collections of shRNAs are used. Recently, high coverage shRNA libraries have been generated containing 25 shRNAs for each gene, increasing the confidence in genes identified in pooled screens [26]. Although the confidence of such screens is higher, the practicality of such an approach to whole genome screening is perhaps limited due to the very large numbers of cells needed for such screens, which is especially limiting in more complicated screening models.

A practical solution is to make use of more focused collections, such as the kinase, phosphatase, epigenetic modifier, RNA binding or DNA damage response gene sets. In addition, subcollections can be generated using specific knowledge of the screening model, for example a list of differentially expressed genes or genes involved in a specific signaling pathway or biological mechanism, such as apoptosis. Focused libraries can be assembled from large collections of individual bacterial stocks from genome-wide collections, but subsets are also commercially available. An alternative method to generate pooled shRNA collections is provided by array-based synthesis of oligonucleotides [26, 27]. This method yields a mixture of shRNA oligonucleotides that can be cloned in a pooled format into a lentiviral expression vector. Because pooled shRNA screens do not require individual shRNA constructs, array based synthesis provides a flexible platform for library composition, but also simplifies their incorporation into several lentiviral vectors carrying different promoters, resistance markers, or genes encoding fluorescent proteins.

Despite the continuous improvement of shRNA design and technologies, relatively little attention has been paid to the development of controls for shRNA screens. Potential negative shRNA controls contain sequences that do not target mammalian genes or are designed against genes that are not expressed in the large majority of cell lines and tissues. Positive shRNA controls are in general more difficult to generate and in many cases are screen specific. Detailed insight into the biological system can provide potential candidate genes as positive controls and these should be validated with the shRNAs present in the screening library. Recently, a general type of positive controls has been described encompassing genes that are straight lethal in a large number of cell lines [28]. These genes are involved in crucial cellular processes, including transcription, translation, the proteasome and cell division. When taking along a control just after infection and puromycin selection ($T=0$), the extent to which shRNAs targeting these essential genes are depleted over time is a coarse, but robust and useful quality measure of any screen.

The protocols described here focus on pooled shRNA screens in cell lines for the purpose of identifying hits in positive and/or negative selection screens. As most of our in-house screening is carried out using the TRC human or mouse shRNA collections, the methods described will be specifically focused on these collections. Importantly, the capture protocol and the PCR primers for the recovery of the shRNA inserts are specifically designed for these collections. Therefore, when using a different shRNA library in a different lentiviral backbone, these steps have to be specifically adapted. Nevertheless, many of the principles described below are applicable to screening with any shRNA collection.

2 Materials

2.1 Cell Culture

1. 6-well tissue culture plates (Corning Costar).

2. 100 mm tissue culture dishes (Corning Falcon).

3. 150 mm tissue culture dishes (Greiner).

4. HEK293T cells (ATCC).

5. HEK293T complete medium: DMEM + 10 % fetal bovine serum + 1 % Pen Strep (Life Technologies).

6. Target cell line.

7. Target cell line growth media.

8. Trypsin.

9. Phosphate buffered saline (PBS).

2.2 Viral shRNA Production and Transductions

1. TRC human or mouse shRNA collections (Dharmacon GE or Sigma-Aldrich).

2. Lentiviral packaging plasmid mix—pRSV-Rev (Addgene), pMDLg/pRRE (Addgene), pCMV-VSV-G (Addgene). Pool equal amounts of plasmid to generate a packaging mix. Add 83 ng (or 1:12) of an EGFP expressing plasmid, such as pCMV-EGFP (Addgene) to every 1 μg of packaging mix to serve as a transfection control.

3. PEI—Polyethylenimine, Linear MW 25,000 (Polysciences Inc.). Suspend the 2 g of powder in 2 L H$_2$O. While stirring, use HCl to adjust pH to 2—at this point the PEI powder will go into solution. Stir for a further 1–2 h. Adjust pH back to 7 using concentrated NaOH. Filter sterilize, aliquot and freeze at −20 °C. Stock remains stable for years at this temperature, while a working aliquot can be stored at 4 °C for months.

4. Polybrene (Hexadimethrine bromide), 8 mg/ml in H$_2$O, sterile filtered (Sigma-Aldrich).

5. Puromycin dihydrochloride, 2 mg/ml in PBS, sterile filtered (Sigma-Aldrich).

2.3 Capture and Next Generation Sequencing of shRNA Inserts

1. NanoDrop (Thermo Scientific) or alternative for determining DNA concentrations.

2. DNeasy Blood & Tissue Kit (Qiagen).

3. CutSmart® buffer (New England Biolabs).

4. AscI enzyme (New England Biolabs).

5. NdeI enzyme (New England Biolabs).

6. BiotinTEG-5′ labeled lentiviral DNA capture oligos (e.g., Integrated DNA Technologies, *see* Table 1 for sequences).

7. Dynabeads® MyOne™ Streptavidin T1 magnetic beads (Life Technologies).

8. DynaMag™-2 magnet rack (Life Technologies).

9. Exonuclease I buffer (New England Biolabs).

10. Exonuclease I (New England Biolabs).

11. Phusion® High Fidelity Polymerase kit (New England Biolabs).

12. dNTPs, 10 mM each (Thermo Scientific).

13. PCR 1 and 2 amplification oligos (e.g., Life Technologies, *see* Table 1 for sequences).

Table 1
Oligo sequences

Oligo name	Oligo sequence (5′–3′)
Lentiviral capture forward	BiotinTEG-TATGCTTACCGTAACTTGAAAGTATTTCGATTTCTTGGCTTTATATATCT
Lentiviral capture reverse	BiotinTEG-CCCTGCTGAGCAGCCGCTATTGGCCACAGCCATGCGGTCGGCGGCGCTG
PCR 1 indexed forward	ACACTCTTTCCCTACACGACGCTCTTCCGATCTXXXXXGGCTTTATATATCTTGTGGAAAGGACG
PCR 1 reverse	GTGACTGGAGTTCAGACGTGTGCTCTTCCGATCTGTGGATGAATACTGCCATTTGTCTC
PCR 2 forward	AATGATACGGCGACCACCGAGATCTACACTCTTTCCCTACACGACGCTCTTCCGATCT
PCR 2 indexed reverse	CAAGCAGAAGACGGCATACGAGATXXXXXXGTGACTGGAGTTCAGACGTGTGCTCTTCCGATCT

Location of the index sequence is indicated in *bold* and can be replaced with any of the 12 Illumina Multiplexing kit indexes

14. Thermal cycler (e.g., Thermo Scientific Arktik™ thermal cycler or Eppendorf Mastercycler nexus thermal cycler).

15. High Pure PCR Purification kit (Roche).

16. Bioanalyser System (Agilent Technologies).

17. DNA 7500 Kit (Agilent Technologies).

3 Methods

Before any screen is started, it is advisable to draw out a setup of the whole screen and determine the number of cells needed at every step. Some screens can become quite large endeavors and it can be helpful to assess their full scale before starting. If we take as an example a negative selection screen using 1000-fold representation and a 4000 vector shRNA library, assuming a transduction efficiency of 20%, we will need $1000 \times 4000/0.2 = 20 \times 10^6$ cells for every arm of the screen. Therefore, such a negative selection screen would require $6 \times 20 \times 10^6$ cells in total to generate enough starting material to set up three replicates of a reference $(T=0)$ and three replicates of a selected $(T=f)$ population.

3.1 Lentivirus Production

Before starting work with lentiviral particles, please consult with your institutional biosafety officer and follow appropriate regulations. Plasmid DNA for the complete shRNA library including any positive and negative controls, is transfected together with the packaging plasmids into HEK293T cells to produce replication deficient lentivirus. Depending on the type of lentiviral backbone, a 2nd or 3rd generation packaging system has to be used.

1. Obtain a plasmid pool for the shRNA library of your interest, either by cherry picking from a genome wide library or by directly obtaining focused sub-pools from a commercial vendor. Ideally, include any additional controls/control pools such as shRNAs targeting the essential and nonessential genes as listed in Table 2. Ensure any combining of pools is done equimolarly per shRNA, to achieve shRNA representations as equal as possible across the entire library (see **Note 1**). Measure the DNA concentration of the shRNA library plasmid pool using a NanoDrop or alternative method.

2. On the day prior to transfection, seed 5×10^6 HEK293T cells/100 mm dish in complete medium and allow them to proliferate for 24 h before transfection. Seed multiple dishes per library transfection (see **Note 2**).

3. The following day, transfect the HEK293T cells, which should be approximately 80% confluent at the time of transfection. Per 100 mm dish to be transfected, combine 5 μg of the shRNA library DNA pool with 5 μg of a lentiviral packaging

Table 2
Essential and nonessential genes utilized as controls for lethality screens

#	Essential genes	Nonessential genes
1	COPA	ABCG8
2	COPB1	ADH7
3	COPS2	CABP5
4	COPS4	CRYGB
5	COPS6	CYP7A1
6	COPS8	DEFB129
7	COPZ1	DMRTB1
8	KPNB1	DMRTC2
9	NUP133	DPCR1
10	NUP205	FAM71B
11	NUP54	FCRL4
12	NUP93	HTR3D
13	NUP98	IL1F10
14	POLA1	IL22
15	POLR2A	KRT25
16	POLR2D	KRT74
17	POLR2F	KRT77
18	PSMA3	KRT9
19	PSMB2	LHX5
20	PSMB3	LUZP4
21	PSMC1	LYZL6
22	PSMC2	MAGEB3
23	PSMC4	MRGPRD
24	PSMD1	NLRP5
25	PSMD11	NPHS2
26	PSMD6	NPSR1
27	PSMD7	OC90
28	RPL11	OLIG2
29	RPL18A	OR12D2
30	RPL19	OR52E8
31	RPL27	OR9Q2

(continued)

Table 2
(continued)

#	Essential genes	Nonessential genes
32	RPL3	OTUD6A
33	RPL30	PIWIL3
34	RPL34	PLA2G2E
35	RPL35A	POTEA
36	RPL36	POU4F2
37	RPL5	RNASE9
38	RPL6	RPTN
39	RPL9	RXFP2
40	RPLP1	SAGE1
41	RPS11	SPATA16
42	RPS13	TAAR1
43	RPS17	TAAR8
44	RPS19	TAS2R13
45	RPS24	TAS2R9
46	RPS27	TGM6
47	RPS3A	TPH2
48	RPS7	TRIM42
49	RPS8	VN1R2
50	RPS9	VN1R5

mix (*see* Subheading 2 for construct information and mix composition), in a total volume of 455 μl of DMEM medium without supplements. Vortex to mix.

4. Add 45 μl of PEI (1 mg/ml stock) to make the volume up to 500 μl, vortex and incubate at room temperature for 5–10 min. Vortex again and add 500 μl per 100 mm dish, dropwise. If transfecting multiple dishes, scale up the transfection mix appropriately. Swirl dishes gently to mix and incubate overnight at 37 °C, 5% CO_2.

5. After 12–18 h, remove transfection medium and replace with 10 ml complete medium per dish.

6. Forty-eight hours after transfection, check the cells under a fluorescent microscope to ascertain that >80% of the cells are GFP positive indicating good transfection efficiency. The supernatant containing the viral particles can then be collected.

7. Pool the supernatant of all transfected dishes and filter through a 0.45 μm filter (*see* **Note 3**).

8. Aliquot the filtered supernatant into sterile cryovials (1 ml per cryovial for titering) and 15 ml tubes (up to 10 ml per 15 ml tube) as screening aliquots. Tubes can be placed directly in a −80 °C freezer for long time storage.

3.2 Optimization of Lentiviral Transduction and Determination of Functional Titer

An important determinant for a successful screen is the fold representation of each shRNA in the infected cell population. Every target cell line is likely to vary in its efficiency of transduction with a given virus preparation. It is therefore important to accurately determine the functional titer for each batch of virus on the target cells, under the same conditions as will be used for the screen.

1. Seed target cells in 2×6 well plates in 2 ml medium per well. Choose a density at which unselected cells will not become over-confluent by the end of the assay.

2. After 24 h, transduce cells with a dilution series of the lentiviral supernatant as follows. Add polybrene to each well of the 2×6 well plates at a final concentration optimized for the cell type being used (*see* **Note 4**).

3. Defrost an aliquot of the viral supernatant and transduce each of the duplicate plates with the following dilution series: Well 1—no virus, Well 2—1:100 dilution (20 μl supernatant), Well 3—1:75 dilution (26.7 μl supernatant), Well 4—1:50 dilution (40 μl supernatant), Well 5—1:25 dilution (80 μl supernatant), Well 6—1:12.5 dilution (160 μl supernatant). Incubate for 24 h.

4. Change media on both transduced plates, to one plate adding an appropriate concentration of puromycin to ensure complete selection against untransduced cells within 48 h (*see* **Note 5**). For most cell types, starting puromycin selection 24 h after infection allows for sufficient puromycin *N*-acetyl-transferase expression to effectively select for transduced cells. In some cases, however, cells may need up to 48 h following transduction to become sufficiently resistant for the selection process to work well.

5. Upon completion of selection, trypsinize and count the cells in each well. Determine the transduction efficiency per virus dilution by dividing the number of cells in the puromycin selected well by the puromycin unselected cell number. Pick a virus dilution that leads to 20–30% transduction efficiency for screening.

3.3 The Primary Pooled Screen

The protocol described below is designed for effective (synthetic) lethality, drug enhancer or drug resistance shRNA screens but can easily be adapted for any positive or negative selection screen. The basic workflow for a pooled shRNA screen is outlined in Fig. 2. Typically, shRNA abundance is determined in an early reference ($T=0$) population and one (in case of screening for direct lethal

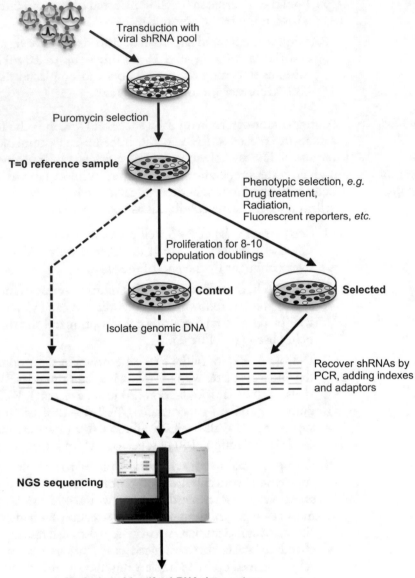

Fig. 2 Schematic of screen workflow. This screen workflow can be applied to a single cell line or multiple cell lines in parallel. Using multiple cell lines may allow for the identification of genes important in a specific tissue type while excluding genes lethal in only a single model system. In the case of synthetic lethality screens, two or more isogenic cell lines with a specific genetic modification are screened in parallel in order to compare vulnerabilities associated with the specific genotype, but absent in the wild-type control. In typical drug enhancer or resistance screen workflow, in addition to collecting $T=0$ control samples, untreated and treated arms are also collected. The difference between resistance and enhancer screens lies in the choice of treatment conditions (drug dose, length of selection) and the analysis output. For drug sensitizers, lower drug doses and shorter time of selection are employed, with analysis output of interest being shRNA dropout. In contrast, enrichment of shRNA representation is of interest in drug resistance screens

genes) or more later time points. In cases where phenotypic selection is part of the screen, both an unselected control and the selected population are harvested at the final time point (T=final, abbreviated T=f). Despite the similarity in workflow, drug enhancer screens are generally preformed using lower drug concentrations and over a shorter length of time than drug resistance screens. Importantly, the absolute parameters of these variables need to be determined empirically for each model cell line and drug combination, but as a broad indication we aim to inhibit long term cell proliferation by approximately 20–30 % during drug enhancer screens, and by approximately 70–80 % during drug resistance screens.

As highlighted throughout this protocol, a major determinant of successful screening is the maintenance of shRNA complexity throughout the screening process, that is, the maintenance of 500- to 1000-fold shRNA representation for negative selection screens and 50- to 100-fold for positive selection screens at all steps including transduction, seeding and reseeding during phenotypic selection, extraction of gDNA, selective capturing, PCR amplification, and high-throughput sequencing.

1. Expand the cells to be used for screening such that you have enough to infect the amount calculated during screen planning. Ideally the whole screen should be replicated several times, but a good alternative is to perform at least three independent infections and keep those as separate replicate samples throughout the whole screening procedure. As an example, in a straight lethality screen, each cell line being screened will require triplicate T=0 and triplicate selected (T=f) samples.

2. Seed target cells in multiple 100 mm or 150 mm dishes, using the same seeding density as used for the lentivirus titration experiment (scaling up the cell number and seeding volume by a factor of 6 for 100 mm dishes, and a factor of 15 for 150 mm dishes). Remember to seed an extra dish for an untransduced, puromycin selection control. Take care to seed cells evenly in the larger dishes to ensure effective puromycin selection of the cells following transduction.

3. After 24 h, add polybrene at a final concentration optimized during the virus titration protocol.

4. Defrost and pool sufficient virus aliquots to transduce all plates seeded. For example, if the titration experiment determined that a 1:50 dilution of the lentiviral supernatant will result in a transduction efficiency of 20–30 %, use 240 µl per 12 ml medium in a 100 mm or 600 µl per 30 ml medium in a 150 mm dish, multiplied by the number of dishes to be transduced.

5. Add virus to each dish and incubate for 24 h.

6. Change media on all plates to complete medium with a concentration of puromycin determined to achieve complete kill of the control untransduced cells in 48 h.

7. Following selection, harvest and pool all transduced cells of each replicate. Determine cell concentration and the total number of cells, making sure that enough cells are available to set up all conditions. If there are excess cells available, setting up extra plates for selection samples and taking extra $T = 0$ reference samples are recommended.

8. Take the cell aliquots for the $T = 0$ replicates—in our example, this would be a minimum of 4×10^6 cells per replicate. Pellet cells by centrifugation (e.g., $400 \times g$ for 4 min), aspirate well and resuspend in 200 μl PBS per replicate (*see* **Note 6**). Transfer to a 1.5 ml tubes and freeze at –20 °C. These samples can be stored until all the selected samples have been collected for gDNA extraction at the same time.

9. Seed out the selection conditions ($T = f$– control and selected arms) per replicate in multiple 100 mm or 150 mm dishes at the correct fold representation of the shRNA library complexity—in our example, three replicates of 4×10^6 cells each for the control and the selected arm. The seeding density will be cell line and length of selection dependent, but for lethality screens, it is advisable to culture the $T = f$ samples for at least eight to ten population doublings to detect strong dropout of essential genes. In contrast, drug dose and length of selection for drug enhancer and drug resistance screens need to be optimized prior to screen set up, ideally using positive control shRNAs that achieve the desired phenotype. It is possible to split dishes if they reach confluence before selection is completed without detrimental effects on reproducibility, as long as the same fold representation is maintained at reseeding.

10. Once selection has been completed, harvest and pool cells from the multiple dishes of each replicate and prepare gDNA extraction samples as for the $T = 0$ condition. Given their extended culture, selected samples will be available in great excess to requirements. Therefore, it is not necessary to keep all the cells, but it is advisable to prepare multiple gDNA samples in case of any losses during extraction.

11. Extract gDNA using the Qiagen DNeasy Blood & Tissue Kit.

3.4 Capture and Next Generation Sequencing of shRNA Inserts

With the availability of next generation sequencing technologies, screening readouts have become high throughput and quantitative, allowing for multiplexed analysis of several samples per lane/run. We routinely use Illumina sequencers, HiSeq or MiSeq, for quantification of shRNA abundance in screen samples. The main consideration when preparing sequencing samples is to use sufficient gDNA as input to maintain the correct fold representation of each shRNA construct in the screening library. As such, for a 4000 shRNA library, gDNA form 4×10^6 cells per sample has to be used for PCR amplification and sequencing. Given that a diploid cell contains 6 pg of DNA, it would be expected that 4×10^6 cells yield

24 µg of gDNA. Keep in mind, however, that many cancer cell lines are hyperdiploid and therefore to maintain the same complexity more genomic DNA will need to be used for PCR amplification. Since a single 50 µl PCR reaction can handle up to approximately 1 µg of genomic DNA before starting to work less efficiently, multiple PCR reactions need to be done on the genomic DNA of a whole screen (*see* **Note 7**). Alternatively, the DNA can first be digested with appropriate restriction enzymes and then biotinylated capture primers can be hybridized specifically to the fragment containing the hairpin and some flanking viral DNA. Magnetic streptavidin beads can then be used to get rid of all the genomic DNA except for the fragments of interest. This allows the PCR based amplification of viral inserts from large amounts of genomic DNA in a single PCR reaction. The capture and amplification protocol described below is presented for 25 µg of gDNA input, but can be scaled to adjust for any screening library size used. As mentioned above, it is imperative to use amplification primers specific for the vector backbone of the library being used. The primers listed in Table 1 and shown schematically in Fig. 3 are specific for

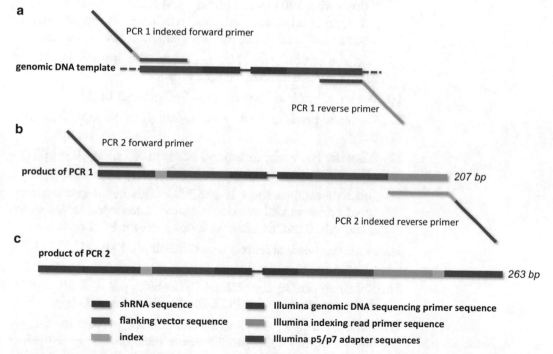

Fig. 3 Schematic of amplification reactions for sequencing library preparation. (**a**) Following capture of the integrated lentiviral shRNA fragment from gDNA samples, the first round of amplification is carried out with primers flanking the hairpin sequence. The PCR 1 forward primer adds an index and the Illumina read 1 primer sequence, while the reverse primer adds the Illumina indexing read primer sequence. (**b**) The second round PCR uses the product of PCR 1 as template to add the p5 and p7 adapters as well as a further optional index in the reverse primer. The final product is a 263 bp fragment containing all the elements required for annealing and sequencing on Illumina high throughput sequencers

amplification of shRNAs from the TRC collection (all currently released versions—1, 1.5 and 2).

1. In a 1.5 ml safelock tube per screen sample, prepare the following reaction mix: 50 μl CutSmart® Buffer; 50 U of AscI enzyme; 50 U of NdeI; 25 μg of gDNA; H$_2$O up to 500 μl.

2. Incubate overnight at 37 °C. To avoid problems with condensation forming in the lid of the tube, do so in an incubator or a water bath rather than a thermoblock.

3. The following day, heat the samples in a thermoblock set at 100 °C for 10 min.

4. Add 500 μl 2 M NaCl, mix and incubate for a further 5 min at 100 °C.

5. Snap freeze tubes in liquid nitrogen.

6. Take samples out of liquid nitrogen and add 10 pmol of each biotinylated capture oligo (see Table 1 for sequences).

7. Place samples in a 60 °C thermoshaker and allow to hybridize overnight.

8. Wash a 20 μl aliquot of Streptavidin T1 Dynabeads per sample 3 times with 500 μl wash buffer (1 M NaCl, 10 mM Tris–HCl, pH 8) in 2 ml tubes. Use the DynaMag™-2 magnet rack to separate the beads from the supernatant between washes.

9. Add the hybridized DNA sample to the washed beads and tumble for 2 h at room temperature.

10. Wash the beads at least twice in 500 μl wash buffer.

11. Wash the beads at least twice in 500 μl of 10 mM Tris–HCl, pH 8.

12. After the last wash, resuspend beads in: 45 μl of 10 mM Tris–HCl, pH 8; 5 μl Exonuclease I buffer; 1 μl Exonuclease I.

13. Incubate samples for 1 h at 37 °C. This will digest any captured primers that have not annealed to lentiviral DNA, which could otherwise interfere with downstream PCR reactions.

14. Wash the beads at least 3 times in 500 μl of 10 mM Tris–HCl, pH 8.

15. Resuspend in 20 μl of 10 mM Tris–HCl, pH 8. Store at 4 °C if not proceeding with PCR amplification immediately.

16. For each sample, as well as a water control, prepare the following 1st round PCR amplification reaction, using a distinct indexed forward primer per sample: 20 μl of captured template on beads or H$_2$O control, 10 μl 5× GC buffer, 1 μl 10 mM dNTP, 2.5 μl 10 μM PCR 1 indexed forward primer, 2.5 μl 10 μM PCR 1 indexed reverse primer, 1.5 μl DMSO, 1 U Phusion polymerase, 12 μl H$_2$O. If more than 12 samples are being processed, indexing in the 2nd round PCR can also be utilized (see Note 8).

17. Run the above reactions in a thermal cycler under the following conditions: (1) 98 °C for 30 s; (2) 20 cycles of 98 °C for 30 s, 60 °C for 30 s, 72 °C for 1 min; (3) 72 °C for 5 min; (4) hold at 4 °C.

18. Use the product of PCR 1 to set up 2nd round PCR reactions as follows, using distinct index primers if multiplexing more than 12 samples (*see* **Note 8**): 2 μl product or H_2O control from PCR 1, 10 μl 5× GC buffer, 1 μl 10 mM dNTP, 2.5 μl 10 μM PCR 2 forward primer, 2.5 μl 10 μM PCR 2 indexed reverse primer, 1.5 μl DMSO, 1 U Phusion polymerase, 30 μl H_2O.

19. Run the above reactions in a thermal cycler under the following conditions: (1) 98 °C for 30 s; (2) 15 cycles of 98 °C for 30 s, 60 °C for 30 s, 72 °C for 1 min; (3) 72 °C for 5 min; (4) hold at 4 °C.

20. To each completed reaction, add 50 μl H_2O and column purify using a Roche High Pure PCR purification kit, eluting in 60 μl kit provided Elution Buffer (EB).

21. Run 5 μl of each sample, including the water control, on a 1% agarose gel to ensure the presence of an appropriately sized product (263 bp) and comparable yield across all samples to be pooled (*see* **Note 9** and Fig. 4a for a typical example).

22. Generate a single sequencing sample by pooling ~10 μl of each individually indexed screen sample, adjusting the volume to compensate for any lower or higher yielding reactions.

23. Run the pooled sequencing sample on a Bioanalyser DNA 7500 chip to accurately determine the concentration of the specific product (*see* **Note 10** and Fig. 4b for a typical example).

24. Run samples on a HiSeq or MiSeq as per manufacturer's instructions for standard DNA sequencing to generate, single-end reads, including an Illumina indexing read if more than one indexed primer was used in the 2nd round PCR reaction (*see* **Note 11** for further tips).

3.5 Analysis and Hit Identification

The results of the DNA sequencing consist of discrete reads and the associated read numbers distributed among the indexes used for the screen. Our analysis pipeline consists of the following steps:

1. The reads are trimmed to the actual shRNA sequence, in case of the TRC collection the 21 bp fragment representing the sense strand of the shRNA.

2. The sequences are mapped to the genome-wide shRNA collection and the library annotations are added (clone ID and gene ID).

3. After this step, it is possible to remove contaminating shRNAs that were not present in the screening library or alternatively apply a low count filter (<10 reads) for the same purpose.

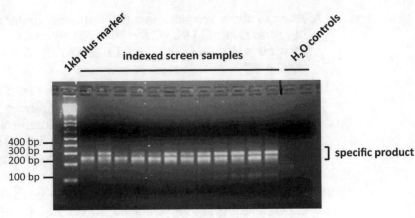

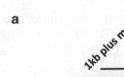

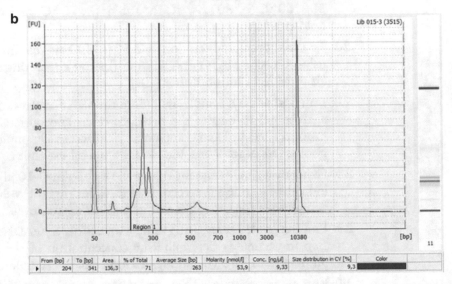

Fig. 4 Typical results of PCR amplifications to generate high throughput sequencing samples. A synthetic lethality screen was carried out in a pair of isogenic cell lines. Genomic DNA from the triplicate $T = 0$ and $T = f$ samples was extracted and PCR amplified. (**a**) A fraction of each individual sample was separated on an agarose gel to compare yield before pooling. (**b**) The final concentration of the pooled sample was determined by analysis on a Bioanalyser DNA 7500 chip by gating on the specific PCR products

4. The read count table can then be used as input for differential analysis of count data. There are several methods available for the analysis of pooled shRNA screens, including the R-package DESeq2 [29] (and **Note 12**). DESeq2 first performs a normalization step after which the normalized counts are used to generate correlation plots for all replicate pairs (Fig. 5a). The package also generates a heatmap of the sample-to-sample distance matrix for all samples included in the analysis (Fig. 5b). The correlation plots and distance matrix are used to assess the quality of the screen and to detect aberrant replicates that could be removed from the analysis at this step.

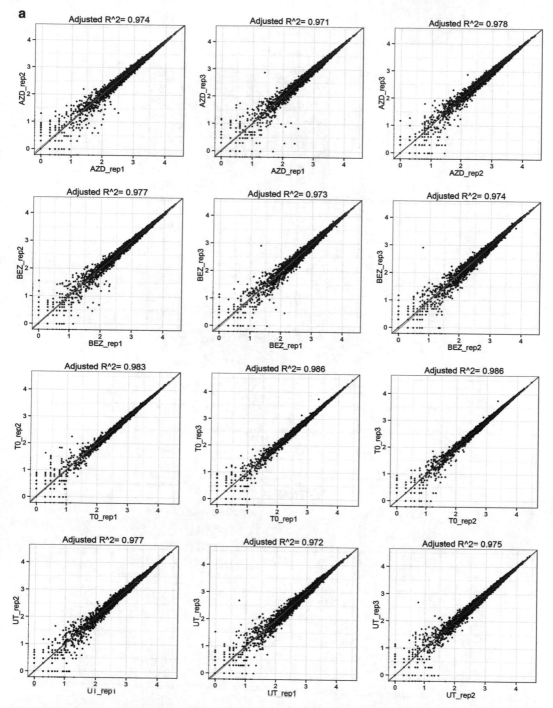

Fig. 5 DESeq2 analysis outputs for a typical screen. DESeq2 analysis is used to generate an output file that includes normalized read counts, log fold change, and an adjusted *P*-value for each shRNA. These outputs can be used to address the quality of the screen and to select shRNAs and their target genes as hits from the screen. (**a**) Correlation plots of the different replicates for each condition. (**b**) Heatmap showing the Euclidian distances between all samples as calculated from the regularized transformation. The *color key* and *histogram* indicates the distance value and frequency. The latter is also depicted in the heatmap.

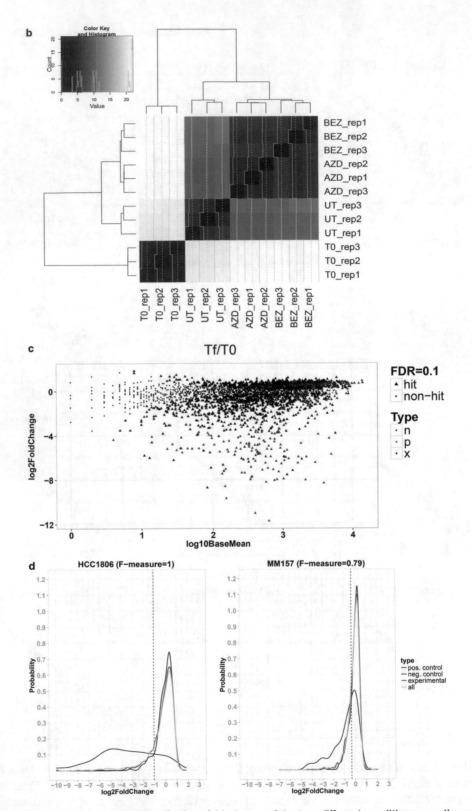

Fig. 5 (continued) (**c**) MA-plot showing the log$_2$-fold change of the two different conditions over the mean of the normalized counts. Each *dot* represents an shRNA, *triangles* represent shRNAs selected as hits (FDR < 0.1). *Colors* indicate the negative (*blue*) and positive (*red*) control shRNAs targeting essential and nonessential genes. (**d**) Density plot of the log$_2$-fold change for all shRNAs in two different cell lines HCC1806 and MDA-MB-157 (MM157). *Colors* indicate the different shRNAs, as described above. The F-measure for each cell line is depicted at the top of each plot

5. DESeq2 allows for paired comparisons, which is used when biological independent replicates have been generated at the lentiviral transduction step of the screening process. From this analysis DESeq2 provides as output the log fold change (LFC) and the associated adjusted p-value (Padj) for each shRNA across the different samples (conditions).

6. These data are used to generate an MA-plot that shows the $\log_2$-fold change between the two different conditions as a function of the mean of the normalized counts (Fig. 5c). For shRNA screens containing sets of shRNAs as positive (essential genes) and negative (nonessential genes) controls, these can be indicated in the MA-plot (Fig. 5c, red dots: positive, blue dots: negative). The shRNAs targeting essential genes should be depleted in the late time point ($T=f$) compared to control ($T=0$).

7. The shRNA controls can be used to generate a density plot for the positive and negative controls (Fig. 5d). Based on the same controls, an F-measure can be calculated as a factor representing the quality of the screen [28]. We consider screens with an F-measure > 0.9 of high quality, between 0.8 and 0.9 sufficient and below 0.8 as low quality screens.

8. A continuing challenge in the interpretation and hit selection of shRNA screens is the presence of off-target effects associated with shRNAs, leading to the detection of false positives. Several approaches have been developed to reduce this type of contamination of screening results including the analysis of the behavior of common seeds shared between different shRNAs [30]. It is also important to include an analytical strategy that incorporates the consistency across multiple shRNAs targeting a gene. Recently, a number of different methods have been developed that allow for the generation of hit-lists based on a gene score, taking into account the effects of the individual shRNAs for each gene. These include MAGeCK [31], HiTSelect [32], and the Bayesian method described by Hart et al. [28]. Each of these methods applies a different approach to eliminate false-positives due to off-target effects, generate a gene-score and a hit list. As a consequence, these different analyses frequently produce different results and therefore validation of the selected hits remains a crucial step in the follow-up of pooled shRNA screening results. This validation includes the reproduction of the phenotype for the selected genes with multiple different shRNAs and the demonstration of effective knockdown. Ideally, the phenotype is also reproduced using other gene-perturbing reagents including CRISPR/Cas9 based technologies or, if available, small molecule inhibitors.

4   Notes

1. To ensure as close to an equimolar representation of each hairpin in the library as possible, it is imperative to pool constructs correctly. As an example, let's take a kinome library containing 4800 hairpins and a control pool with hairpins against essential genes of 384 hairpins that need to be combined at an equimolar ratio. To do so, one will need to add $12.5 \times$ the amount of DNA for the kinome library than for the 384 hairpin control pool—i.e., 1 µg of the 4800 clone kinome pool and 80 ng of the 384 control clone pool.

2. Seeding multiple plates for transfection is recommended. The exact number of plates is dependent on the size of the screening library, the intended screen design and number of cell lines to be screened, but in general, $5–10 \times 100$ mm dishes will generate a sufficient amount of virus for several "standard" screens. Virus will be frozen after production, so that any excess supernatant can be stored and used for later screens.

3. Vacuum pump-driven aspirators are often not permitted in lentiviral facilities due to health and safety regulations. In those cases it is necessary to filter rather large volumes of virus using a syringe-fitted 0.45 µm filter. It is not uncommon for the filter to become clogged, so it is useful to have several filters on hand and change them regularly as supernatant flow stops.

4. Polybrene is a cationic polymer used to increase the efficiency of transduction of cells with retroviruses [33, 34]. Although not frequent, prolonged exposure to polybrene can be toxic to some cells. The optimal concentration of polybrene can range from 2 to 10 µg/ml depending on cell type, although 4–8 µg/ml is commonly used. If polybrene has not previously been used on the cells of interest, a simple dilution series (0, 2, 4, 6, 8, 10 µg/ml) can be performed to determine if any toxic effects are seen over a period up to 48 h.

5. Before virus titration and screening is carried out, a puromycin titration experiment needs to be performed to determine a concentration of puromycin that kills all untransduced cells within 48 h of exposure. This should be done under conditions closely resembling those of the subsequent titration and screen. Thus, cells seeded in a 6 well plate, at the same density as for the titration protocol, should be grown for 48 h before treatment with a range of puromycin doses (0, 0.5, 1, 2, 4 and 8 µg/ml). Following a further 48 h of culture, cells should be assessed by microscopy to determine the lowest dose of puromycin at which all cells have been killed.

6. The Qiagen DNeasy Blood & Tissue Kit for gDNA extraction recommends processing no more than 5×10^6 cells per column.

If the cells used for screening are polyploid, the number of cells extracted per column should be reduced to avoid overloading and clogging the column. Cell suspensions prepared and frozen in 200 μl PBS, once defrosted, can be processed following the standard Qiagen kit protocol. It is imperative to fully solubilize the lysates before loading on the column. Furthermore, it is important to keep in mind that some loss of gDNA may occur during extraction; therefore, it is wise to prepare excess samples in order to be able to keep representation in the subsequent capture and PCR at the appropriate fold representation.

7. If you opt to prepare sequencing samples without capturing the lentiviral insert DNA first, it is necessary to carry out multiple 1st round PCR reactions per sample, each containing a maximum of 1 μg gDNA as input. As an illustration, for each sample generated with a 4000 shRNA construct library, at a 1000-fold representation, this will mean 24×1 μg reactions. Thus, to prepare sequencing samples for a nine condition screen, it will be necessary to set up 216 PCR reactions. Following the first round PCR, all replicate reactions per sample should be pooled and a 2 μl aliquot used as template in the 2nd round PCR.

8. It is possible to multiplex screen samples for simultaneous sequencing on a single lane of a flow cell. For this we use 12 standard Illumina multiplexing indexes integrated into either the PCR 1 indexed forward primer or the PCR 2 indexed reverse primer as indicated in Table 1. By combining indexes this way, up to 144 samples can be multiplexed in a single sequencing run. During sequencing, the PCR 1 index will form the beginning of each read, not only allowing tracking of which sample the subsequent shRNA sequence originates from, but also providing nucleotide diversity in the first 6 rounds of the sequencing round. The latter is imperative for efficient deconvolution of individual clusters being sequenced on the Illumina flow cell. As such, at least six indexed samples should be pooled per lane to ensure maximal yield from the sequencing run. The index used for PCR 2 amplification can be read with the standard Illumina indexing read, which is only necessary when more than 12 samples are being sequenced simultaneously.

9. We often observe a doublet of the specific product, the lower band running at the expected size, while the higher band running just below the 300 bp marker. The latter is likely a result of heteroduplex formation at the end of a PCR and in our experience does not affect the quality of sequencing results.

10. In our experience, minor levels of lower and higher molecular weight products are often observed in the sequencing sample, but do not interfere with the efficiency of high throughput sequencing. Nevertheless, it is possible to further purify the pooled sample using gel extraction or an alternative size selection technique.

11. Although standard 50 nt reads would just fall short of reading the 21 nt of specific shRNA sequence, we standardly achieve high quality 65 nt read lengths using 50 nt sequencing chemistry. Again, in order to achieve sufficient depth of reads per sample, we aim to obtain the same fold representation per shRNA construct per condition as calculated earlier. Therefore, for a screen with nine conditions (triplicate samples of each $T = 0$, control and selected conditions) generated with a library of 4000 shRNA constructs, we would require 2.4×10^7 reads. This will easily be achieved on a single HiSeq lane (expected number of reads per lane being $\sim 2 \times 10^8$) or two runs of a MiSeq (expected number of reads per run being $\sim 2.5 \times 10^7$).

12. The DESeq2 package is available at http://www.bioconductor.org/packages/release/bioc/html/DESeq2.html

Acknowledgements

This work was supported by a NWO grant to the Cancer Systems Biology Center. We thank Cor Lieftink, Tao Chen, and members of the Bernards and Beijersbergen labs for input and discussions.

References

1. Elbashir SM, Harborth J, Lendeckel W et al (2001) Duplexes of 21-nucleotide RNAs mediate RNA interference in cultured mammalian cells. Nature 411:494–498. doi:10.1038/35078107

2. Brummelkamp TR, Bernards R, Agami R (2002) A system for stable expression of short interfering RNAs in mammalian cells. Science 296:550–553. doi:10.1126/science.1068999

3. Winzeler EA, Shoemaker DD, Astromoff A et al (1999) Functional characterization of the S. cerevisiae genome by gene deletion and parallel analysis. Science 285:901–906

4. Lum PY, Armour CD, Stepaniants SB et al (2004) Discovering modes of action for therapeutic compounds using a genome-wide screen of yeast heterozygotes. Cell 116:121–137

5. Wright R, Parrish ML, Cadera E et al (2003) Parallel analysis of tagged deletion mutants efficiently identifies genes involved in endoplasmic reticulum biogenesis. Yeast 20:881–892. doi:10.1002/yea.994

6. Giaever G, Chu AM, Ni L et al (2002) Functional profiling of the Saccharomyces cerevisiae genome. Nature 418:387–391. doi:10.1038/nature00935

7. Berns K, Hijmans EM, Mullenders J et al (2004) A large-scale RNAi screen in human cells identifies new components of the p53 pathway. Nature 428:431–437. doi:10.1038/nature02371

8. Cowley GS, Weir BA, Vazquez F et al (2014) Parallel genome-scale loss of function screens in 216 cancer cell lines for the identification of context-specific genetic dependencies. Sci Data 1:140035. doi:10.1038/sdata.2014.35

9. Marcotte R, Brown KR, Suarez F et al (2012) Essential gene profiles in breast, pancreatic, and ovarian cancer cells. Cancer Discov 2:172–189. doi:10.1158/2159-8290.CD-11-0224

10. Silva JM, Marran K, Parker JS et al (2008) Profiling essential genes in human mammary cells by multiplex RNAi screening. Science 319:617–620. doi:10.1126/science.1149185

11. Luo B, Cheung HW, Subramanian A et al (2008) Highly parallel identification of essential genes in cancer cells. Proc Natl Acad Sci U S A 105:20380–20385. doi:10.1073/pnas.0810485105

12. Luo J, Emanuele MJ, Li D et al (2009) A genome-wide RNAi screen identifies multiple synthetic lethal interactions with the Ras oncogene. Cell 137:835–848. doi:10.1016/j.cell.2009.05.006

13. Brummelkamp TR, Fabius AWM, Mullenders J et al (2006) An shRNA barcode screen provides insight into cancer cell vulnerability to MDM2 inhibitors. Nat Chem Biol 2:202–206. doi:10.1038/nchembio774

14. Prahallad A, Sun C, Huang S et al (2012) Unresponsiveness of colon cancer to BRAF(V600E) inhibition through feedback activation of EGFR. Nature 483:100–103. doi:10.1038/nature10868

15. Huang S, Hölzel M, Knijnenburg T et al (2012) MED12 controls the response to multiple cancer drugs through regulation of TGF-β receptor signaling. Cell 151:937–950. doi:10.1016/j.cell.2012.10.035

16. Bric A, Miething C, Bialucha CU et al (2009) Functional identification of tumor-suppressor genes through an in vivo RNA interference screen in a mouse lymphoma model. Cancer Cell 16:324–335. doi:10.1016/j.ccr.2009.08.015

17. Rudalska R, Dauch D, Longerich T et al (2014) In vivo RNAi screening identifies a mechanism of sorafenib resistance in liver cancer. Nat Med 20:1138–1146. doi:10.1038/nm.3679

18. Chen T, Heller E, Beronja S et al (2012) An RNA interference screen uncovers a new molecule in stem cell self-renewal and long-term regeneration. Nature 485:104–108. doi:10.1038/nature10940

19. Possemato R, Marks KM, Shaul YD et al (2011) Functional genomics reveal that the serine synthesis pathway is essential in breast cancer. Nature 476:346–350. doi:10.1038/nature10350

20. Zhou P, Shaffer DR, Alvarez Arias DA et al (2014) In vivo discovery of immunotherapy targets in the tumour microenvironment. Nature 506:52–57. doi:10.1038/nature12988

21. Carette JE, Guimaraes CP, Wuethrich I et al (2011) Global gene disruption in human cells to assign genes to phenotypes by deep sequencing. Nat Biotechnol 29:542–546. doi:10.1038/nbt.1857

22. Akhtar W, de Jong J, Pindyurin AV et al (2013) Chromatin position effects assayed by thousands of reporters integrated in parallel. Cell 154:914–927. doi:10.1016/j.cell.2013.07.018

23. Klemm S, Semrau S, Wiebrands K et al (2014) Transcriptional profiling of cells sorted by RNA abundance. Nat Methods 11:549–551. doi:10.1038/nmeth.2910

24. Knott SRV, Maceli AR, Erard N et al (2014) A computational algorithm to predict shRNA

potency. Mol Cell 56:796–807. doi:10.1016/j.molcel.2014.10.025

25. Kampmann M, Horlbeck MA, Chen Y et al (2015) Next-generation libraries for robust RNA interference-based genome-wide screens. Proc Natl Acad Sci U S A 112:E3384–E3391. doi:10.1073/pnas.1508821112

26. Bassik MC, Lebbink RJ, Churchman LS et al (2009) Rapid creation and quantitative monitoring of high coverage shRNA libraries. Nat Methods 6:443–445. doi:10.1038/nmeth.1330

27. Cleary MA, Kilian K, Wang Y et al (2004) Production of complex nucleic acid libraries using highly parallel in situ oligonucleotide synthesis. Nat Methods 1:241–248. doi:10.1038/nmeth724

28. Hart T, Brown KR, Sircoulomb F et al (2014) Measuring error rates in genomic perturbation screens: gold standards for human functional genomics. Mol Syst Biol 10:733–733. doi:10.15252/msb.20145216

29. Love MI, Huber W, Anders S (2014) Moderated estimation of fold change and dispersion for RNA-seq data with DESeq2. Genome Biol 15:550. doi:10.1186/s13059-014-0550-8

30. Marine S, Bahl A, Ferrer M, Buehler E (2012) Common seed analysis to identify off-target effects in siRNA screens. J Biomol Screen 17:370–378. doi:10.1177/1087057111427348

31. Li W, Xu H, Xiao T et al (2014) MAGeCK enables robust identification of essential genes from genome-scale CRISPR/Cas9 knockout screens. Genome Biol 15:554. doi:10.1186/s13059-014-0554-4

32. Diaz AA, Qin H, Ramalho-Santos M, Song JS (2015) HiTSelect: a comprehensive tool for high-complexity-pooled screen analysis. Nucleic Acids Res 43:e16. doi:10.1093/nar/gku1197

33. Manning JS, Hackett AJ, Darby NB (1971) Effect of polycations on sensitivity of BALD-3T3 cells to murine leukemia and sarcoma virus infectivity. Appl Microbiol 22:1162–1163

34. Davis HE, Morgan JR, Yarmush ML (2002) Polybrene increases retrovirus gene transfer efficiency by enhancing receptor-independent virus adsorption on target cell membranes. Biophys Chem 97:159–172

Chapter 6

A Protocol for a High-Throughput Multiplex Cell Viability Assay

Daniel F. Gilbert and Michael Boutros

Abstract

High-throughput cell viability assays are broadly used in RNAi and small molecule screening experiments to identify compounds that selectively kill cancer cells or as counter screens to exclude the compounds that have a generic effect on cell growth. While there are several assaying techniques available, cellular fitness is often assessed on the basis of one single and often rather indirect physiological indicator. This can lead to inconsistencies and poor correspondence between cell viability screening experiments, conducted under comparable conditions but with different viability indicators. Multiplexing, i.e., the combination of different individual assaying techniques in one experiment and subsequent comparative analysis of multiparametric data can decrease inter-assay variability and increase dataset concordance. Here, we describe a protocol for a multiplexing approach for high-throughput cell viability screening to address the issues encountered in the classical strategy using a single fitness indicator described above. The method combines a biochemical, luminescence-based approach and two fluorescence-based assay types. The biochemical method assesses cellular fitness by quantifying intracellular ATP concentration. Calcein labeling reflects cell fitness through membrane integrity and indirect measurement of ATP-dependent enzymatic esterase activity. Hoechst DNA stain correlates cell fitness with cellular DNA content. The presented multiplexing approach is suitable for low, medium and high-throughput screening and has the potential to decrease inter-assay variability and increase dataset concordance as well as reproducibility of experimental results.

Key words High-throughput screening, Cell-based assays, Multiplexing, Cell viability, Cell fitness, RNAi screening, Drug discovery, Target validation, In vitro toxicity screening

1 Introduction

Cell-based viability or fitness screening has become a widely used method in assessing a vast range of biological questions, including in cancer research, drug discovery, and in vitro toxicity. The spectrum of available cell fitness indicators as well as the cellular and physiological parameters assessed by individual indicators is large: common assay types assess for instance metabolic activity (e.g., reductase-enzyme product, ATP content or esterase activity), cell proliferation (e.g., nucleus stain), cellular integrity (e.g., membrane integrity), or cell morphology (e.g., impedance) [1–4]. Despite this

David O. Azorsa, Shilpi Arora (eds.), *High-Throughput RNAi Screening: Methods and Protocols*, Methods in Molecular Biology, vol. 1470, DOI 10.1007/978-1-4939-6337-9_6, © Springer Science+Business Media New York 2016

vast variety of available viability indicators, cell fitness screening is typically conducted based on a single indicator, providing very limited information on the cell fitness phenotype and only partially and indirectly reflecting cellular viability. As a consequence, screening experiments conducted even under comparable conditions—in terms of used cell lines, culture conditions and reagents, e.g., drugs—but with different viability indicators, can reveal discordant results. An example of poor correlation between screening experiments has recently been discussed [5]. In this study, the authors compared two recently published large-scale pharmacogenomic studies addressing gene expression and metabolic drug response in a panel of several hundred cancer cell lines [6, 7]. While gene expression was well correlated between studies, there were apparent discrepancies in drug sensitivity, possibly because different indicators of metabolic activity, reductase-enzyme product (CellTiter 96 Aqueous One Solution Cell Proliferation Assay) [6] and ATP content (CellTiter-Glo Luminescent Cell Viability Assay Kit) [7] were used in both studies for measuring drug response.

To overcome the issues encountered in the classical assaying methods described above, we have established an assay to assess cellular viability by a "multiplexing" approach combining different methods in one experiment [8]. Multiplexing, i.e., the combination of various approaches in the same experiment, typically run individually and in serial mode, can decrease inter-assay variability and increase dataset concordance as well as reproducibility of experimental results. Our method combines a biochemical, luminescence-based approach (CellTiter-Glo Luminescent Cell Viability Assay Kit, Promega) and two fluorescence-based assay types (Calcein-AM and Hoechst 33342 DNA stain).

The luminescence-based method (CellTiter-Glo Luminescent Cell Viability Assay Kit, Promega) reflects cellular fitness by quantifying the intracellular ATP level [ATP]i. [ATP]i is an energy carrier driving virtually all cellular functions and it has been a long-serving indicator of cellular viability. However, solely relying on [ATP]i as a measure of cell fitness can be misleading as [ATP]i varies markedly during cell differentiation [9], with circadian rhythm [10] and even within populations of genetically identical eukaryotic cells due to inhomogeneous distribution of mitochondria during cell division [11].

One fluorescence-based assay employs Calcein as indicator of cell viability through membrane integrity and indirect measurement of ATP-dependent enzymatic esterase activity. The nonfluorescent uncharged and hydrophobic acetoxymethyl ester molecule Calcein-AM can permeate cell membranes and accumulate inside the cell, where it is hydrolyzed by intracellular ATP-dependent esterases. The hydrophilic strongly fluorescent product Calcein remains inside the cell, reflecting both, an intact membrane and esterase activity. Due to its low cytotoxicity Calcein-AM is considered a well-suited fluorescent viability probe and is commonly employed in cell fitness screening [12]. However, the indicator reflects fitness based on cellular metabolism and ATP content, thus analysis and interpretation of quantification data requires careful consideration in analogy to measuring intracellular ATP content for assessment of cellular viability. In general, measurements based fluorescent probes can be compromised by extrusion pumps, which remove fluorophores from the cytoplasm [13].

Hoechst 33342, the second fluorescent indicator employed in the described multiplexing approach, quantifies nuclear DNA content. The fluorescent probe exhibits distinct fluorescence emission upon binding into the minor groove of DNA and stains condensed as well as normal chromatin of living or dead cells. The indicator's fluorescence intensity is directly proportional to nuclear DNA content and has therefore been proposed as a measure of cellular viability [14]. Despite its simple handling and a broad spectrum of applications, the use of Hoechst 33342 and similar probes in assessment of cellular viability is limited as co-labeling of living and dead cells can yield inaccurate results.

The present protocol provides detailed instructions for multiplexed cell fitness screening. It also demonstrates strategies and offers tools for comparative analysis of multiparametric data and quantification of phenotype intersection as a basis of hit confirmation. While this protocol describes an HTS RNAi screening experiment in HEK293 cells, the protocol is also adaptable for other cells and screening approaches, such as small molecule or combined RNAi and small molecule as well as in vitro toxicity screening with different cell lines. The overall experimental workflow is shown in Fig. 1.

2 Materials

2.1 siRNA Reagents

1. siRNA pools of four synthetic siRNA duplexes siGENOME (Dharmacon, Life Technologies).
2. RNAse-free water.
3. RPMI-1640.
4. Dharmafect1 (Dharmacon, Life Technologies).
5. Reverse transfection medium: 15 µl RPMI-1640 with 0.05 µl Dharmafect1 added per well of a 384-well plate.

2.2 Multititer Plates

1. 384-well multititer plates: Sterile, with lid, white with transparent bottom (BD Falcon/Corning). Aluminum seal.

2.3 Cell Culture, Harvesting and Counting

1. HEK293 cells (CRL-1573™, ATCC).
2. T75 flasks with filter cap.

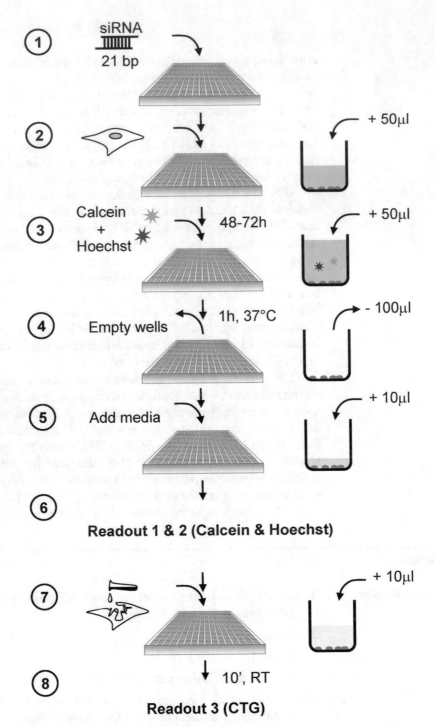

Fig. 1 Experimental work flow of the cell fitness multiplexing approach. Prior to high-throughput cell fitness screening, siRNA pools consisting of four individual siRNAs are distributed into 384-well multititer plates (1) and stored at −20 °C until the experiment. In a next step cells are seeded into the wells of multititer plates at defined concentration (2) and are reversely transfected for 72 h at 37 °C and 5 % CO_2. Upon reverse transfection the fluorescence indicators Hoechst 33342 and Calcein-AM are added to the cells and incubated for the indicated times (3). To minimize background fluorescence and signal-to-noise ratio the staining solution is completely removed from the wells (4) and replaced by 10 μl cell culture medium (without phenol-red) (5). Calcein and Hoechst fluorescence signals are measured using a plate reader (6). For analysis of cellular fitness based on metabolic activity and intracellular ATP concentration CellTiter-Glo Luminescent Cell Viability Assay Kit (CTG) is added to the cells and incubated at room temperature for 10 min (7). Upon cell lysis, luminescence intensity is recorded using a plate luminometer. Reproduced from (8), published under an open access license (CC-BY)

3. Culture expansion medium: Dulbecco's Modified Eagle's Medium (DMEM), 10 % fetal bovine serum (FBS), 100 U/ml penicillin, 100 mg/ml streptomycin.

4. Culture screening medium: DMEM, 10 % FBS.

5. Phosphate-buffered saline (PBS): Sterile Ca^{2+}- and Mg^{2+}-free phosphate buffered saline.

6. Harvesting medium: 0.05 % trypsin containing 0.025 % EDTA.

7. Hemocytometer.

2.4 Cell Fitness Screening

Protect all fluorescence and luminescence indicators from light

1. DMEM without phenol-red.

2. Dimethyl sulfoxide (DMSO).

3. Hoechst 33342.

4. Hoechst 33342 stock solution: 10 mM in RNAse-free water.

5. Calcein-AM.

6. Calcein-AM stock solution: 10 mM in 100 % DMSO.

7. Hoechst 33342/Calcein-AM staining solution: 20 μM Hoechst 33342, 20 μM Calcein-AM in DMEM.

8. CellTiter-Glo Luminescent Cell Viability Assay Kit (CTG, Promega).

9. CTG solution: 1:1 mixture of CTG and DMEM without phenol-red.

10. 24-channel wand.

3   Methods

Prepare all solutions with ultrapure RNAse-free water and analytical grade reagents. Prepare stock solutions at room temperature and store all reagents at –20 °C unless indicated otherwise. All steps and incubations are performed at room temperature unless indicated otherwise. *See* Fig. 1 for screening workflow. Conduct screening experiments in duplicate or in more replicates.

3.1 Preparation of siRNAs

1. Dissolve siRNA pools of four synthetic siRNA duplexes (*see* **Note 1**) as described by the manufacturer's instructions and dilute stock solutions for RNAi screening to a concentration of 200 nM in ultrapure RNAse-free water (*see* **Note 2**).

2. Distribute 5 μl of 200 nM sample and control siRNAs (*see* **Notes 3** and **4**) in white 384-well multititer plates with transparent bottom (*see* **Note 5**) manually or using a liquid-handling system. Cover the plates with aluminum seal and store until the experiment at –20 °C.

3.2 Cell Culture, Harvesting and Counting

1. Expansion: Seed 10^6 cells, suspended in 10 ml culture expansion medium in T75 (75 cm^2 growth area) flasks and culture cells at 37 °C, 5 % CO_2 in a humidified incubator according to standard procedures. Replace medium every 2–3 days. Use cells in RNAi screening experiments when approximately 80 % confluent (*see* **Note 6**).

2. Harvesting: To collect cells, remove the medium and wash cells gently with 5 ml PBS. Remove PBS and replace with 2 ml harvesting solution. Incubate cells for 2–4 min. Add 8 ml culture screening medium and dislodge cells from the flask by pipetting approx. 10 times up and down using a 10 ml serological pipet (*see* **Note 7**).

3. Counting: Dilute cell suspension 1:10 in culture screening medium. Add 10 µl diluted cell suspension to both compartments of a hemocytometer and count the number of cells in each of the eight (2×4) grids (*see* **Note 8**). Calculate the concentration of cells per ml using the following formula. Cells per ml = (cell count in eight squares/8) × dilution factor × 10^4. Where: dilution factor = 10; 10^4 = dilution factor of the hemocytometer as directed by the manufacturer.

4. Adjust the cell concentration to 1.3×10^5 cells per ml with culture screening medium (*see* **Note 9**).

3.3 siRNA Transfection

1. Thaw frozen siRNAs. Prior to removing the aluminum seal briefly centrifuge the 384-well plates to remove drops from the foil and to prevent cross contamination of different siRNA pools.

2. Prepare reverse transfection medium: For each well of a 384-well plate prepare 15 µl RPMI-1640 and add 0.05 µl Dharmafect1. Incubate for 10 min at room temperature (*see* **Note 10**).

3. Add 15 µl reverse transfection medium to each well containing 5 µl siRNA solution and incubate for 30 min at room temperature (*see* **Note 11**).

4. Add 30 µl cell suspension (adjusted to 1.3×10^5 cells per ml in culture screening medium) to each well (containing 5 µl siRNA pool and 15 µl reverse transfection medium) and allow the cells to sediment for 5 min (*see* **Note 12**).

5. Put plate in incubator and incubate for 72 h at 37 °C, 5 % CO_2 (*see* **Note 13**).

3.4 Cell Fitness Multiplexing

1. To assess cell fitness using fluorescence reporters, add 50 µl Hoechst 33342/Calcein-AM staining solution to each well of a 384-well plate and incubate for 1 h at 37 °C, 5 % CO_2 (*see* **Note 14**).

2. Empty wells using a 24-channel wand. If a 24-channel wand is not available, turn the plate upside-down onto a stack of tissue and leave for approx. 30 s until the solution is entirely removed from the wells.

3. Add 10 μl DMEM without phenol-red.

4. Immediately after solution exchange, measure fluorescence intensity of Hoechst stain using a plate reader with 355 nm excitation and 460 nm emission filter set.

5. Record Calcein fluorescence using the same plate reader with 485 nm excitation and 535 nm emission filter set (*see* **Note 15**).

6. Add 10 μl CTG solution (*see* **Note 16**) and incubate for 10 min at room temperature and protected from light.

7. Measure luminescence intensity with the same plate reader as used for quantification of fluorescence intensity.

3.5 Data Analysis and Normalization Using cellHTS2 or web cellHTS2

1. Analyze your data using *cellHTS2* (offline, *see* **Note 17**) or *web cellHTS2* (online, *see* **Note 18**)

2. When using the online tool, upload your data of Hoechst 33342, Calcein AM and CTG luminescence reading individually to http://web-cellhts2.dkfz.de/.

3. Download analysis results from the online analysis and unpack the archives. Click on the file 'index.html' to open an offline browser-based report of your experiment, including information on plate configuration and sample annotation, quality control data (e.g., replicate correlation, dynamic range of the assay) and a color-coded visualization of scored values providing an intuitive summary of your screening results.

4. Navigate to the subfolder named 'in'. The file 'toptable.txt' lists all raw and analysis data including normalized and scored values. Use data listed in the columns named 'median_ch1' and 'median_ch2' for subsequent analysis and assessment of phenotype intersection form the different fitness indicators.

5. Normalize plate reader data generated from individual fitness indicators and replicates on the plate median.

3.6 Analysis of Phenotype Intersection

1. Calculate the arithmetic mean of the normalized plate replicates.

2. Rank cell fitness phenotypes in increasing order. Top ranking mean values indicate lowest cell fitness and strongest phenotypes.

3. Calculate the intersection of a defined number of top ranking phenotypes. You may decide to consider selecting hits from your list based on the degree of intersecting phenotypes.

4 Notes

1. Any type of single or pooled siRNA duplexes can be used in the method.

2. Experimentally optimize the siRNA concentration prior to RNAi screening based on the instructions and concentration range given by the manufacturer. The siRNA concentration can vary depending on the used siRNA. Higher siRNA concentrations may result in an increased number of off-targets.

3. For negative control use for example a single or pooled non-targeting siRNAs. As further technical negative controls you might consider replacing siRNA and/or transfection reagents with water. We recommend using multiple negative controls, for example in duplicates to quadruplicates.

4. As a positive control use a single or pooled siRNA inducing a strong cellular phenotype, such as cell death, e.g., single or pooled WEE1, PLK1 or COPB2 siRNA. For example, the gene WEE1 plays a key role in cell cycle and causes cell death when silenced by RNAi [15]. Frequent hitters can also be retrieved from the database GenomeRNAi [16]. Additional technical positive controls to be considered might be functionally relevant single or pooled siRNAs, empty wells or wells of the multititer plate not equipped with cells in the course of the protocol.

5. For the described method, we recommend using white plates with transparent bottom to allow both bottom reading of fluorescence signal and top treading of luminescence signal. You may also consider using other plate types such as transparent or black plates with transparent bottom. Transparent plates are usually cheaper compared to white or black plates but may also result in comparably lower reproducibility of screening results due to co-illumination and increased photo bleaching of Calcein in adjacent wells during fluorescence reading. Nevertheless, when indicators with relatively robust fluorescence signal such as GFP or YFP variants are to be employed, e.g., in multiplexing approaches assessing the functional properties of ion channels [17–20] transparent plates should be suitable. When transparent plates are used with luminescence-based readouts such as the employed CellTiter-Glo Luminescent Cell Viability Assay Kit, emitted luminescence light from adjacent wells may interfere with the luminescence reading and result in poor reproducibility of screening results. Black plates are well suited for fluorescence indicators due to low auto fluorescence and reflective properties but are not optimal for luminescence based assaying approaches. We recommend experimental evaluation and optimization depending on the indicators used in the assaying technique.

6. The initial cell number for maintenance and expansion of cells as well as the frequency of medium exchange strongly depends on the used cell line, the cycling time and the age, i.e., the passage number of the cell culture. Refer to the supplier's instructions and recommendations regarding the cell line's characteristics and culture method.

7. Some cell lines require a different detachment procedure and involve other methods such as scratching or other reagents. Refer to the supplier's instructions and recommendations for the appropriate method.

8. For a newly established cell culture and when there is no experience regarding the characteristics of the cells, it is recommended to quantify the proportion of viable cells prior reseeding cells in culture flasks or multititer plates, e.g., with trypan blue. Trypan blue is a stain used to selectively color dead cells. When using trypan blue for counting viable cells, follow the manufacturer's instructions with regard to dye concentration and incubation time and count unstained cells only.

9. The cell concentration strongly depends on the cell line, the size of the cells, the cyling time, the culture plastic ware, the culture conditions, and the duration of the assay and requires individual and specific experimental optimization. Very low cell numbers may result in a small dynamic range of the assay as well as strong intra- and inter-multiwell plate variations. Very high cell numbers may cover small effects or result in overgrown monolayer cultures with altered characteristics.

10. The ratios of medium and transfection reagent as well as the incubation time and temperature require experimental optimization. Refer to the manufaturer's recommendations and individually optimize the conditions for different cell lines and RNAi reagents including siRNAs.

11. The incubation time has been experimentally optimized. Refer to the manufaturer's recommendations and individually optimize the conditions for different cell lines and RNAi reagents.

12. The given cell concentration has exclusively been optimized for the described method based on the mentioned reagents, plastic ware, and laboratory-specific reading infrastructure. We strongly recommend individual experimental and laboratory-specific optimization.

13. The duration of incubation may be shortened or extended depending on the assaying parameters, in particular the efficiency of gene knockdown, that for the listed reagents is reported to be highest after approx. 72 h upon reverse siRNA transfection.

14. The listed concentrations and incubation times have been optimized for HEK293 cells but should yield comparable results with other mammalian cell lines.

15. The order of Hoechst and Calcein measurement could be reversed if required by infrastructure.

16. Keep CTG solution on ice and protected from light at all times.

17. cellHTS2 provides an end-to-end analysis of cell-based high-throughput screening experiments [21]. Download and documentation are available at http://www.bioconductor.org/packages/release/bioc/html/cellHTS2.html

18. web cellHTS2 [22] is a front end for cellHTS2 and provides all features of cellHTS2. Web cellHTS2 guides the user through all analysis options and outputs a HTML file including a full quality control report and a ranked hit list. A detailed tutorial as well as a manual is available at http://web-cellhts2.dkfz.de/.

References

1. Sekhon BK, Roubin RH, Tan A et al (2008) High-throughput screening platform for anticancer therapeutic drug cytotoxicity. Assay Drug Dev Technol 6:711–721

2. Cai XY, Xiong LM, Yang SH et al (2014) Comparison of toxicity effects of ropivacaine, bupivacaine, and lidocaine on rabbit intervertebral disc cells in vitro. Spine J 14:483–490

3. Laurenza I, Pallocca G, Mennecozzi M et al (2013) A human pluripotent carcinoma stem cell-based model for in vitro developmental neurotoxicity testing: effects of methylmercury, lead and aluminum evaluated by gene expression studies. Int J Dev Neurosci 31:679–691

4. Wiezorek C (1984) Cell cycle dependence of Hoechst 33342 dye cytotoxicity on sorted living cells. Histochemistry 81:493–495

5. Haibe-Kains B, El-Hachem N, Birkbak NJ et al (2013) Inconsistency in large pharmacogenomic studies. Nature 504:389–393

6. Barretina J, Caponigro G, Stransky N et al (2012) The Cancer Cell Line Encyclopedia enables predictive modelling of anticancer drug sensitivity. Nature 483:603–607

7. Garnett MJ, Edelman EJ, Heidorn SJ et al (2012) Systematic identification of genomic markers of drug sensitivity in cancer cells. Nature 483:570–575

8. Gilbert DF, Erdmann G, Zhang X et al (2011) A novel multiplex cell viability assay for high-throughput RNAi screening. PLoS One 6, e28338

9. Womac AD, Burkeen JF, Neuendorff N et al (2009) Circadian rhythms of extracellular ATP accumulation in suprachiasmatic nucleus cells and cultured astrocytes. Eur J Neurosci 30:869–876

10. Ataullakhanov FI, Vitvitsky VM (2002) What determines the intracellular ATP concentration. Biosci Rep 22:501–511

11. das Neves RP, Jones NS, Andreu L et al (2010) Connecting variability in global transcription rate to mitochondrial variability. PLoS Biol 8, e1000560

12. Braut-Boucher F, Pichon J, Rat P et al (1995) A non-isotopic, highly sensitive, fluorimetric, cell-cell adhesion microplate assay using calcein AM-labeled lymphocytes. J Immunol Methods 178:41–51

13. Graca da Silveira M, Vitoria San Romao M, Loureiro-Dias MC et al (2002) Flow cytometric assessment of membrane integrity of ethanol-stressed Oenococcus oeni cells. Appl Environ Microbiol 68:6087–6093

14. Larsson R, Nygren P (1989) A rapid fluorometric method for semiautomated determination of cytotoxicity and cellular proliferation of human tumor cell lines in microculture. Anticancer Res 9:1111–1119

15. Mollapour M, Tsutsumi S, Neckers L (2010) Hsp90 phosphorylation, Wee1 and the cell cycle. Cell Cycle 9:2310–2316

16. Horn T, Arziman Z, Berger J et al (2007) GenomeRNAi: a database for cell-based RNAi phenotypes. Nucleic Acids Res 35:D492–D497

17. Gilbert DF, Wilson JC, Nink V et al (2009) Multiplexed labeling of viable cells for high-throughput analysis of glycine receptor function using flow cytometry. Cytometry A 75:440–449

18. Talwar S, Lynch JW, Gilbert DF (2013) Fluorescence-based high-throughput functional profiling of ligand-gated ion channels at the level of single cells. PLoS One 8, e58479

19. Gebhardt FM, Mitrovic AD, Gilbert DF et al (2010) Exon-skipping splice variants of excitatory amino acid transporter-2 (EAAT2) form heteromeric complexes with full-length EAAT2. J Biol Chem 285:31313–31324

20. Gilbert D, Esmaeili A, Lynch JW (2009) Optimizing the expression of recombinant alphabetagamma GABAA receptors in HEK293 cells for high-throughput screening. J Biomol Screen 14:86–91

21. Boutros M, Bras LP, Huber W (2006) Analysis of cell-based RNAi screens. Genome Biol 7:R66

22. Pelz O, Gilsdorf M, Boutros M (2010) web cellHTS2: a web-application for the analysis of high-throughput screening data. BMC Bioinformatics 11:185

Chapter 7

RNAi Screening of Leukemia Cells Using Electroporation

Anupriya Agarwal and Jeffrey W. Tyner

Abstract

RNAi-mediated screening has been an integral tool for biological discovery for the past 15 years. A variety of approaches have been employed for implementation of this technique, including pooled, depletion/enrichment screening with lentiviral shRNAs, and segregated screening of panels of individual siRNAs. The latter approach of siRNA panel screening requires efficient methods for transfection of siRNAs into the target cells. In the case of suspension leukemia cell lines and primary cells, many of the conventional transfection techniques using liposomal or calcium phosphate-mediated transfection provide very low efficiency. In this case, electroporation is the only transfection technique offering high efficiency transfection of siRNAs into the target leukemia cells. Here, we describe methods for optimization and implementation of siRNA electroporation into leukemia cell lines and primary patient specimens, and we further offer suggested electroporation settings for some commonly used leukemia cell lines.

Key words siRNA screening, Leukemia, Electroporation

1 Introduction

Since the inception of RNAi, a number of techniques have emerged that employ the ubiquitous gene-silencing capacity of short interfering RNA (siRNA) and short hairpin RNA (shRNA) to functionally assess the biological relevance of genes in a variety of contexts, including many of the functional screens that have been conducted for target discovery in cancer [1–15]. There are two basic strategies for these screens depending on whether the siRNA or shRNA are delivered together in a single pool to the target cells, or whether they are segregated and delivered individually. In the former strategy, a panel of shRNAs coupled to identifiable barcodes in lentiviral vectors is delivered as a single pool to target cells. By comparing the initial frequency of each shRNA barcode with the frequency after a treatment or culture period (or comparing pools of cells where shRNA expression has been induced versus uninduced), target genes that are biologically important for the cellular phenotype under interrogation can be elucidated. In the latter, segregated

David O. Azorsa, Shilpi Arora (eds.), *High-Throughput RNAi Screening: Methods and Protocols*, Methods in Molecular Biology, vol. 1470, DOI 10.1007/978-1-4939-6337-9_7, © Springer Science+Business Media New York 2016

strategy, a panel of siRNAs is distributed across multi-well plates where each well contains siRNA targeting a single gene. These siRNAs are then batch transfected into target cells that are subsequently cultured to allow for biological examination of the impact of each siRNA on the cellular phenotype in question (cell growth, survival, differentiation, etc.).

Both of these screening modalities have been successfully used to drive many important biological discoveries. Here we will focus on the segregated screening approach, and specifically on the methods for application of this approach on difficult-to-transfect leukemia cells (both cell lines and primary cells). Because leukemia cells are recalcitrant to transfection with standard liposomal or calcium phosphate methods, we have extensively used electroporation as a technique for delivery of both individual siRNAs as well as panels of siRNAs into leukemia cell lines and primary patient specimens. This chapter will describe the methodologies that we have developed for optimization of electroporation settings to balance the highest possible transfection efficiency with robust cell viability and growth post-electroporation [3–5, 16–18]. We additionally provide settings we have determined using this optimization approach for a variety of commonly used leukemia cell lines as well as primary patient specimens.

2   Materials

1. *siRNA reconstitution buffer*: dilute 5× siRNA buffer (GE Dharmacon) with Nuclease Free water.

2. *Lyophilized siRNA library* (e.g. siGENOME SMARTPool library from GE Dharmacon) in 96-well plates: Library plates are commonly comprised of siRNAs targeting 94 individual genes, one nonsilencing siRNA, and one well kept empty for a no cell, blank control (*see* **Note 1**).

3. *Culture media for cells*: For cell lines: use media according to the specific culture requirements of each cell line.

   For primary myeloid leukemia samples: RPMI with 10% FBS, 2 mM L-glutamine, 100 U/mL penicillin, 100 µg/mL streptomycin + βME.

   For primary B-cell lymphoid leukemia samples: RPMI with 20% FBS, 2 mM L-glutamine, 100 U/mL penicillin, 100 µg/mL streptomycin + βME.

   For primary T-cell lymphoid leukemia samples: Same as B-cell lymphoid sample media with the addition of 1× Insulin Transferrin Selenium.

   βME concentration is 10^{-4} M (dilute 3 µl of βME into 500 ml media); no βME is required for cell lines.

4. 96-well tissue culture plates.

5. 96-well PCR plates with conical bottom.

6. 200 μl filtered tips.

7. 10–20 μl filtered tips.

8. Adhesive breathable plate seals to cover 96-well plates and to avoid edge effect due to evaporation.

9. Multichannel pipettes.

10. Plastic trough for multichannel pipetting.

11. Cell strainer (40 μm).

12. Phosphate-buffered saline (PBS).

13. 96-well electroporation plates (Bio-Rad).

14. 96-well electroporation machine (such as Bio-Rad Gene Pulser MXCell).

15. Centrifuge to spin 96-well plates.

16. CellTiter 96® AQueous One Solution Cell Proliferation Assay reagent (Promega).

17. Cell viability reagent (e.g. propidium idodide, trypan blue).

18. Spectrophotometric plate reader.

19. Optional: Use an automated liquid handler to aliquot siRNA library and prepare media plates (Such as Epimotion, Eppendorf; Multidrop, ThermoScientific; etc.).

20. siPORT Buffer Recipe: The recipe for the siPORT buffer is listed in Table 1.

Table 1
siPORT buffer recipe

Components	Stock (M)	Dilution	Final (mM)	For 250 ml	For 500 ml
Trehalose	1.2	0.1	120	25	50
HEPES	1	0.02	20	5	10
Myo-Inositol	0.1	0.01	1	2.5	5
KCl	0.1	0.01	1	2.5	5
$MgCl_2$	0.1	0.01	1	2.5	5
K_2HPO_4	0.1	0.01	1	2.5	5
KH_2PO_4	0.04	0.01	0.4	2.5	5
KOH	0.214	0.01	2.14	2.5	5
Glutathione	0.1	0.01	1	2.5	5
Water				202.5	405

3   Methods

Perform all the steps at room temperature unless specified.

3.1 Reconstitute Library

1. Make 7.5 ml siRNA reconstitution buffer per one 96-well plate containing 1 nmol siRNA per well (mix 1.5 ml 5× siRNA buffer with 6 ml Nuclease Free water).

2. Spin down 96-well plate containing lyophilized 1 nmol siRNA library for 30 s at $2000 \times g$ at room temperature.

3. Aliquote 54 µl reconstitution buffer per well in 96-well master siRNA plate, resulting in a stock siRNA concentration in each well of ~18.5 µM (*see* **Note 1**).

4. Vortex briefly (using Eppendorf MixMate or similar product) and let it sit at 4 °C for 10 min, vortex again and then spin before aliquoting.

5. Next from each plate aliquot 6 µl/well into seven skirted PCR plates using multichannel pipette or automated liquid transfer device. Master plate will be saved as 8th plate. Thus, a single siRNA masterplate containing 1 nnol per well siRNA library will create eight daughter libraries.

6. Seal the plates with PCR plate transparent seals and store at −80 °C until ready to use.

3.2 Optimization of Electroporation Protocol

Before performing siRNA screening, optimize electroporation conditions for each new cell line or type of cells (Fig. 1).

1. Spin down 1×10^5 cells per condition for leukemia cell lines or 3×10^5 cells per condition for primary leukemia cells at $350 \times g$, for 5 min.

2. Resuspend in 1 ml PBS.

3. Spin down again.

4. Resuspend in 100 µl siPORT Buffer per condition.

5. Optional—if you have a known positive control target gene that will reduce growth/viability of target cells ("killer siRNA") add to a final concentration of 1 µM nonspecific or killer siRNA per condition (6 µl of 18.5 µM siRNA + 100 µl of cells in siPORT buffer). In the absence of a known target gene, PLK1 siRNA can be used as a generic killer siRNA.

6. Save unelectroporated cells (equivalent to one condition) for control.

7. Transfer to 96-well electroporation plates with gap width of 4 mm (cuvettes of varying gap width can also be used, however, changing cuvette gap width will dramatically alter the effective pulse lengths).

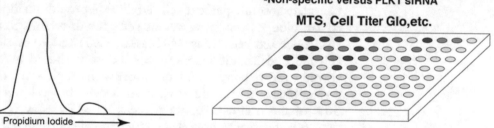

a Electroporate Target Cells with Variety of Voltages and Pulse Lengths
-4 wells are electroporated at once
-Positive control (killer) siRNAs can be used, if available (e.g. ABL1 siRNA for CML cells)
-In absence of cell line-specific killer siRNA, PLK1 can be used

Voltage (Volts)	200	200	200	200	300	300	300	300	400	400	400	400
Pulse Length (msec)	3.5	4.0	4.5	5.0	3.5	4.0	4.5	5.0	3.5	4.0	4.5	5.0

Culture 2-4 Days

b Evaluate Absolute Cell Viability Percent
-PI Exclusion, Trypan Blue, etc.

Propidium Iodide

c Evaluate Relative Cell Growth/Viability
-Non-specific versus cell-specific Killer siRNA
-Non-specific versus PLK1 siRNA

MTS, Cell Titer Glo,etc.

d Select Optimal Settings, Test Knockdown (qPCR, Immunoblot), Perform Screen

Fig. 1 Workflow for optimization of electroporation conditions for leukemia cells. (**a**) To determine optimal electroporation conditions, incubate cells with nonspecific siRNA or siRNA targeted to a gene that is necessary for maintenance of the growth/viability of the cells of interest. In the absence of a gene target that is specific to the cell line of interest, siRNA targeting PLK1 can be used as a generic "killer siRNA". Electroporate cells using a variety of different voltages and pulse lengths, a good starting range for voltage is 150–450 V. Pulse length will vary widely depending on the gap width of cuvettes being used. For standard 4 mm gap width, a good starting range is 1.5–5.0 ms. (**b**) After electroporation, culture for 2 days and determine the percent cell viability using a method such as PI exclusion. (**c**) In parallel, plate cells in 96-well plates to conduct a proliferation/cell viability assay after 4 days using a tetrazolium-based assay, such as MTS. (**d**) To select the optimal conditions for electroporation, several factors must be balanced including PI exclusion cell viability readings exceeding at least 80 %, MTS cell viability readings of at least 60 % of unelectroporated control cells, and maximal impact of killer siRNA on cell viability compared with nonspecific control

8. Electroporate using Square Wave protocol using a combination of different voltages and pulse lengths, ranging from 150 to 450 V and 1.5–5.0 ms, respectively (Fig. 1) (*see* **Note 2**).

9. Transfer 10–12 µl electroporated cells in triplicate in a 96-well plate containing 90 µl media/well to perform MTS analysis at 96 h and culture left over cells in a 24-well plate with culture media in 1:10 ratio to analyze cell viability at 48 h (*see* **Note 3**).

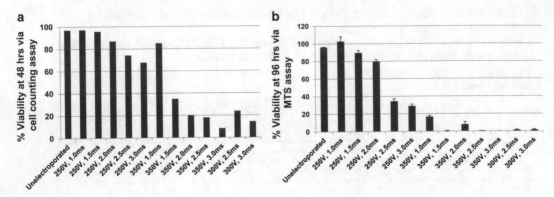

Fig. 2 Exemplary PI exclusion and MTS cell viability readings from electroporation optimization experiments. MOLT-4 cells (1×10^5 cells/well) were electroporated using a square wave protocol with indicated voltages and pulse lengths for two pulses. 12 μl of electroporated cells were transferred to 90 μl of culture media for assessment of cell viability by PI exclusion at 48 h (**a**) and by MTS assay at 96 h in triplicate (**b**)

10. Compare absolute percent cell viability via propidium idodide, tyrpan blue, or similar as well as cell growth relative to non-electroporated cells using MTS assay, CellTiterGlo or similar (Figs. 1 and 2). Electroporation conditions should maintain absolute cell viability at 80 % or higher with propidium iodide/ trypan blue and reduction in growth should be no lower than 50 % of the non-electroporated cells by MTS assay (greater than 60 % relative to non-electroporated cells is preferred) (*see* **Note 4**, Table 2).

3.3 Library Screening with siRNA in Leukemia Cells

1. Prepare three 96-well plates with 90 μl of appropriate culture media in each well and store in incubator at 37 °C with 5 % CO_2 until use.

2. Reconstitute 3×10^7 cells from a primary patient or 1×10^7 cells from a cell line in 50 ml PBS for each 96-well plate siRNA library.

3. Spin the cells at $350 \times g$ for 10 min.

4. During the spin, thaw an aliquot of the 6 μl siRNA library. Once thawed, spin at $2800 \times g$ for 15 s. leaving centrifuge break off and let slow down while waiting for cells to finish spinning.

5. Resuspend cells in 10.5 ml cold siPORT Buffer, mix the single cell suspension by pipetting and passing through a 40 μm nylon cell strainer.

6. Transfer the cell suspension as quickly as possible to a disposable trough. Aliquot 100 μl into each well of the siRNA library (except A1, blank well), making sure to mix thoroughly. Addition of 100 μl of cells to the 6 μl siRNA in each well results in a final siRNA concentration of ~1 μM.

7. Transfer the entire contents from each well of the PCR plate to electroporation plate with multi-channel pipette set at 150 μl.

Table 2
Suggested electroporation conditions for several leukemia cell lines

Cell line	Electroporation condition	% viability via cell counting	% viability via MTS assay
MOLT4	250 V, 2.0 ms	86	79
JURKAT	200 V, 2.5 ms	81	62
GDM-1	250 V, 4.0 ms	95	63
Kasumi-2	200 V, 4.0 ms	81	53
LOUCY	250 V, 4.0 ms	83	87
MOLT-16	250 V, 2.0 ms	N/A	75
UT-7	350 V, 1.0 ms	N/A	77
SUPT-13	200 V, 4.5 ms	N/A	81
HBPALL	250 V, 3.5 ms	N/A	85
SKW-3	200 V, 4.5 ms	N/A	75
PEER	200 V, 4.5 ms	N/A	90
CCRF	250 V, 3.0 ms	N/A	89
RPMI-8402	250 V, 3.0 ms	N/A	60
PF-382	250 V, 3.0 ms	N/A	70
AML-1	250 V, 3.0 ms	N/A	53
ML-1	250 V, 3.0 ms	N/A	72
HL-60	250 V, 3.0 ms	N/A	63
TF-1	250 V, 3.0 ms	N/A	62
HT-93	300 V, 3.0 ms	N/A	80
Primary myeloid cells	275 V, 5.0 ms		
Primary lymphoid cells	250 V, 4.0 ms		

Note: The electroporation conditions might slightly vary from above suggested conditions because of variation in cell clones. Therefore it is recommended to optimize own conditions around the above-given parameters

8. Add 106 μl of blank siPORT buffer to well A1 of the electroporation plate.

9. Inspect the plate to make sure the bottom of each well is fully covered in liquid by gently shaking plate; pop any remaining bubbles with pipette tips.

10. Select the appropriate protocol for electroporation as optimized in Subheading 3.2:

11. Place the plate in the plate handler, making sure to push down on plate until it is fully inserted. Leave the plate lid on and close the lid of the plate handler.

12. When ready, press pulse using the optimized electroporation program.

13. Remove the three plates with media from the incubator. For each row, mix thoroughly using a P200 multi-channel pipette set at 50 μl and then transfer 12 μl (*see* **Note 5**) from electroporation plate into each of the three plates with media using a P20 multi-channel pipette.

14. Seal all plates with adhesive and breathable plate sealer.

15. Incubate the plates at 37 °C for 4 days (96 h).

16. At day 4, add 20 μl of MTS reagent to every well (including A1). Plates should be monitored throughout the day with readings taken when media is changing from yellow to brown. Generally with patient samples, plates should be visually checked after 1–2 h. If visible color change has occurred, then a reading should be taken. If not, take a longer reading (4–8 h later) and then it is a good idea to take another reading the next morning. Absorbances in the 0.1–1.0 range are preferred. If a sample has already achieved readings above 0.2, no further readings are needed.

17. For data analysis, subtract the blank well absorbance value from the individual well value. Take the full plate median and normalize each well absorbance value to the full plate median to calculate % growth. Then calculate the mean and standard deviation across all data points on the plate. Any siRNA conditions with values lower than two standard deviations below the plate mean are candidate hits. Carefully examine data from all three plates for consistency and accuracy (*see* **Note 6**).

3.4 Electroporation Plate Cleaning Protocol

Electroporation plates can be reused up to four times after following an extensive cleaning protocol as described below

1. Immediately after transferring electroporated cells to warmed media, shake the remaining liquid out of the electroporation plate.

2. Wash the plate twice with MiliQ water making sure to shake the water out of the plate after each wash.

3. Place in a tub with MiliQ water for 5–10 min.

4. Shake out the water and then place in a tub with 0.2 M HCl for 5–10 min (making sure not to leave the plate in for longer because the acid can corrode the metal).

5. Shake out the acid above the container and then wash with MiliQ water.

6. Using a 70% EtOH spray bottle, spray each row and column at least 3 times.

7. Place the plate in the hood and let air dry.

8. Once dry, expose the plate and lid to a cell culture hood UV light source for 15 min; cover the plate with the lid and return to the original plate packaging until the next use.

4   Notes

1. Use A1 corner well of a 96-well plate as a blank well and check orientation of plates while aliquoting the library. Additionally after aliquoting, check if each well contains siRNA. For consistency the library aliquoting could be performed using a liquid handler such as EpMotion.

2. On a 96-well electroporation plate there are a total of 24 well sets, each well set comprises four wells. All four wells in an individual well set will always be electroporated with the same electroporation condition. Therefore, a total of 24 electroporation conditions can be tested simultaneously. It is recommended to optimize at least 12 electroporation conditions for a new cell line. Also, it is not necessary to use the whole plate at the same time and unused well sets can be utilized for later experiment. For example four cell lines can be tested using half of a plate or eight cell lines can be tested using a whole plate with 12 different electroporation conditions (though only half this number would be possible if using a nonspecific and killer siRNA or each cell line as this would require two rows for each cell line).

3. Once cells are reconstituted in siPORT buffer and electroporated, cells need to be transferred to their destination plates immediately and quickly as prolonged exposure to siPORT buffer can have cytotoxic effects.

4. If using a positive control siRNA, then the percent reduction in viability relative to the nonsilencing control should be used as an additional factor for selecting the optimal electroporation condition. The knockdown of the target can be validated by quantitative PCR and/or immunoblot. If utilizing fluorescently tagged siRNA, then the shift in mean fluorescent intensity of electroporated versus non-electroporated conditions (as assessed by flow cytometry) can be used in addition to cell growth/viability readings to select optimal conditions.

5. For slow growing cells, up to 18 µl of electroporated cells per well can be transferred from the electroporation plate into the final cell culture plates containing cell culture media.

6. For data analysis, in addition to normalization of individual well values to plate median, values can also be normalized to the mean of each respective row and column. This can be done for each well for every row and column to eliminate positional artifacts and reduce run deviation.

References

1. Ngo VN, Davis RE, Lamy L et al (2006) A loss-of-function RNA interference screen for molecular targets in cancer. Nature 441:106–110

2. Westbrook TF, Martin ES, Schlabach MR et al (2005) A genetic screen for candidate tumor suppressors identifies REST. Cell 121:837–848

3. Tyner JW, Walters DK, Willis SG et al (2008) RNAi screening of the tyrosine kinome identifies therapeutic targets in acute myeloid leukemia. Blood 111:2238–2245

4. Tyner JW, Deininger MW, Loriaux MM et al (2009) RNAi screen for rapid therapeutic target identification in leukemia patients. Proc Natl Acad Sci U S A 106:8695–8700

5. Agarwal A, MacKenzie RJ, Eide CA et al (2014) Functional RNAi screen targeting cytokine and growth factor receptors reveals oncorequisite role for interleukin-2 gamma receptor in JAK3-mutation-positive leukemia. Oncogene 34:2991–2999

6. Bric A, Miething C, Bialucha CU et al (2009) Functional identification of tumor-suppressor genes through an in vivo RNA interference screen in a mouse lymphoma model. Cancer Cell 16:324–335

7. Hu G, Kim J, Xu Q et al (2009) A genome-wide RNAi screen identifies a new transcriptional module required for self-renewal. Genes Dev 23:837–848

8. Luo J, Emanuele MJ, Li D et al (2009) A genome-wide RNAi screen identifies multiple synthetic lethal interactions with the Ras oncogene. Cell 137:835–848

9. Schlabach MR, Luo J, Solimini NL et al (2008) Cancer proliferation gene discovery through functional genomics. Science 319:620–624

10. Ebert BL, Pretz J, Bosco J et al (2008) Identification of RPS14 as a 5q-syndrome gene by RNA interference screen. Nature 451:335–339

11. Lam LT, Davis RE, Ngo VN et al (2008) Compensatory IKKalpha activation of classical NF-kappaB signaling during IKKbeta inhibition identified by an RNA interference sensitization screen. Proc Natl Acad Sci U S A 105:20798–20803

12. Silva JM, Mizuno H, Brady A et al (2004) RNA interference microarrays: high-throughput loss-of-function genetics in mammalian cells. Proc Natl Acad Sci U S A 101:6548–6552

13. Zender L, Xue W, Zuber J et al (2008) An oncogenomics-based in vivo RNAi screen identifies tumor suppressors in liver cancer. Cell 135:852–864

14. Hannon GJ, Rossi JJ (2004) Unlocking the potential of the human genome with RNA interference. Nature 431:371–378

15. Paddison PJ, Silva JM, Conklin DS et al (2004) A resource for large-scale RNA-interference-based screens in mammals. Nature 428:427–431

16. Bicocca VT, Chang BH, Masouleh BK et al (2012) Crosstalk between ROR1 and the pre-B-cell receptor promotes survival of t(1;19) acute lymphoblastic leukemia. Cancer Cell 22:656–667

17. Maxson JE, Gotlib J, Pollyea DA et al (2013) Oncogenic CSF3R mutations in chronic neutrophilic leukemia and atypical CML. N Engl J Med 368:1781–1790

18. Sanda T, Tyner JW, Gutierrez A et al (2013) TYK2-STAT1-BCL2 pathway dependence in T-cell acute lymphoblastic leukemia. Cancer Discov 3:564–577

Chapter 8

Self-Assembled Cell Microarray (SAMcell) for High-Throughput RNAi Screening

Hanshuo Zhang and Juan Li

Abstract

RNAi has now become a valuable research tool for cell-based high-throughput screening. However, traditional RNAi high-throughput methods are based on multi-well plates, relying on expensive instruments and complicated operations. In this chapter, we describe a method termed self-assembled cell microarray (SAMcell), which integrates micro-fabrication, reverse transfection, and RNAi technologies and allows for cell behavior investigations to be performed directly on the cell chip. This method has been successfully employed to perform large-scale functional screening assays to identify gene modulators of cell migration, cell proliferation, and cellular apoptosis.

Key words RNAi, High-throughput screening, SAMcell, Chip, Cell behavior

1 Introduction

RNAi is a biological process in which RNA molecules inhibit gene expression, typically by degradation of messenger RNA (mRNA) molecules with specific sequences. In 2006, Andrew Fire and Craig C. Mello shared the Nobel Prize in Physiology or Medicine for their work on RNA interference in the nematode worm *C. elegans* [1]. There are two types of small ribonucleic acid (RNA) molecules that play central roles in RNAi process, microRNA (miRNA) and small interfering RNA (siRNA). According to the central dogma, RNA transcripts are the direct products of genes, and mRNAs guide the protein translation [2]. These small RNAs can bind to target mRNA molecules containing complementary sequence and can decrease their activity, either by inducing cleavage of mRNAs or by preventing mRNAs from producing proteins [3].

RNAi has now become a valuable research tool, and large-scale RNAi-based screening allows for the identification of the genetic components necessary for a particular cellular process such as cell proliferation and cell migration [4, 5], by systematically knocking down each gene in the cell. The RNAi high-throughput screening

David O. Azorsa, Shilpi Arora (eds.), *High-Throughput RNAi Screening: Methods and Protocols*, Methods in Molecular Biology, vol. 1470, DOI 10.1007/978-1-4939-6337-9_8, © Springer Science+Business Media New York 2016

(HTS) technology allows for genome-wide loss-of-function screening and is broadly used to identify genes associated with specific biological phenotypes [6]. This technology has been hailed as the second genomics wave, following the first genomics wave of gene expression microarray and single-nucleotide polymorphism (SNP) platforms [6]. One of the major advantages of the RNAi HTS technology is the ability to simultaneously test thousands of genes, which lead to an explosion in the rate of generating data.

Traditional RNAi HTS methods are mainly based on multi-well plates, including cell seeding, transfection, incubation, assay treatment, and data processing procedures, relying on expensive instruments and complicated operations. To systematically investigate functional genes on a large scale, we developed a novel on-chip method, SAMcell (self-assembled cell microarray) [7]. This method was demonstrated to be particularly suitable for high-throughput RNAi screening because of its unique advantages, including lower costs of reagents (transfection reagents, RNAs, antibodies, or dyes), decreased likelihood of cross-contamination, increased throughput, and increased reliability and accuracy of the data. Due to a thermally responsive polymer, this microarray has additional key features, such as tailored cell patterns, as well as a clear cell boundary and hence no interference from neighboring cells.

The cell chip is an open system and retains ease of conduct as the procedures are conducted once contrasting a well-by-well method.

This cell chip is an open system and easy to use and all of the procedures are performed only once. Cells are cultured on a chip and treated with the same condition, which results in low variation. We demonstrated this method to investigate miRNAs involved in cell migration and cell apoptosis at first. Furthermore, it will be readily adapted to perform large-scale screening of functional genes regulating other phenotypes, such as cell proliferation and cell autophagy [7–11].

2 Materials

2.1 Micro-Fabrication

1. Glass slides: Size of glass slide is 2.2 cm × 2.2 cm. Slides were washed with detergent, milli-Q water (Millipore), and ethanol. Slides are dried using a blower.

2. 6% Poly (N-isopropylacrylamide) (PNI) solution: PNI (Sigma-Aldrich) is dissolved in ethanol and stored at 4 °C.

3. Shadow mask: Silicon slide etched using a laser to form round holes with a diameter of 0.8 mm, and distance to adjacent holes at 2.25 mm (center to center).

4. Oxygen plasma machine (Beijing Technology).

2.2 Reverse Transfection	1. siRNA oligonucleotides (Ambion); dissolved in DEPC water and stored at −80 °C.
	2. Lipofectamine 2000 (Invitrogen).
	3. 0.4 M Sucrose in OptiMEM (Invitrogen).
	4. 0.2 % Gelatin solution: Dissolve gelatin powder (Type B, Sigma-Aldrich) in milliQ water (Millipore) at 56 °C for 20 min. After cooling to room temperature, add human fibronectin (Sigma-Aldrich) to a concentration of 0.01 % (v/v). Filter sterilize using a 0.45 μm filter.
	5. 384-Well low-volume plates (RNase-free, Axygen).
	6. Automated liquid-handling robot (Bravo, Agilent).
	7. Nano-dispenser (Phoenix, Art Robbins Instruments).
2.3 Cell Culture	1. Cell petri dish (3.5 cm, BD Falcon).
	2. HeLa cervical carcinoma cells (ATCC).
	3. Growth media: Dulbecco's modified Eagle medium (Gibco) containing 10 % fetal bovine serum, 100 U/ml penicillin, and 0.1 mg/ml streptomycin.
	4. PBS buffer: 137 mM NaCl, 2.7 mM KCl, 10 mM Na_2HPO_4, and 2 mM KH_2PO_4 dissolved in ddH_2O. pH 7.4. Sterilized by autoclaving.
	5. Trypsin solution: 0.25 g Trypsin powder (Amresco) dissolved in 100 ml PBS buffer and filter sterilize using a 0.22 μm filter.
	6. CO_2 incubator.
2.4 Cellular Assays	1. 4 % Paraformaldehyde (PFA) solution: Dissolve 4 g paraformaldehyde powder (Amresco) in 100 ml PBS buffer.
	2. Hoechst 33342 dye solution (Sigma).
	3. High-throughput microscope system (Image Xpress, Molecular Devices).
	4. Cell proliferation assay kit: Cell-Light™EdU DNA Cell Proliferation Kit (Guangzhou RiboBio).
	5. Cell apoptosis assay kit: Annexin-V-FLUOS Staining Kit (Roche).

3 Methods

3.1 Fabrication of SAMcell (Self-Assembled Cell Microarray)	1. Glass slides are covered with poly (N-isopropylacrylamide) dissolved in ethanol (6 % w/v).
	2. The slides are etched via a shadow mask by oxygen plasma for 5 min at 200 W.
	3. For reverse transfection, 3 μl of OptiMEM and 2.5 μl Lipofectamine™ 2000 are transferred to each tube and mixed

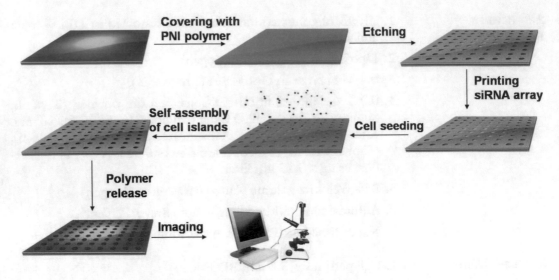

Fig. 1 Construction of the self-assembled cell microarray

thoroughly. Then, 2 µg siRNA or 1 µg plasmid is added to each tube and the mixture is incubated for 20 min at room temperature. Finally, 7.25 µl of a 0.2 % (w/v) gelatin solution is added to each tube and mixed thoroughly.

4. After UV sterilization, the reverse transfection reagent is printed on the chip via a nano-dispenser. Pre-fabricated siRNA arrays can be used without loss of transfection efficiency at least up to 6 months after printing.

5. The chips are fixed in a 3.5 cm petri dish by melted wax.

6. 1–5×10^5 Hela cells in about 3 ml of media at 37 °C are transferred to the petri dish containing a siRNA-printed SAMcell chip. The dish is then incubated at 37 °C.

7. About 24–48 h later, cells self-assemble to form cell islands (*see* **Note 1**). The dish is moved to room temperature for 5 min and washed three times with PBS to ensure the total removal of the polymer (*see* **Note 2**) (Fig. 1).

3.2 Cross-Contamination Detection (Optional)

Considering that the SAMcell chip is an open system, cross-contamination is a concern. Cross-contamination of the SAMcell chip can be tested for by using a GFP plasmid.

1. A GFP-plasmid-printed SAMcell chip is used where the plasmid is alternatively spotted onto 10×10 arrays in the microarray (Fig. 2).

2. Cells are added to the array as described above.

3. After removal of the PNI polymer, a high-throughput microscope system is used to capture images.

Schematic diagram   **Fluorescent microscopic images**

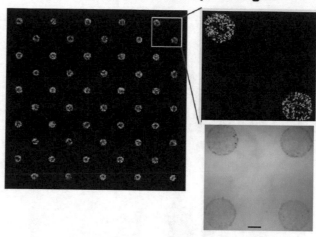

● GFP plasmid ● NC plasmid

Fig. 2 No detectable cross-contamination in neighboring diagonal positions. A green fluorescent protein-expressing plasmid is alternatively spotted on 10 × 10 arrays in the microarray. Schematic diagram and fluorescent microscopic images are shown in the *left* and *right* panels, respectively. Scale bar, 500 μm

3.3 Cell Migration Assay

1. A siRNA-printed SAMcell chip is used and with selected siRNA (*see* **Note 3**) the cells are added as described above. Four repeats are performed in each group.

2. After removal of the PNI polymer, a high-throughput microscope system is used to record cell island images and calculate cell island areas at 0 and 10 h (*see* **Note 4**) (Fig. 3).

3.4 Cell Proliferation Assay

1. A siRNA-printed SAMcell chip is used (*see* **Note 5**) and cells are added as described above.

2. After removal of the PNI polymer, the cells are treated with PFA buffer and stained with Hoechst.

3. The Cell-Light TMEdU DNA Cell Proliferation Kit is used to detect cell proliferation activity (Fig. 4).

4. A high-throughput microscope system is used to record images.

3.5 Cell Apoptosis Assay

1. A siRNA-printed SAMcell chip is used (*see* **Note 6**) and cells are added as described above.

2. After removal of the PNI polymer, Annexin V FLUOS Staining Kit is used to detect cell apoptosis activity (Fig. 5).

3. A high-throughput microscope system is used to record images.

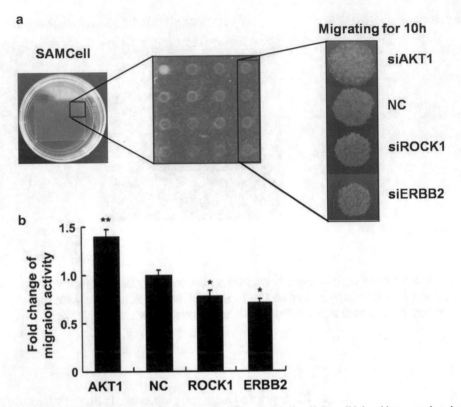

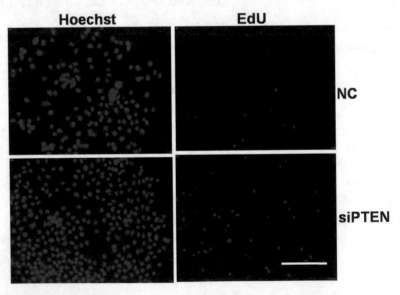

Fig. 3 Use of SAMcell for the study of cell migration. (**a**) Representative Hela cell island images showing migration phenotypes. Scale bar: 500 μm. (**b**) Statistical results are shown in histogram. $N = 4$

Fig. 4 Use of SAMcell for the study of cell proliferation. *Blue*: Hoechst. *Red*: EdU. Scale bar: 500 μm

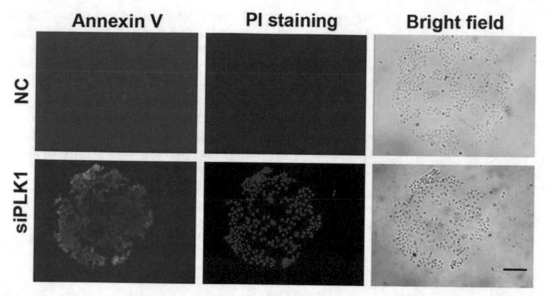

Fig. 5 Use of SAMcell for the study of cell apoptosis. *Green*: Annexin V-FITC. *Red*: PI. Scale bar: 500 µm

4   Notes

1. Cells self-assemble within each circle as they grow well on the glass slide, but rather poorly on PNI.

2. PNI has been previously demonstrated to have a sharply lower critical solution temperature, ~32 °C [12], indicating that PNI undergoes a solid–liquid-phase transition as it is cooled below 32 °C, and dissolves in the surrounding aqueous medium. Therefore, the subsequent removal of the dissolved polymer results in the formation of individual cell islands, enabling the cells the freedom to move.

3. siRNA sequences for cell migration assay include the following: NC: UUCUCCGAACGUGUCACGUtt (sense), ACGUGAC ACGUUCGGAGAAtt (anti-sense). siAKT1: GCGUGACCAU GAACGAGUUtt (sense), AACUCGUUCAUGGUCACGC gg (antisense). siROCK1: GGUUAGAACAAGAGGUAAAtt (sense), UUUACCUCUUGUUCUAACCgt (anti-sense). siER BB2: GGAGACCCGCUGAACAAUAtt (sense), UAUUGU UCAGCGGGUCUCCat (antisense).

4. The areas of the cell islands on the SAMcell chip were increasing as a linear function of time within a certain period so that the slopes could represent the migratory activities. Consequently, we used a formula to calculate the cell island's migration speed, $MS = \dfrac{A_f - A_i}{T}$, where A_f is the final area, A_i is the initial area, and T is the time of the process. The migra-

tion speed treated with one specific siRNA was normalized to that treated with scrambled siRNA which is used as the negative control. Finally, the normalized migration speed, which is equal to fold change, could represent the migratory activity influenced by the siRNAs [10].

5. siRNA sequences for cell proliferation assay include the following: NC: UUCUCCGAACGUGUCACGUtt (sense), ACGUGACACGUUCGGAGAAtt (antisense).siPTEN: CAC CGCAUAUUAAAACGUAtt (sense), UACGUUUUAAUA UGCGGUGcc (antisense).

6. siRNA sequences for cell apoptosis assay include the following: NC: UUCUCCGAACGUGUCACGUtt (sense), ACGUGA CACGUUCGGAGAAtt (antisense).siPLK1: GCAAUUACAU GAGCGAGCAtt(sense),UGCUCGCUCAUGUAAUUGCgg (antisense).

Acknowledgement

We thank Suzhou Genoarray Biotech Co. Ltd. (Suzhou, China) for contributing to industrialization of SAMcell technology. This work was supported by projects of NSFC (Grant No. 81030040), MOST (Grant No. 2008ZX09401-002, 2011CB809106), and NSFC (20733001, 30600142) and Coulter Foundation Seed Grant.

References

1. Fire A, Xu S, Montqomery MK et al (1998) Potent and specific genetic interference by double-stranded RNA in Caenorhabditis elegans. Nature 391:806–811

2. Crick F (1970) Central dogma of molecular biology. Nature 227:561–563

3. Ahlquist P (2002) RNA-dependent RNA polymerases, viruses, and RNA silencing. Science 296:1270–1273

4. Simpson KJ, Selfors LM, Bui J et al (2008) Identification of genes that regulate epithelial cell migration using an siRNA screening approach. Nat Cell Biol 10:1027–1038

5. Whitehurst AW, Bodemann BO, Cardenas J et al (2007) Synthetic lethal screen identification of chemosensitizer loci in cancer cells. Nature 446:815–819

6. Matson RS (2005) Applying genomic and proteomic microarray technology in drug discovery. CRC Press, Boca Raton, FL, USA

7. Zhang H, Hao Y, Yang J et al (2011) Genome-wide functional screening of miR-23b as a pleiotropic modulator suppressing cancer metastasis. Nat Commun 2, e554

8. Zhang H, Li J, Hou S et al (2014) Engineered TAL Effector modulators for the large-scale gain-of-function screening. Nucleic Acids Res 42, e114

9. Rong Y, Liu M, Ma L et al (2012) Clathrin and phosphatidylinositol-4,5-bisphosphate regulate autophagic lysosome reformation. Nat Cell Biol 14:924–934

10. Zhang H, Wu PY, Ma M et al (2013) An integrative approach for the large-scale identification of human genome kinases regulating cancer metastasis. Nanomedicine 9:732–736

11. Wang Z, Huang H, Zhang H et al (2012) A magnetic bead-integrated chip for the large scale manufacture of normalized esiRNAs. PLoS One 7, e39419

12. Xi J, Schmidt JJ, Montemagno CD et al (2005) Self-assembled microdevices driven by muscle. Nat Mater 4:180–184

Chapter 9

In Vitro-Pooled shRNA Screening to Identify Determinants of Radiosensitivity

Alessandro Ceroni, Geoff S. Higgins, and Daniel V. Ebner

Abstract

Short hairpin RNA (shRNA)-pooled screening is a valuable and cost-effective tool for assaying the contribution of individual genes to cell viability and proliferation on a genomic scale. Here we describe the key considerations for the design and execution of a pooled shRNA screen to identify determinants of radiosensitivity.

Key words shRNA, Lentivirus, Pooled library, Genomic screening, Radiosensitivity

1 Introduction

High-throughput RNA interference screens have been employed for the last decade to identify genetic markers responsible for a variety of biological processes and pathways [1, 2]. RNAi has enabled researchers to systematically probe the function of individual proteins across the entire genome yielding an astonishing amount of information not only on the function of individual proteins, but also on the cellular processes [3], gene networks [4], protein/protein interactions [5], and protein/drug interactions [6] to name a few. Additionally, the development of genome-wide genomic tools has enabled research scientists to probe cellular processes involved in the pathology of disease in order to more accurately define potent targets for drug development [7].

Small interfering RNA (siRNA) and short hairpin RNA (shRNA) molecules are able to suppress gene expression by using cellular microRNA pathways inducing mRNA degradation upon binding of the short single-stranded DNA oligo within the multi-protein RNA-induced silencing complex (RISC). However, the experimental procedures for executing a high-throughput screen using either shRNA or siRNA are fundamentally different with each technique having its own merits when considering issues such

David O. Azorsa, Shilpi Arora (eds.), *High-Throughput RNAi Screening: Methods and Protocols*, Methods in Molecular Biology, vol. 1470, DOI 10.1007/978-1-4939-6337-9_9, © Springer Science+Business Media New York 2016

as experimental design, screening rationale/goals, cell types, readouts, and available laboratory instrumentation. siRNAs are characterized by an optimized chemistry and are usually delivered to cells using lipid-based transfection reagents which enables efficient silencing activity. They are generally understood to be experimentally easier to use when cells can be readily transfected with commercial transfection agents, and are typically used in arrayed formats. One of the main disadvantages, however, is that siRNAs allow only a short-term gene silencing, typically 3–5 days, and some cell lines (such as primary cells) are difficult to transfect. On the other hand, the shRNA is characterized by a lentivirus system delivery which makes it compatible with almost any cellular type, including primary and transformed cells; thus, the permanent integration of the shRNA into the cellular genome enables sustained gene silencing. However, these integrations into the genome are random and it is possible that they may disrupt the expression of other genes. Importantly, one major advantage of shRNA screening is that it can also be carried out in vivo [8].

In terms of experimental procedure, both siRNA and shRNA libraries can be used in an arrayed format (96- and 384-well format) where unique RNAi molecules are distributed across individual wells and phenotypic changes are determined by simple cell viability assays, and colony formation assays, or with more sophisticated methods, such as high-content imaging to capture more detailed information. The advantage of the arrayed format is the potential for lower downstream costs for the readout (especially when miniaturized to 384-well format); however, the library construction or purchase of commercial arrayed libraries can entail significant costs.

Pooled shRNA libraries are an alternative screening format where multiple shRNAs targeting the entire genome or specific gene families are grouped together and used to infect the cell lines of interest [9]. Since not all shRNA sequences provide efficient knockdown of their target gene and constructs may have sequence-specific off-target effects, shRNA libraries are designed to include several unique constructs targeting the same gene. Furthermore, pooled screening enables genome-wide screening without the need for expensive robotics or high-throughput imaging systems. The principal limitation of this approach is that it affords a limited number of phenotypic readouts.

Perhaps the most widely used readout for pooled shRNA screening is cell viability/proliferation, particularly in the field of cancer genomics. In this case, the long-term knockdown achieved by viral integration means that pooled screening offers advantages in viability screening as compared with siRNA screening. Since the growth period can be long, perturbations with modest effects on cell proliferation can be detected, as the effect is enhanced with every population doubling. This is particularly beneficial since RNAi frequently causes only partial silencing of gene expression. Initially, pooled screens used microarray technology to assess the abundance of individual shRNA at the beginning and end of the experiment; however, the decreasing costs of next-generation sequencing (NGS) means that this is now the most common method to assess hairpin abundance using the sequence of the shRNA itself as a "barcode" to identify and count each cell [1].

In general, the experimental design of a pooled shRNA loss-of-function genetic screen follows a standard protocol. To start, a cell population is infected with an shRNA pool, and the positively transduced cells are selected by the antibiotic resistance, which is acquired upon cellular transduction; upon antibiotic selection, a reference sample is collected and used to identify those genes whose disruption causes cell death (with or without treatment) or alternatively treatment resistance. An important aspect of this type of screen is that shRNAs have to be used in a 1:1 ratio with cells (shRNA:cell ratio) to ensure that any phenotypic effect is due to one shRNA construct and not a combination of multiple shRNAs. Next, the cell population is divided into two sub-pools, one of which is treated with drugs/compounds, radiation, or other relevant treatment (e.g., hypoxic growing conditions) while the other sub-pool is left untreated. After incubating the sub-pools for a number of population doublings, cells are collected and genomic DNA is isolated from all conditions. PCR reactions are then used to amplify the integrated shRNA of interest and the depletion or accumulation of individual shRNA within the cellular genome is assessed by next-generation sequencing. This screen can lead to the identification of genes responsible for increasing sensitivity or resistance to treatment such as irradiation (Fig. 1a).

Another approach is to start with two defined cell lines, for example harboring wild-type and mutated copies of a gene of interest. Carrying out the screen with the same procedure described above can lead to the identification of any synthetically lethal interactions, such as genes responsible for cellular depletion in combination with a particular genetic lesion. Additionally each cell line can also be treated with compounds or radiation in order to understand differential response to treatments when the studied mutation is present (Fig. 1b).

In vitro-pooled shRNA screening is now a well-established method for conducting an unbiased integration of the entire genome. It is comparatively inexpensive in terms of cost and labor and is therefore an attractive alternative to arrayed RNAi screening. The methodology can be employed by almost any laboratory and has the potential to yield novel results which would otherwise be difficult to achieve for many laboratories without substantial resources.

Here, we describe a pooled shRNA screening approach to identify determinants of radiosensitivity in cancer cells but generally this methodology can be applied to treatments with other agents such as drugs/compounds or to study synthetically lethal interactions. As radiotherapy remains a key treatment option in the

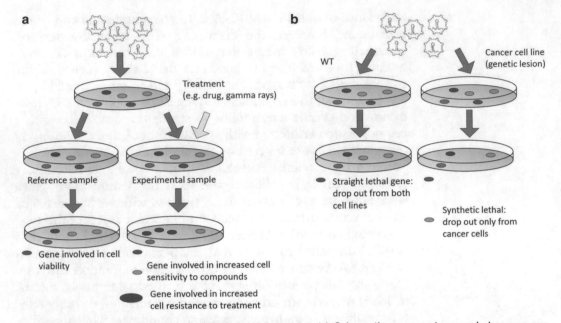

Fig. 1 Schematic representation of shRNA-pooled screens. (**a**) Schematic represents a pooled screen performed to identify genes that cause increased cell sensitivity/resistance to treatments such as irradiation. (**b**) Schematic represents a pooled screen performed to identify genes that cause cell death in combination with other genes (synthetic lethality)

curative management of solid tumors, identifying therapeutically relevant targets for drug development could significantly improve the efficacy of radiotherapy if tumors could be rendered more sensitive to radiation without altering the sensitivity of normal cells. Historically, radiosensitization screens have been limited by the sensitivity of the screen readout [7] and limited to cell types that are relatively radioresistant, and easy to transfect, and form tight colonies. However, because shRNA screens have the advantage of long-term knockdown achieved by viral integration, perturbations with modest effects on cell proliferation can be detected more easily and this means that pooled shRNA screening can overcome previously observed technical difficulties with no real limitation to the cell types that can be screened.

2   Materials

1. Polybrene stock solution at 8 mg/mL in deionized, sterile water, filtered through a 0.22 μm filter. Aliquot 100 μL into sterile microtubes and store them at −20 °C for long-term storage (*see* **Note 1**).

2. Antibiotic stock solution at 1 mg/mL in deionized, sterile water, filtered through a 0.22 μm filter. Aliquot 100 μL into sterile microtubes and store them at −20 °C for long-term storage.

3. Media: Depending on cell lines of interest; "complete media" refers to penicillin/streptomycin-containing media (*see* **Note 2**).

4. Polystyrene CellSTACK®—10 Chambers with Vent Caps (Corning).

5. Decode Pooled Human GIPZ Whole Genome Library (viral particles) (GE Life Sciences).

6. Phusion Hot Start II DNA Polymerase (2 U/μL) (Thermo Fisher Scientific).

7. 10 mM dNTP Set and dNTP Mix, PCR Grade (Qiagen).

8. Betaine solution 5 M, PCR Reagent (Sigma-Aldrich).

9. Illumina-adapted Decode Forward and Reverse Indexed PCR primers (GE Life Sciences).

3   Methods

In the application of this methodology a working knowledge of tissue culture techniques is required. The full methodology is carried out in a category II safety cabinet, and the lab should obtain appropriate permissions to work with lentiviral material prior to commencing the screen including the Risk Assessment and COSHH forms. To obtain a successful and robust pooled shRNA screen, there are many steps that require careful attention and optimization.

3.1 shRNA Library

1. The shRNA libraries can be purchased for a relatively low cost from commercial sources (such as GE and Sigma) which will provide sequenced high-titer viral particles covering a large variety of gene families. Alternatively, lentiviral shRNA libraries can be produced using standard protocols including bacterial culture of individual shRNAs in growth media in a 96-deep-well block followed by plasmid DNA isolation using midi or maxi preparation kits.

2. Packaging of the lentiviral particles is carried out via co-transfection of the packaging cell line (usually HEK293T) with the transfer vectors (represented by multiple shRNAs) along with the packaging plasmids psPAX2 and pMD2.G.

3. Forty-eight hours post-transfection the viral supernatant is collected and filtered through a 0.22 μm PES filter and, if highly concentrated viral particles are required, ultracentrifuged at $24,000 \times g$ for 2 h.

4. The pellet is then resuspended in 1/20th of the original volume in the resuspension solution (0.5 % BSA in PBS).

3.2 Cell Density and Growth Kinetics

When shRNA-pooled screens are carried out using multiple cell lines, it is very important that growth kinetics are measured. Ideally two or more cell lines used in the screen should be characterized by the same growth rate in order to simplify the screen and remove variability at every screen step (i.e., avoid passaging one cell line more frequently than the other one). When cell lines are mutated and a specific gene of interest is knocked-in/out or mutated (such as in order to study synthetically lethal interactions) it is critical that the wild-type (WT) and mutated cell lines are tested for cellular growth rate (*see* **Note 3**).

1. Seed 5.0×10^3 cells are seeded per well in a 96-well plate (three technical replicates) and incubated for 24 h at 37 °C.

2. For radiosensitization screening, the cells are treated with a single dose of radiation. The relative biologic effectiveness (RBE) of gamma rays/X-rays produced by most laboratory irradiation systems is usually equivalent to that used to treat patients and is therefore clinically relevant. Irradiation exposure is designed to kill 50–75 % of cells when screening to identify determinants of radiosensitivity in cancer cells. As there is significant variation in the intrinsic radiosensitivity of cell lines, the radiation dose required to reduce the screen cell type by 50 % should be determined experimentally but in the case of most cancer cells, this is typically between 2 and 10 Gy.

3. Incubate the cells for 48 h at 37 °C.

4. After 48 h, stain the cells with DAPI (used according to standard protocols) to assess cell number using a high-content imaging scanner, or counted using a cell counter.

3.3 Cell Tolerance to Polybrene

Hexadimethrine bromide (Polybrene) is added to the cell lines of interest to enhance lentiviral transduction, thereby improving viral particle binding to the cell surface. It is important to empirically determine the final concentration of Polybrene to maximize transduction efficiency with minimal cytotoxicity. Testing several concentrations for each cell line, ranging from 0 to 16 μg/mL, is recommended (*see* **Note 4**).

1. Seed 5.0×10^3 cells per well in a 96-well plate (three technical replicates) and incubate for 24 h at 37 °C.

2. The next day, prepare 350 μL of each solution of Polybrene (e.g., 16, 14, 12, 10, 8, 4, 2, 1, and 0 μg/mL) in antibiotic-free media.

3. Replace media with 100 μL of Polybrene solution at several concentrations and incubate the plate for 24 h at 37 °C.

4. The next day, replace the media with complete media (containing Pen/Strep) and incubate for 48 h at 37 °C.

5. After 48 h, visually inspect the cells or stain with DAPI (used according to standard protocols) to assess viability compared to mock treatment (0 μg/mL Polybrene).

3.4 Antibiotic Kill Curve

The majority of the shRNA vector backbones used to produce pooled libraries contain an antibiotic resistance cassette that confers antibiotic resistance to cells that have integrated the shRNA construct. Depending on the screen layout, antibiotic selection can start early, 24 or 48 h post-transduction, or at later time, such as 72 h post-transduction and should last between 2 and 5 days (*see* **Note 5**). Testing several concentrations for each cell line, ranging from 0 to 5 μg/mL, is recommended in order to find the lowest concentration that results in 100% cell death of non-transduced cells within the desired time frame. It is very important that cells do not reach 90% confluency during this time, as this may compromise antibiotic activity during cell selection.

1. Seed 5.0×10^3 cells per well in a 96-well format plate (three technical replicates) and incubate for 24 h at 37 °C.

2. The next day, prepare 350 μL of each solution of antibiotic (e.g., 5, 4, 3, 2, 1, 0.5, and 0 μg/mL) in media (no Pen/Strep).

3. Replace media with 100 μL of antibiotic solution at several concentrations and incubate the plate for 24 h at 37 °C.

4. The next day, inspect the cells for viability and further inspection is carried out over the next few days.

5. After 24 h (or alternative designated time), visually inspect the cells to assess viability compared to mock treatment (0 μg/mL antibiotic) (*see* **Note 6**).

3.5 Viral Titration and Functional Titer

When an shRNA screen is carried out on multiple cell lines it is important to define the viral titer as well as the functional titer, which is an empirical measure of the transduction efficiency established experimentally, is established. When viral particle pools are purchased from companies, the viral titer indicated on the information sheet is usually determined using the packaging cell line (typically HEK293T cells). As each cell line used in the screen could be less or more prone to being efficiently transduced than HEK293T, the functional titer has to be determined empirically within the cell line(s) of interest. When the differential transduction efficiency is found, a correction factor can be determined and subsequently universally applied any time this specific cell line is used in screens (*see* **Note 7**).

The following method to identify the functional titer applies when the vector backbone contains a fluorescent reporter gene that can be visualized using a high-content imaging scanner but it can be adjusted when a fluorescent reporter gene is not expressed in the positively transduced cells. In the latter case, cells will be selected with antibiotic after transduction for 2 days and stained with DAPI (used according to standard protocols). Cell number will be assessed using a high-content imaging scanner and compared to the untreated control in order to determine the percentage of positively transduced cells.

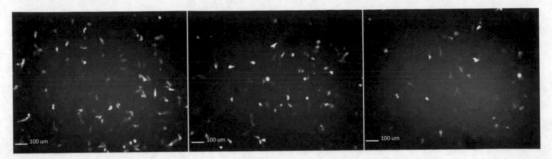

Fig. 2 HEK293T cells were transduced with serial dilution of viral particles and GFP-positive cells are identified using a high-content imaging scanner, i.e., Operetta (PerkinElmer)

1. Seed 5.0×10^3 cells per well in a 96-well format plate (three technical replicates) and incubate for 24 h at 37 °C.

2. The next day, prepare viral stock dilutions (from neat concentration to $1:10^6$) in Polybrene-containing media (Polybrene concentration measured in Subheading 3.2) with no Penn/Strep (*see* **Note 8**). Depending upon the initial concentration of the viral stock dilutions must include low multiplicity of infection (MOI) < 0.3 to reach less than 20–25 % of positivity.

3. Replace media with 100 µL of virus solution at several concentrations and plate is incubated for 24 h at 37 °C.

4. The next day, replace media with fresh complete media and incubated for 24 h at 37 °C.

5. After 24 h, cells are visually inspected to assess fluorescent reporter gene expression. Positive cells/colonies are counted using a high-content imaging scanner and used to measure the viral titer in each cell line using the following formula (Fig. 2):

$$\text{Transducing unit per mL} = (\text{colonies counted} \times \text{dilution factor}) / \text{volume of virus added (mL)}$$

For example: Assuming that in the dilution corresponding to 1:1000, 150 positive colonies are identified, the unit per mL will be as follows:

$$\text{TU per mL} = 150 \times 1000 / 0.100\,\text{mL} = 1.5 \times 10^6\,\text{TU} / \text{mL}$$

3.6 Cell Seeding

Based on the size and morphology of the cell line(s) used, appropriate numbers of cells must be seeded into the flasks. Different cell lines require different seeding densities to grow at an exponential rate. Cells should never reach confluency, and when this is not possible, they have to be passaged in order to keep the cells growing in the exponential phase. This ensures that a correct selection of shRNAs is carried out and that shRNA representation is reflecting the natural selection due to gene knockdown (*see* **Note 9**).

Due to 75% cell death upon antibiotic selection when using an MOI of 0.3, four times the number of cells required will have to be seeded. To calculate the cells required for each library at the time of transduction, we must know the doubling time of the cells and the total number of cells necessary at the time for transduction, usually 24 h post-cell seeding. For example when an shRNA pool contains 10,000 hairpins and the coverage/shRNA representation used is 500, 2.0×10^7 cells will be required on the day of transduction ($10,000 \times 500 \times 100/25 = 2.0 \times 10^7$ cells required). The number of cells required at seeding time will be 50% of the total at 24 h if cells double every 24 h and then half this value will need to be seeded, which is approximately 1.0×10^7 cells. This will require several T175 flasks so that the cells reach optimal confluency for transduction after 24 h.

1. Day 0—Seed cells in T175 flasks. In total, if the previous example is used, five flasks will be required with 2.5×10^6 cells in each with 20 mL media. Four flasks will be transduced while one flask will not be transduced and be used for antibiotic selection control.

2. Day 1—Estimated total cells would now be 2.5×10^7 ($4 \times$ T175 flasks with 5.0×10^6 each flask for the screen plus $1 \times$ T175 flask with 5.0×10^6 as control). Remove media and replace with 13 mL fresh media containing lentivirus in flasks at the correct dilution to give MOI of 0.3 based on titration optimization (*see* Subheading 3.8). Different cells may require different amounts of lentivirus. For control flask replace media with 13 mL fresh media containing Polybrene alone.

3.7 shRNA Coverage and Transduction

A key parameter in pooled shRNA screens is the shRNA coverage used and maintained during the screen. Here, shRNA coverage represents the number of cells that are transduced with an individual shRNA construct during an experiment and a high coverage or shRNA representation, typically between 250 and 500 cells per shRNA for each step throughout the duration of the screen, will result in more power to detect changes in representation over time, particularly when focusing on hairpin depletion. Coverage for each cell line subjected to a treatment, in this case irradiation, is important because we expect 50% cell death upon treatment and in order to maintain shRNA representation (coverage) sufficient for adequate statistical analysis the cell loss due to the treatment must be accounted for at this step.

The recommended coverage is not always experimentally feasible. There are a few parameters to consider when deciding which one to choose. When the shRNA pool is large, choosing a large coverage may lead to an unmanageable screen, due to cell number, costly consumables, and other resources and potentially more operators to complete the screen. An alternative is to perform multiple biological replicates at lower shRNA representation although it must be understood that a higher coverage is more powerful in detecting new hits than increasing the number of biological replicates [10].

The length of viral infection is another parameter that must be considered. It can vary between 5 and 24 h and, based on the length of infection, FBS content must be adjusted accordingly. Although a lower amount of FBS is recommended for an efficient transduction, this can be applied only for short-term infections to avoid cell cycle arrest and/or cell death, while for a long infection FBS is required for cell growth. Ideally, when a cell line is easily transducible, we recommend reducing the time of transduction and when this is not possible we advise reducing the FBS to a minimum.

3.8 Multiplicity of Infection

The MOI is the ratio of viral particles to cells and represents the total number of viral particles that are added to a pool of cells. In pooled shRNA screening, it is crucially important that each cell in the pool is transduced with only one shRNA construct to ensure that the observed phenotype per cell (e.g., cell death) is the result of one viral particle integration into the cellular DNA and not multiple integrations within one cell. However, by reducing the MOI the number of non-transduced cells increases; therefore, together with the "coverage" the MOI has to be carefully decided in advance in order to keep the screen manageable.

To avoid the integration of multiple hairpins, we recommend using a low MOI of 0.3 which as shown in Table 1 results in 25% of positive transduced cells.

1. For example: in a library composed of 10,000 individual shRNAs and a desired screen coverage of 500 cells/shRNA construct, it will be necessary to infect 2.0×10^7 cells with 5.0×10^6

Table 1
The table shows the number of cells with the number of integrant(s) when a specific MOI is used. For example, when MOI = 0.3 is used, 22% of the cells will contain one integrant, and 3% will contain two integrants

	Number of lentiviral integrants per cell				
MOI	*0*	*1*	*2*	*3*	*4*
0.1	0.9	0.09	0.00	0.00	0.00
0.2	0.82	0.16	0.02	0.00	0.00
0.3	0.74	0.22	0.03	0.00	0.00
0.4	0.67	0.27	0.05	0.01	0.00
0.5	0.61	0.3	0.08	0.01	0.00
0.6	0.55	0.33	0.1	0.02	0.00
0.7	0.5	0.35	0.12	0.03	0.00

number of viral particles ($10,000$ shRNA$\times 500$ coverage$= 5.0 \times 10^6$ viral particles).

2. For each condition only 25 % of cells will be positive; therefore we will require 5.0×10^6 cells$\times 4 = 2.0 \times 10^7$ cells to be transduced to maintain the correct representation.

3. In order to take into account any unforeseen cell loss we further increase the seeded cells by 20 %, and consequently the amount of virus used to maintain the shRNA representation.

3.9 Screen Production

Following cell seeding (Subheading 3.6) and transduction (Subheadings 3.7 and 3.8) cells will be treated as follows:

1. Day 2—Twenty-four hours post-transduction, replace the media with 20 mL antibiotic-containing media (antibiotic-containing media could also be added 48 h post-transduction, *see* Subheading 3.4) and incubate for at least 48 h (this time is measured in Subheading 3.4 and depends on cell lines and concentration of the antibiotic used) or until the cells in the control flask are dead.

2. Day 5—When the antibiotic selection is completed, irradiate two T175 flasks at the desired dose.

3. Return irradiated flasks to the cell incubator. Unirradiated (untreated) T175 flasks are left in the incubator.

4. Day 7—Rinse cells from all the flasks with fresh media to remove dead cells and trypsinize the flask.

5. Collect 5×10^6 cells from the unirradiated flask, wash in PBS, and freeze to use as a reference sample. The reference sample will be used to assess the heterogeneity of the shRNAs integrated into transduced cells and any shRNA depletion and enrichment when compared to the samples collected at the end of the screen. For example when an shRNA pool contains 10,000 hairpins and the coverage/shRNA representation used is 500, 5.0×10^6 cells will be required for the reference sample. As we account for gDNA extraction kit, it is advisable to save 30 % more cells.

6. Seed 5.0×10^6 cells for each arm of the screen (irradiated vs. untreated) into two CellSTACK® (5.0×10^6 cells from the two irradiated flasks and 5.0×10^6 cells from the unirradiated flasks) in 1.3 L of complete media and incubated for 9 days at 37 °C (until day 16).

   For example, if radiation treatment kills 50 % of the cells, then $5.0 \times 10^6 \times 100/50 = 1.0 \times 10^7$ cells have to be used for the treated sample in order to maintain the correct number of cells throughout the screening and have enough cells for analysis.

7. Days 11 and 14—Change media with 1.3 L of complete media (follow the manufacturer's instruction for changing media in the CellSTACK®).

8. Day 16—Collect 5.0×10^6 cells from each CellSTACK®; it is advisable to save 30 % more cells.

The screen layout relies on the choice of multiple key parameters. The size of the shRNA pools, cell growth kinetics, virus incubation time, treatment, antibiotic selection time, coverage, etc. are affecting the size of the screen and thus its final cost. In addition to this, using top-scale parameters (high coverage, long incubation time) may result in an unmanageable screen. To overcome these problems, but still maintaining high-quality screen parameters, our laboratory uses CellSTACK® and/or multilayer flasks. They enable screens with large numbers of cells (up to 6.0×10^8 cells each CellSTACK®) with reduced amount of media and make the screen manageable by one operator, especially when the incubation time is long and frequent cell passages may otherwise be required (*see* **Note 10**).

3.10 Genomic DNA Extraction

1. Collect cells from each condition of the screen and wash in PBS twice, in order to remove the media and trypsin residues using standard centrifugation protocols (i.e., $300 \times g$, 5 min at 4 °C). The number of cells for each condition is determined based on the size of the shRNA pool and coverage. For example: Assuming that the library is composed of 10,000 individual shRNA and the screen coverage is 500, for each condition we will require 5×10^6 cells to use for subsequent gDNA isolation diluted in the appropriate volume of PBS according to the gDNA extraction kit used (*see* **Note 11**).

2. Extract genomic DNA using mini, midi, or maxi preparation kits according to the manufacturer's protocol. The number of cells processed will vary based on the complexity of the library and the coverage maintained during the screen. It is vital that shRNA representation is maintained and a minimal number of cells corresponding to the desired number of integrants is used during gDNA isolation.

3. gDNA is quantified using a spectrophotometer to assess purity by measuring absorbance at 260 nm, 280 nm, and 230 nm and relative ratios A260/A280 (ideally between 1.8 and 2.0) and A260/A230 (ideally > 2.0).

3.11 PCR Amplification and Amplicon Purification

Genomic DNA extracted from each condition is independently amplified by PCR. This step requires thorough optimization and it is advisable to follow the shRNA library manual instructions. Additionally, it is likely that libraries from different vendors will employ a different high-fidelity polymerase which can alter several experimental parameters as well as specific sets of primers which are usually compatible with the sequencer recommended. Many parameters have to be optimized, such as the amount of gDNA template to use in each reaction, the number of PCR cycles, the number of polymerase units, and the number of reactions per condition. As a general rule of thumb, the amount of template should be calculated to maintain the desired coverage, assuming that only one shRNA is integrated in one cell when optimized transduction conditions are used. A diploid cell contains on average 6.6 pg of gDNA, and the number of reactions required to maintain the shRNA representation is as follows:

1. Assuming that the library is composed of 10,000 individual shRNA and the screen coverage is 500, for each condition 5×10^6 cells are required to maintain the correct representation.

2. The total gDNA amount to use as template will be 5×10^6 cells $\times 6.6$ pg $= 3.3 \times 10^7$ pg (33 µg).

3. The DECODE shRNA-pooled library uses 0.825 µg per reaction; therefore in the previous example four PCR reactions will be necessary to cover the whole library representation (33 µg/0.825 µg $=$ 40 PCR).

4. Calculate the total number of PCR reactions accounting also for the number of conditions used in the screen. For example, if the screen is composed of three conditions, then the final number of reaction will be 40 PCR $\times$ 3 conditions $=$ 120 PCR.

The number of required PCR reactions will depend on the amount of template used. For several shRNA pooled libraries available, PCR conditions have been optimized, including the amount of template, number of cycles, and reagents used (e.g., polymerase). We also recommend using PCR-enhancing agents, such as betaine or DMSO for the amplification of targets to reduce the formation of secondary structures, especially G-C-rich sequences, which can result in poor PCR yields.

The following settings are used for the DECODE shRNA-pooled library (Tables 2 and 3) (*see* **Note 12**).

When a screen is composed of multiple experimental conditions (arms) or treatments, it is possible and advisable to use unique indexing primers for each condition in order to group several conditions together during sequencing to maximize the output of each flow cell lane. The indexes can then be used to de-convolute each experimental condition during NGS analysis and separate each back to the original condition. Maximizing the flow cell will substantially reduce the cost of NGS.

Indexing primers compatible with different sequencing platforms are commercially available. The Decode pooled shRNA library uses PCR primers incorporating Illumina adaptors for use with Illumina sequencers. The final choice of primers will depend upon the sequencer available, or the company providing the sequencing service, and it is best to discuss the PCR step with the

Table 2
PCR reagents for hairpin amplification

	×1 Rxn (µL)	× 4 Rxns (µL)
5× Phusion HF buffer (final 1×)	10	40
10 mM dNTPs (final 200 nM)	1	4
Decode forward primer (50 µM → 0.5 µM)	0.5	2
Decode reverse primer (50 µM → 0.5 µM)	0.5	2
5 M Betaine (final 0.5 M)	5	20
gDNA (825 ng/µL)	1.0	4.0
Phusion 2 U/µL	2	8
H_2O	30.0	120.0

Table 3
PCR conditions for the thermal cycler

98 °C	× 3 min	
98 °C	*× 10 s*	*23 cycles*
57 °C	*× 15 s*	
72 °C	*× 15 s*	

sequencing facility, including primer design, and PCR protocols, early in the experimental design process.

PCR reactions are subsequently purified using commercial kits and modified manufacturer's instructions. It is important to adjust the protocol to the higher than normal volume of PCR reactions (*see* **Note 13**).

4 Notes

1. Polybrene stock solutions may be stored at –20 °C for up to 1 year. Do not freeze/thaw the stock solution more than three times as this may result in a loss of activity. The working stock may be stored at +4 °C for up to 2 weeks.

2. Purchase all reagents at once in order to use the same batches of media, FBS, and plasticware.

3. This test is carried out in a 96-well format plate; each cell line is tested with complete media in three technical replicates. The goal is to define the growth rate of the cell lines used in the screen. When two cell lines have different cell growth kinetics it is important to adjust the screening parameters in order to maintain the same coverage for both cell lines. Varying growth rates can be compensated for by performing a faster/slower antibiotic selection, passaging the cell lines at different times, or employing a larger amount of consumables.

4. This test is carried out in a 96-well format plate; each cell line is tested with several solutions at different concentrations of Polybrene in three technical replicates. The goal is to define the highest amount of Polybrene resulting in no cytotoxicity. In our experiments, a final concentration of 4–8 µg/mL is generally used.

5. This test is carried out in a 96-well format plate; each cell line is tested with several solutions at different concentrations of antibiotic in three technical replicates. The goal is to define the lowest amount of antibiotic to use that results in cell death within the designated timeframe. When early antibiotic selection is required (within 24–48 h post-transduction) for the screen, we recommend using a lower dose at selection day 1, and an increased dose at selection day 2. For late selection (after 48–72 h post-transduction), use higher concentrations of antibiotic as, at this stage, all cells that have integrated constructs will express the antibiotic-resistant cassette.

6. For the majority of our screens, we aim at selecting the positive cells 48 h post-transduction and we carry out the first 24-h selection in 0.5 µg/mL increasing after 24 h to 1 µg/mL. During the screen, when cells are transduced with the pooled library and positive cells are selected with antibiotic, remember to keep non-transduced cells growing and treat them with antibiotic to determine when the selection process is complete.

7. This test is carried out in a 96-well format plate; each cell line is tested with several solutions at different dilutions of virus in three technical replicates. The goal is to confirm the viral titer using HEK293T cells and the functional titer in the cell line(s) of interest. It is important that the virus stock is diluted enough to obtain less than 25 % of positive cells after transduction; when a higher number of positive cells is achieved, this may be the result of multiple shRNA integration into one cell and may make it difficult to calculate the true viral titer. When testing the functional titer it is important to use the same conditions as for the screen (including, media composition, Polybrene concentration, transduction duration, cell density at transduction, etc.).

8. It is important in this step to use a large range of dilutions in order to be able to count the positive cells/colonies (between 1 and 10^6 is recommended). When a high titer is used, we encounter two problems: (a) the high-content imaging scanner may not be able to count all the positive cells correctly, and (b) multiple shRNAs may have integrated into one cell. When lower viral concentration is used the probability of having 1:1 shRNA-to-cell ratio is higher, a condition necessary for determining the correct viral titer.

9. Prior to each shRNA pool screen, we bank multiple vials of each cell line. When a large screen is divided into multiple sub-screens due to the size and number of the pools, frozen cell vials will be thawed and passaged for 2 weeks before the screen starts in order to keep the status of the cells consistent for each library pool used.

10. When considering what plasticware to use in the screen it is important to define the length of the screen. For a synthetic lethality interaction and dropout screens, we recommend incubating the cell lines for at least 8 days after antibiotic selection. This applies when the cell lines of interest double their number in 24 h. For slow-growing cells, incubation time may increase in order to complete shRNA depletion.

11. DNA extraction kits are not 100% efficient. To account for this inefficiency it is advisable to increase the cell number by 30% when isolating gDNA. For example: Assuming that the library is composed by 10,000 individual shRNA and the screen coverage is 500, for each condition we will require 5×10^6 cells to maintain the correct representation. We recommend using $5 \times 10^6 \times 30/100 = 6.5 \times 10^6$ cells for genomic DNA isolation (30% increase). Remember to elute the gDNA in EDTA-free buffer to avoid inhibition of following PCR reactions. We also recommend banking multiple cells aliquots in case further gDNA isolation is required.

12. Before a large number of PCR reactions are performed, it is recommended to test PCR conditions, including appropriate positive and negative controls, and then apply those conditions to the large number of technical replicates.

13. Additional amount of buffers may have to be ordered to cope with large volumes of amplified DNA as the kits are generally used with small reaction volumes (usually 50 μL/reaction, while in a screen hundreds of reactions may be necessary); it is also important to verify the binding capacity of the purification column and ensure that the predicted mass of amplicons can be purified using a number of columns minimizing the loss of amplified DNA.

References

1. Berns K, Hijmans EM, Mullenders J et al (2004) A large-scale RNAi screen in human cells identifies new components of the p53 pathway. Nature 428(6981):431–437

2. Whitehurst AW, Bodemann BO, Cardenas J et al (2007) Synthetic lethal screen identification of chemosensitizer loci in cancer cells. Nature 446(7137):815–819

3. Herr P, Lundin C, Evers B et al (2015) A genome-wide IR-induced RAD51 foci RNAi screen identifies CDC73 involved in chromatin remodeling for DNA repair. Cell Discovery 1 (15034):1–16

4. Dopie J, Rajakyla EK, Joensuu MS et al (2015) Genome-wide RNAi screen for nuclear actin reveals a network of cofilin regulators. J Cell Sci 128:2388–2400

5. Tu Z, Argmann C, Wong KK et al (2009) Integrating siRNA and protein–protein interaction data to identify an expanded insulin signaling network. Genome Res 19:1057–1067

6. Mendes-Pereira AM, Sims D, Dexter T et al (2012) Genome-wide functional screen identifies a compendium of genes affecting sensitivity to tamoxifen. Proc Natl Acad Sci U S A 109(8):2730–2735

7. Tiwana GS, Prevo R, Buffa FM et al (2015) Identification of vitamin B1 metabolism as a tumor-specific radiosensitizing pathway using a high-throughput colony formation screen. Oncotarget 6(8):5978–89

8. Gargiulo G, Serresi M, Cesaroni M et al (2014) In vivo shRNA screens in solid tumors. Nat Protoc 9(12):2880–2902

9. Brummelkamp TR, Fabius AWM, Mullenders J et al (2006) An shRNA barcode screen provides insight into cancer cell vulnerability to MDM2 inhibitors. Nat Chem Biol 2(4):202–206

10. Strezoska Ž, Licon A, Haimes J et al (2012) Optimized PCR conditions and increased shRNA fold representation improve reproducibility of pooled shRNA screens. PLoS One 7(8):e42341

Chapter 10

Three-Dimensional Spheroid Cell Culture Model for Target Identification Utilizing High-Throughput RNAi Screens

LaKesla R. Iles and Geoffrey A. Bartholomeusz

Abstract

The intrinsic limitations of 2D monolayer cell culture models have prompted the development of 3D cell culture model systems for in vitro studies. Multicellular tumor spheroid (MCTS) models closely simulate the pathophysiological milieu of solid tumors and are providing new insights into tumor biology as well as differentiation, tissue organization, and homeostasis. They are straightforward to apply in high-throughput screens and there is a great need for the development of reliable and robust 3D spheroid-based assays for high-throughput RNAi screening for target identification and cell signaling studies highlighting their potential in cancer research and treatment. In this chapter we describe a stringent standard operating procedure for the use of MCTS for high-throughput RNAi screens.

Key words siRNA, High throughput, Robotics, Lipid transfection, Spheroid

1 Introduction

1.1 3D vs. 2D Cell Cultures

Although the establishment of cancer cell lines has enabled researchers to significantly advance the understanding of cancer biology, the harsh reality is that many findings have not been successfully translated into clinical practice. Commonly used in vitro testing methods typically involve growing cancer cell lines in 2-dimensional (2D) monolayer cell culture systems on plastics. It is now accepted that 2D monolayer cell culture models have intrinsic limitations. Essential cellular functions that are present in the three-dimensional (3D) tumor microenvironment are missed by "petri dish-based" 2D monolayer cell cultures which limits their potential to predict the cellular responses of real organisms [1–3]. The intrinsic limitations associated with 2D monolayer cell culture systems have prompted the development of 3D models. Studies by Bissell et al. [4] and others [1, 2] spanning more than two decades have shown that growing cells within 3D scaffolds reduces the gap between cell cultures and physiological tissues. At the present time, the most commonly used 3D model is the 3D multi-cellular tumor

David O. Azorsa, Shilpi Arora (eds.), *High-Throughput RNAi Screening: Methods and Protocols*, Methods in Molecular Biology, vol. 1470, DOI 10.1007/978-1-4939-6337-9_10, © Springer Science+Business Media New York 2016

spheroid (MCTS) model. The 3D MCTS model has biological outcomes of intermediate complexity between monolayer cultures and in vivo tumors and displays characteristics close to those of experimental tumors in mice and natural tumors in humans, before the development of neo-vascularization [5, 6]. Importantly, similar to solid tumors, 3D MCTS also exhibits oxygen gradients that result in hypoxia and thus heterogeneous growth rates of the cells within the 3D MCTS [6–11].

1.2 Screening Using 3D MCTS Models

The sequencing of the human genome resulted in the development of genome-wide siRNA libraries that, through their use in high-throughput RNAi screens, opened up an enormous opportunity for the discovery of novel molecular mechanisms mediating the onset and progression of cancer. High-throughput screening (HTS) siRNA screens have played a significant part in furthering our understanding of cancer biology and treatment. The biological alterations associated with the loss of gene function have permitted a reliable interpretation of the function of the targeted gene. Typically, high-throughput screens are conducted on two-dimensional monolayer cell cultures due to the ease and convenience of performing these studies. Data generated from high-throughput screens utilizing two-dimensional cell culture models have no doubt contributed to furthering our understanding of cancer. However, these models do not recapitulate the complexity of the 3D tumor microenvironment, and the associated physiological outcomes, signaling profiles, and heterogeneity. Three-dimensional (3D) models, on the other hand, recapitulate many aspects of the tumor microenvironment and serve as relevant preclinical models to generate data with high clinical relevance as confirmed in follow-up in vivo animal models [8, 12–15]. The 3D MCTS model thus bridges the gap between cell culture and living tissues [14, 16]. Studies have demonstrated an overlap in gene expression profiles between 3D MCTS and the related cancer [17]. This is not the case in parallel studies performed utilizing two-dimensional monolayer cultures generated from the same cancer cell line used to generate the 3D MCTS [8, 12, 14, 18]. Interestingly, the genes that are up-regulated in the spheroids are also up-regulated in tumors [1, 19]. These findings have resulted in the increasing popularity of 3D high-throughput/high-content screening. The improved capabilities of high-content screening (HCS) have contributed to the use of 3D MCTS cell culture models in these types of screens as it provides an added dimension for data analysis based on morphological readouts [13, 20, 21].

Most studies utilizing 3D cultures are oriented toward cancer treatment since these models bring new insights into the identification of druggable targets within molecular mechanisms known to regulate cancer proliferation, invasion, and metastasis [6, 22, 23]. Three-dimensional models have also been used to study cell metabolism [24], morphology, cell-cell communication/ adhesion [23, 25–27], the microenvironment [13, 16, 26, 28–30], polarity [31], hypoxia [8], angiogenesis [30, 32], and drug efficacy and resistance to radiation and chemotherapeutics [13, 15, 30, 32–35]. The morphologies of 3D systems are dependent on the method utilized for their generation. These methods include the use of poly(lactide-co-glycolide) (PLG) [32] or poly (-caprolactone) (PCL) scaffolds [28, 30], spinner flasks [8, 16], roller tubes or bottles, gyratory shakers [35], micro-printing [14, 16], hollow fiber cultures and hanging drop models [36–38], collagen gel models [38, 39], microfluidic channel-based models [40], co-cultures [15, 26, 35], and multi-cellular tumor spheroid cell culture models [30, 41, 42]. Advantages and disadvantages of these models have been well described in the review by Jong Bin Kim and colleagues [43]. It is therefore imperative that when selecting a 3D cell culture model for a study, the model selected recapitulates the biological outcomes relevant for the study [14].

1.3 Characteristics of 3D MCTS Growth

MCTS cell culture models were adapted for cancer research in the early 1970s by Sutherland and Associates [15, 44] and take advantage of the natural tendency of host cells to aggregate into microscale spherical clusters. There are three main phases in the development of compact spheroids [41, 45]. During the first phase, the cells migrate and aggregate. Aggregates are used to describe loose packages of host cells [12, 14, 41]; thus, aggregates posses a three-dimensionally organized complex network displaying cell-to-cell and cell-to-matrix interactions [16]. They are nearly spherical and may easily fall apart if advanced analytical processing is required and may not express all physiological characteristics known to be present in compact multi-cellular tumor spheroids [35]. In the second phase, the number of host cells increases and chemical gradients develop in which two cellular layers gradually appear [41]. Cells located on the periphery reflect actively dividing cells that are adjacent to capillaries, whereas innermost cells are quiescent which eventually die due to the lack of nutrients and oxygen, resulting in apoptosis or necrosis [14, 30, 46, 47]. The third phase is characterized by a decline in growth rate until it reaches a plateau [41]. In this chapter, we discuss in detail the methodology of a high-throughput/high-content siRNA synthetic lethal screen using a 3D MCTS model of Ewing sarcoma (ES) (Fig. 1), the second most common pediatric bone cancer [28, 30].

In order to perform high-throughput siRNA screens with a high degree of efficiency utilizing 3D cell culture models, it is essential to use matrix-free plates to generate the 3D MCTS. One such system utilized at our facility is a plate whose base contains a non-matrix transparent cycloolefin resinous sheet comprising nanoscale indented patterns with a 500 nm line width, 1 mm line depth, and 10 mm to 500 nm line spacing [42] (Fig. 2). Use of

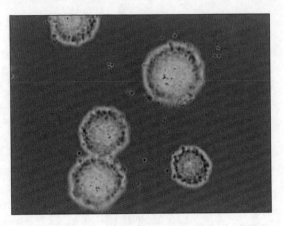

Fig. 1 3D MCTS of TC-71 Ewing sarcoma cells. The cells were grown in a 96-well low-attachment plate (MBL International) and imaged (GE INCELL 6000)

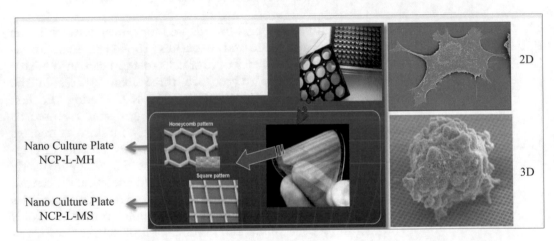

Fig. 2 Plates containing a matrix-free nanomaterial scaffold. The nanomaterial scaffolds are printed in two patterns: a hexagonal pattern (NCP-L-MH) and square pattern (NCP-L-MS). Images provided by the plate manufacturer—MBL International

matrix-based systems might interfere with transport of the siRNA/lipid complex into the host cells, thus reducing transfection efficacy [30] and affecting cell viability [42]. We have developed a robust and reproducible standard operating procedure (SOP) that has permitted us to successfully perform high-throughput siRNA screens using 3D MCTS models. Described below is the procedure for a screen performed on the Ewing sarcoma cell line TC-71. Although this procedure will apply for most cell types, minor changes might be required to optimize the transfection of the particular 3D MCTS model being used.

2   Materials

2.1   Cell Culture and Assay Development

1. TC-71 Ewing sarcoma cell line.
2. T-25 cell culture flask (CELLSTAR).
3. 96-Well plate (Greiner Bio-One).
4. 384-Well plate (Greiner Bio-One).
5. MycoAlert Mycoplasma Detection Kit (Lonza).

2.2   High-Throughput/High-Content Screening

1. 384-Well low-attachment nano-culture plate MBL International.
2. 96-Well low-attachment Nano-Culture plate MBL International.
3. Phosphate-buffered saline (PBS; HyClone).
4. Trypsin (0.25%), 2.21 mM ethylenediamine tetraacetic acid (EDTA) (Corning).
5. Growth media: RPMI-1640 with L-glutamine (Corning) supplemented with 10% fetal bovine serum (Sigma Aldrich).
6. Opti-MEM (Gibco).
7. Negative, non-targeting, control siRNA—ON-TARGETplus Non-Targeting siRNA #1 (Dharmacon).
8. Positive targeting, control siRNA (SMARTPOOL:COPB2 siRNA) (Dharmacon).
9. Cell Titer Glo® Luminescent Kit (Promega).
10. Cell Titer Blue® Cell Viability Assay (Promega).

2.3   Instrumentation

1. XR Vi-Cell Cell Viability Analyzer (Beckman Coulter).
2. BioMek® FX Automation Workstation (Beckman Coulter).
3. BioMek® 3000 Automation Workstation (Beckman Coulter).
4. INCELL Analyzer 6000 Automated Cellular and Subcellular Confocal Imaging System (GE Healthcare Life Sciences).
5. SCREEN Cell³iMager (SCREEN Holdings Co., Ltd).
6. Maxi Rotator (Lab-Line).
7. PHERAstar FS Multifunctional Microplate Reader (BMG LabTech).

3   Methods

3.1   Preliminary Meeting

The preliminary meeting is the most important step in a high-throughput/high-content screen as we have come to realize that a successful high-throughput siRNA screen is a team-driven process. This team comprises the investigator, the biostatistician, and the screening facility. During these meetings, we discuss the SOP of the siRNA facility, which includes our ability to optimize the assay in our platform, any limitations with utilizing our platform, as well as the objectives and goals of the screen, and the study will generate data that is statistically significant.

3.2 Mycoplasma Testing

Mycoplasma is a bacterium lacking a cell wall, serving as the smallest free-living, self-replicating organism, usually attached to the external surface of the host cell membrane. Their presence on human skin makes them a common source of contamination, especially in cases of poor cell culture techniques. Mycoplasma can cause stress to the host cell line at the time of transfection leading to poor transfection efficiency and potential false positives from cell death due to stress; therefore mycoplasma-infected cell lines are not suitable models for high-throughput/high-content screening (*see* **Note 1**).

1. Remove 2 ml media from a T-25 cell culture flask of host cells that are >90 % confluent.

2. Centrifuge the sample at $1789 \times g$ for 4 min.

3. Plate 100 µl of the sample into a 96-well plate in triplicate.

4. Using the MycoAlert Mycoplasma Detection Kit, dispense 100 µl of Reagent "A" and incubate at room temperature for 5 min.

5. Read the luminescence reading on the microplate reader.

6. Using the MycoAlert Mycoplasma Detection Kit, dispense 100 µl of Reagent "B" and incubate at room temperature for 10 min.

7. Read the luminescence reading on the microplate reader.

Calculate the amount of mycoplasma present by dividing the luminescence reading "B" by reading "A" and take the average (*see* **Note 2**).

3.3 Determination of Growth Characteristics

When growing cells in a 2D monolayer cell culture in a standard 384-well plate, we typically plate between 500 and 1200 cells per well. For purposes of growing cells as 3D MCTS we utilize 384-well low-attachment nano-culture plate, and typically plate between 1000 and 5000 cells per well. Cells are observed over a period of 7 days to determine their ability to form spheroids, the time taken to form compact distinct spheroids, and the best starting cell density needed to generate the 3D MCTS (*see* **Note 3**). Morphological changes are determined by imaging the cells daily using our INCELL Analyzer 6000 and parameters such as area, volume, diameter, and viability determined daily by scanning the plates using The SCREEN Cell³iMager (SCREEN Holdings Co. Ltd.), a bright-field spheroid scanner.

1. Remove the T-75 cell culture flask.

2. Carefully remove the media and wash with 1× PBS.

3. Add 1 ml of trypsin-EDTA to the flask.

4. Deactivate the trypsin by adding 10 ml growth media.

5. Count cells using the Vi-Cell cell viability analyzer.

6. In a low-attachment 96-well Scivax Nano-Culture plate, dispense cell densities at various concentrations (1000–5000 cells per well) in 50 µl of cell/media solution per well.

7. Incubate at 37 °C, 5 % CO_2, and >95 % humidity.

8. Image daily using the INCELL Analyzer 6000 Automated Cellular and Subcellular Confocal Imaging System and scan plates daily using the SCREEN Cell³iMager.

3.4 Optimizing Transfection Efficiency

Success of a high-throughput/high-content siRNA screening requires the efficient uptake of siRNA into the host cell to knock down the targeted gene. Highly charged RNA cannot penetrate the cellular lipid membrane and are rapidly degraded by endogenous enzymes resulting in unsuccessful gene silencing [41, 48–50]; thus the siRNAs must be transported into the host cells. Our group at the MD Anderson Cancer Center siRNA Core Facility prefers to use lipids to deliver siRNAs into the host cells due to the ease, convenience, and sensitivity to the host cell. To identify the optimum transfection conditions with minimum toxicity for each cell line, we have developed an in-house plate termed the "Assay Development Plate." The Assay Development Plate consists of a 384-well plate that has nine negative, non-targeting, control siRNA and four positive, targeting, control siRNA arrayed using the Beckman Coulter FX Automation Workstation. The controls are then tested against a panel of eight lipid reagent (Fig. 3). This plate permits us to simultaneously determine the optimal transfection conditions of a cell line using viability as the readout (*see* **Note 4**). The use of the Assay Development Plate also yields important information about the reproducibility, robustness, and ease of the assay, as well as identifies conditions for minimal lipid toxicity [41].

1. Pre-made 384-well assay development plates consisting of 10 µl 200 nM control siRNAs are removed from the −20 °C freezer and thawed to room temperature (*see* **Note 5**).

2. Plates are spun down at $252 \times g$ for 5 min.

3. Prepare diluted lipid at a dilution of 7 µl lipid reagent in 1 ml volume of Opti-MEM

4. Add the lipid/ Opti-MEM mixture to the Assay Development Plate, using the liquid dispenser.

5. Complex the siRNA/lipid mixture by rotating on the Maxi Rotator at room temperature for 30 min.

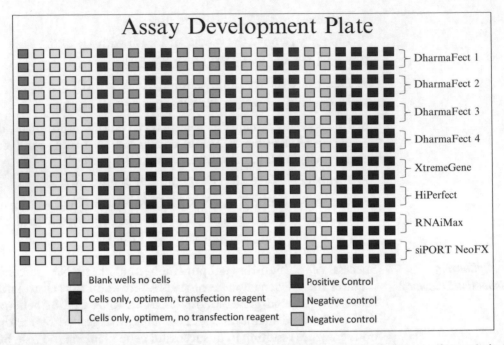

Fig. 3 Assay development plate format. The well design for this plate consists of nine negative controls, four positive controls (Dharmacon.com), and eight lipid reagents used to optimize transfection conditions (DharmaFECT 1-4 (Dharmacon.com), Xtreme Gene (Roche.com), Lipofectamine RNAiMax (Life Technologies), HiPerfect (Qiagen. Com), siPORT NeoFX (Life Technologies))

6. Prepare cells by removing the media and washing with 1× PBS.

7. Add 1 ml of EDTA and incubate at 37 °C for 5 min.

8. Deactivate the trypsin by adding 10 ml growth media.

9. Count cells using the Vi-Cell cell viability analyzer.

10. Dispense the desired concentration of cells in 30 μl growth media per well, using the liquid dispenser (*see* **Note 6**).

11. Incubate at 37 °C, 5 % CO_2, and >95 % humidity for 120 h.

12. For viability readout, dispense CellTiter Blue at the manufacturer's recommendations using the liquid dispenser (*see* **Note 7**).

13. Read the fluorescence on the microplate reader

3.5 Dose–Response Curve

Dose–response curves are generated when performing "Synthetic Lethal" high-throughput/high-content screens (if there are no chemotherapeutic agents involved in the HTS, this step is skipped). Synthetic lethal high-throughput/high-content screens are used to identify target genes whose silencing sensitizes host cells to the therapeutic agent being studied [51]. As lipid transfections sensitize host cells to these therapeutic agents, it is imperative that a dose–response curve be performed on lipid-transfected host cells. The MD Anderson Cancer Center siRNA Core Facility generates

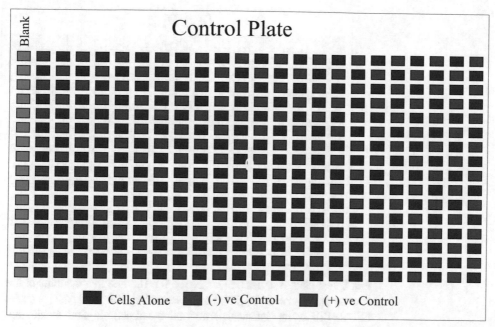

Fig. 4 TC-71 dose–response using Drug X. Cells were transfected with the negative control siOP1 and treated with increasing concentrations of Drug X (columns 1–4 0.05 % DMSO (solvent), columns 5–8 1 nM Drug X, columns 9–12 5 nM Drug X, columns 13–16 10 nM Drug X, columns 17–20 50 nM Drug X, columns 21–24 100 nM Drug X), 48 h post-plating, and imaged after 120 h

in-house "Control Plates" consisting of positive and negative controls (identified in Subheading 3.3) arrayed across a 384-well Scivax nano-culture plate using the BioMek FX Automation Workstation (Fig. 4).

1. "Dose Response" plates are arrayed using the BioMek FX Automation Workstation prior to transfection with 10 μl of 200 nM control siRNAs in a 384-well Scivax Nano-Culture plate on the day of transfection.

2. Prepare diluted lipid at a concentration of 0.07 μl per well in 10 μl per well volume of Opti-MEM.

3. Add the lipid/Opti-MEM mixture to the Assay Development Plate using the liquid dispenser.

4. Complex the siRNA/lipid mixture by rotating on the Maxi Rotator at room temperature for 30 min.

5. Prepare cells by removing the media from the T-75 culture flask and wash the monolayer with 1× PBS.

6. Add 1 ml of trypsin-EDTA.

7. Deactivate the trypsin by adding 10 ml growth media.

8. Count cells with Vi-Cell Cell viability analyzer.

9. Dispense the desired concentration of cells in 30 μl media per well using the liquid dispenser.

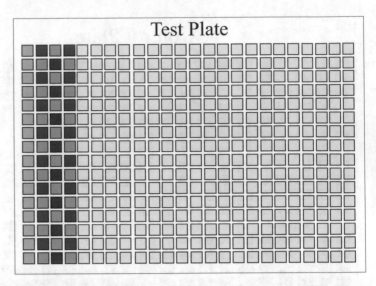

Fig. 5 Test plate well design (*see* **Note 9**). The first four columns of the plate contain the "in-house" controls (negative control siOP1 and positive control siG-ENOME COPB2) for statistical normalization and plate-to-plate monitoring

10. Incubate at 37 °C, 5 % CO_2, and >95 % humidity for 48 h.

11. Dispense 10 μl per well of the desired therapeutic agent at defined increasing concentrations with the vehicle as a control.

12. Incubate at 37 °C, 5 % CO_2, and >95 % humidity for an additional 72 h.

13. For viability readout, dispense Cell Titer Glo luminescent substrate at the manufacturer's recommendations using the liquid dispenser.

14. Read the luminescence reading on the microplate reader.

3.6 Primary High-Throughput Screening

The optimum conditions identified during the assay development phase are used for the primary screen. All siRNA screens are performed in 384 nano-culture plates (*see* **Note 8**). Each plate is arrayed with 10 μl of test siRNA (200 nM) using the BioMek FX Automation Workstation such that the first four columns of each plate remain empty on the day of transfection (Fig. 5).

1. Test plate consisting of 200 nM target siRNAs is spun down at $252 \times g$ for 5 min.

2. The positive and negative controls identified in Subheading 3.3 are introduced into the same well of each test plate within the first four empty columns using Biomek 3000. This control set is used to determine transfection efficiency within each test plate. In a similar manner, if available, assay-specific negative and positive control plates will be introduced into designated wells of each test plate within the first four empty columns using the Biomek 3000.

3. Ten microliters of the lipid reagent (0.07 μl lipid reagent in 10 μl Opti-MEM) is added into each well of the test plate using the liquid dispenser.

4. The plates are placed on a Maxi Rotator at room temperature and gently rotated for 30 min to permit complexing of the siRNA/lipid mixture.

5. Prepare cells by removing the media from the T-75 culture flask and washing with 1× PBS.

6. Add 1 ml of trypsin-EDTA.

7. Deactivate the trypsin by adding 10 ml growth media.

8. Count cells with Vi-Cell Cell Viability Analyzer.

9. Dispense the desired concentration of cells in 30 μl media per well using the liquid dispenser.

10. Divide the test plates into two sets: the "un-treated' set in which 10 μl of the solvent is dispensed to every well and the "treated" set in which 10 μl of the desired drug concentration (identified during the dose–response phase) is dispensed to every well 48 h post-transfection using the liquid dispenser.

11. Incubate at 37 °C, 5 % CO_2, and >95 % humidity for 120 h.

12. For viability readout, dispense Cell Titer Glo luminescent substrate at the manufacturer's recommendations using the liquid dispenser.

13. Read the luminescence reading on the microplate reader.

3.7 Statistical Analysis and Validation

Statistical normalization is a vital component of a successful high-throughput/high-content screen. We typically use an "in-house" normalization that serves as a guideline for potential targets. In-house controls are arrayed in the first [4] columns of each test plate containing target siRNAs. The targeting siRNA of each plate is then normalized to the average of the negative controls of that plate. The median of each set of triplicate values is used as a measure to rank the targets, identifying possible "weak" targets while still capturing "strong" targets, minimizing false positives and outliers more effectively than using mean standard deviations.

3.8 Image Analysis

One major difference in data analysis between high-throughput two-dimensional monolayer cell cultures and high-throughput/high-content multi-cellular tumor spheroid cell culture models is morphology. High-throughput/high content MCTS screens illustrate a range of morphologies among transfected host cells [41]. The INCELL Analyzer 6000 Automated Cellular and Subcellular Confocal Imaging System is a laser-based confocal imaging platform used in most high-content assays and screens as a source for image-based readouts. Multiple images are captured for each well and scored in terms of phenotypic descriptors, including degree of hypoxia, volume, and morphology that is analyzed based on the type of assay and screening mode [41]. The INCELL Analyzer 6000 allows for images to be captured at planes of various depths within the sample known as z-stacks in which each slice can be processed by the INCELL Developer Toolbox, the INCELL Investigator Image Analysis Software, or the INCELL Miner High-Content Manager (HCM) Data Management System.

1. Image processing: Image preprocessing includes operations for improving image quality. Image data acquired from the INCELL Analyzer 6000 are initially preprocessed to correct possible homogeneities in illumination and contrast and the next step is cell segmentation. Segmentation is one of the most significant steps in the analysis of image data serving as a method for detecting and isolating the target set in the image, segregating cellular regions from the background [41].

2. Clustering/classification of phenotypes: Clustering algorithms are routinely used to group image features into clusters. Each cluster defines a group of wells or targeted genes from the screen whose image measurements are similar. Visually examining the clusters allows for the revelation of the phenotypes of interest [41].

3. Multiple tools for 3D image analysis range from Volocity (Perkin Elmer-www.perkinelmer.com), Bitplane (www.bitplane.com), INCELL Developer (www.ge.com), Pipeline Pilot (www.accelrys.com), and Definiens (www.definiens.com) to open-source tools like ImageJ (http://rsb.info.nih.gov/ij/), CellClassifier (http://acc.ethz.ch/), OMero (http://www.openmicroscopy.org/site/products/omero), CellProfiler (http://www.cellprofiler.org/), and V3D (http://vaa3d.org) [41].

4. Another method of 3D high-throughput/high-content image analysis is the use of the SCREENCell^{3}iMager, a bright-field spheroid counter that allows for high-speed well plate scanning and automatic measuring. This scanner scans various 3D culture plates in approximately 1 min per plate and prepares a recipe for measuring based on the scanned images. Each recipe allows investigators to make fine adjustments.

3.9 Hit Validation

The idea of off-target effects highlights the need for validating a selected target. Validation utilizes the identical conditions for the primary screen. During the validation stage, the pooled siRNA or candidate hit is then deconvoluted and each individual siRNA is tested separately. If two or more of the individual siRNAs lead to the phenotype of interest, this candidate is deemed validated. This is then followed up by Western Blot analysis to identify expression levels and qRT-PCR to confirm gene knockdown [41].

4 Notes

1. According to Lonza.com, mycoplasma is the most common contaminant present in cell culture affecting 15–35 % of all continuous cell cultures which can be spread by untested infected host cell lines and contaminating supplies or are directly contaminated from the researcher themselves. Mycoplasma does not kill the host cells but rather affects cellular parameters including an increase in sensitivity to apoptotic inducers, inhibiting cell growth and metabolism or causes chromosomal aberrations, and interferes with transfection efficiencies.

2. Readings greater than 1.2 are deemed mycoplasma positive and therefore not used in the high-throughput/high-content screen.

3. Not all host cell lines form compact spheroids and not all host cell lines prefer the same nano pattern. Scivax Corp has two different nano-culture plates with different patterns, hexagonal and honeycomb. Test the host cell line on each plate to identify the correct nano-culture plate.

4. To optimize transfection efficiency and minimize any variation, an z-factor score is utilized. The z-factor is a calculation that considers the dynamic range of the assay as well as data variability based on the measured value for positive and negative controls producing a "quality" score [41].

5. Assay development is conducted on Greiner 384-well plates, which allows for assay plates to be pre-made, sealed, and stored for later use. But SCIVAX plates have a nano-scale grid pattern that has the potential of being destroyed during freezing and thawing which can interfere with the migration of the host cell; therefore, any assays conducted moving forward are arrayed on the day of transfection.

6. The final concentration of the siRNA duplex is 40 nM.

7. CellTiter-Blue Cell Viability Assay provides a homogeneous, fluorescent method for monitoring cell viability based on the ability of living cells to convert a redox dye (resazurin) into a fluorescent end product (resorufin). Nonviable cells rapidly lose metabolic capacity and thus do not generate a fluorescent signal.

8. The purpose of generating a dose–response curve is to identify a drug concentration between the IC10 and IC30 that will synergistically be used with the targeted siRNAs to identify genes, which when silenced will sensitize the host cell to the therapeutic agent. The rationale behind using a range between IC10 and IC30 is that the increased cell death that would occur at the higher concentrations of the drug would mask the sensitization of the host cell to the therapeutic agent following gene silencing.

Readout is based on (1) viability and (2) morphology—to determine changes in morphology of the spheroids.

9. Primary screens are performed in triplicate.

References

1. Pampaloni F, Reynaud EG, Stelzer EH (2007) The third dimension bridges the gap between cell culture and live tissue. Nat Rev Mol Cell Biol 8(10):839–845

2. Hess MW et al (2010) 3D versus 2D cell culture implications for electron microscopy. Methods Cell Biol 96:649–670

3. Lee J, Cuddihy MJ, Kotov NA (2008) Three-dimensional cell culture matrices: state of the art. Tissue Eng Part B Rev 14(1):61–86

4. Bissell MJ, Hall HG, Parry G (1982) How does the extracellular matrix direct gene expression? J Theor Biol 99(1):31–68

5. Sutherland RM (1988) Cell and environment interactions in tumor microregions: the multicell spheroid model. Science 240(4849):177–184

6. Desoize B (2000) Contribution of three-dimensional culture to cancer research. Crit Rev Oncol Hematol 36(2-3):59–60

7. Friedrich J et al (2007) A reliable tool to determine cell viability in complex 3-d culture: the acid phosphatase assay. J Biomol Screen 12(7):925–937

8. Friedrich J, Seidel C, Ebner R, Kunz-Schughart LA (2009) Spheroid-based drug screen: considerations and practical approach. Nat Protoc 4(3):309–324

9. Mueller-Klieser W (1987) Multicellular spheroids. A review on cellular aggregates in cancer research. J Cancer Res Clin Oncol 113(2):101–122

10. Jiang Y, Pjesivac-Grbovic J, Cantrell C, Freyer JP (2005) A multiscale model for avascular tumor growth. Biophys J 89(6):3884–3894

11. Stein AM, Demuth T, Mobley D, Berens M, Sander LM (2007) A mathematical model of glioblastoma tumor spheroid invasion in a three-dimensional in vitro experiment. Biophys J 92(1):356–365

12. Abbott A (2003) Cell culture: biology's new dimension. Nature 424(6951):870–872

13. Elliott NT, Yuan F (2011) A review of three-dimensional in vitro tissue models for drug discovery and transport studies. J Pharm Sci 100(1):59–74

14. Hirschhaeuser F et al (2010) Multicellular tumor spheroids: an underestimated tool is catching up again. J Biotechnol 148(1):3–15

15. Kunz-Schughart LA, Freyer JP, Hofstaedter F, Ebner R (2004) The use of 3-D cultures for high-throughput screening: the multicellular spheroid model. J Biomol Screen 9(4):273–285

16. Kim JB (2005) Three-dimensional tissue culture models in cancer biology. Semin Cancer Biol 15:365–377

17. Zietarska M et al (2007) Molecular description of a 3D in vitro model for the study of epithelial ovarian cancer (EOC). Mol Carcinog 46(10):872–885

18. Grun B et al (2009) Three-dimensional in vitro cell biology models of ovarian and endometrial cancer. Cell Prolif 42(2):219–228

19. Ghosh S et al (2005) Three-dimensional culture of melanoma cells profoundly affects gene expression profile: a high density oligonucleotide array study. J Cell Physiol 204(2):522–531

20. Justice BA, Badr NA, Felder RA (2009) 3D cell culture opens new dimensions in cell-based assays. Drug Discov Today 14(1):102–107

21. Bullen A (2008) Microscopic imaging techniques for drug discovery. Nat Rev Drug Discov 7(7):54–67

22. Bissell MJ, Rizki A, Mian IS (2003) Tissue architecture: the ultimate regulator of breast epithelial function. Curr Opin Cell Biol 15(6):753–762

23. Mroue R, Bissell MJ (2013) Three-dimensional cultures of mouse mammary epithelial cells. Methods Mol Biol 945:221–250

24. Rodriguez-Enriquez S et al (2008) Energy metabolism transition in multi-cellular human tumor spheroids. J Cell Physiol 216(1):189–197

25. Cukierman E, Pankov R, Stevens DR, Yamada KM (2001) Taking cell-matrix adhesions to the third dimension. Science 294(5547):1708–1712

26. Chambers KF et al (2011) Stroma regulates increased epithelial lateral cell adhesion in 3D culture: a role for actin/cadherin dynamics. PLoS One 6(4), e18796

27. Weaver VM et al (1997) Reversion of the malignant phenotype of human breast cells in three-dimensional culture and in vivo by integrin blocking antibodies. J Cell Biol 137(1):231–245

28. Fong EL et al (2013) Modeling Ewing sarcoma tumors in vitro with 3D scaffolds. Proc Natl Acad Sci U S A 110(16):6500–6505

29. Nichols GL et al (1994) Identification of CRKL as the constitutively phosphorylated

39-kD tyrosine phosphoprotein in chronic myelogenous leukemia cells. Blood 84(9):2912–2918

30. Lamhamedi-Cherradi SE et al (2014) 3D tissue-engineered model of Ewing's sarcoma. Adv Drug Deliv Rev 79–80:155–171

31. Vidi PA, Bissell MJ, Lelievre SA (2013) Three-dimensional culture of human breast epithelial cells: the how and the why. Methods Mol Biol 945:193–219

32. Fischbach C et al (2007) Engineering tumors with 3D scaffolds. Nat Methods 4(10):855–860

33. Ansari N, Muller S, Stelzer EH, Pampaloni F (2013) Quantitative 3D cell-based assay performed with cellular spheroids and fluorescence microscopy. Methods Cell Biol 113:295–309

34. Ivascu A, Kubbies M (2006) Rapid generation of single-tumor spheroids for high-throughput cell function and toxicity analysis. J Biomol Screen 11(8):922–932

35. Friedrich J, Ebner R, Kunz-Schughart LA (2007) Experimental anti-tumor therapy in 3-D: spheroids—old hat or new challenge? Int J Radiat Biol 83(11-12):849–871

36. Kelm JM, Timmins NE, Brown CJ, Fussenegger M, Nielsen LK (2003) Method for generation of homogeneous multicellular tumor spheroids applicable to a wide variety of cell types. Biotechnol Bioeng 83(2):173–180

37. Timmins NE, Dietmair S, Nielsen LK (2004) Hanging-drop multicellular spheroids as a model of tumour angiogenesis. Angiogenesis 7(2):97–103

38. Tung YC et al (2011) High-throughput 3D spheroid culture and drug testing using a 384 hanging drop array. Analyst 136(3):473–478

39. Lee GY, Kenny PA, Lee EH, Bissell MJ (2007) Three-dimensional culture models of normal and malignant breast epithelial cells. Nat Methods 4(4):359–365

40. Huh D, Hamilton GA, Ingber DE (2011) From 3D cell culture to organs-on-chips. Trends Cell Biol 21(12):745–754

41. Bartholomesuz G, Rao A (2014) A three dimensional spheroid cell culture model for robust high throughput RNA interference screens. In: Trip RA, Karpilow J (eds) Frontiers in RNAi, vol 1. Bentham Science Publishers, pp 215–231

42. Yoshii Y et al (2011) The use of nanoimprinted scaffolds as 3D culture models to facilitate spontaneous tumor cell migration and well-regulated spheroid formation. Biomaterials 32(26):6052–6058

43. Kim JB, Stein R, O'Hare MJ (2004) Three-dimensional in vitro tissue culture models of breast cancer—a review. Breast Cancer Res Treat 85(3):281–291

44. Sutherland RM, McCredie JA, Inch WR (1971) Growth of multicell spheroids in tissue culture as a model of nodular carcinomas. J Natl Cancer Inst 46(1):113–120

45. Dubessy C, Merlin JM, Marchal C, Guillemin F (2000) Spheroids in radiobiology and photodynamic therapy. Crit Rev Oncol Hematol 36(2-3):179–192

46. Kunz-Schughart LA, Kreutz M, Knuechel R (1998) Multicellular spheroids: a three-dimensional in vitro culture system to study tumour biology. Int J Exp Pathol 79(1):1–23

47. Kunz-Schughart LA (1999) Multicellular tumor spheroids: intermediates between monolayer culture and in vivo tumor. Cell Biol Int 23(3):157–161

48. Li CX et al (2006) Delivery of RNA interference. Cell Cycle 5(18):2130–2139

49. Zhang S, Zhao B, Jiang H, Wang B, Ma B (2007) Cationic lipids and polymers mediated vectors for delivery of siRNA. J Control Release 123(1):1–10

50. Whitehead KA, Langer R, Anderson DG (2009) Knocking down barriers: advances in siRNA delivery. Nat Rev Drug Discov 8(2):129–138

51. Whitehurst AW et al (2007) Synthetic lethal screen identification of chemosensitizer loci in cancer cells. Nature 446:815–819

Chapter 11

In Vitro High-Throughput RNAi Screening to Accelerate the Process of Target Identification and Drug Development

Hongwei Yin and Michelle Kassner

Abstract

High-throughput RNA interference (HT-RNAi) is a powerful tool that can be used to knock down gene expression in order to identify novel genes and pathways involved in many cellular processes. It is a systematic, yet unbiased, approach to identify essential or synthetic lethal genes that promote cell survival in diseased cells as well as genes that confer resistance or sensitivity to drug treatment. This information serves as a foundation for enhancing current treatments for cancer and other diseases by identifying new drug targets, uncovering potential combination therapies, and helping clinicians match patients with the most effective treatment based on genetic information. Here, we describe the method of performing an in vitro HT-RNAi screen using chemically synthesized siRNA.

Key words High-throughput, RNA interference (RNAi), siRNA, Target discovery, Drug development, Drug sensitizer, Gene knockdown, Functional genomics, Gene silencing, Essential gene, Synthetic lethal

1 Introduction

RNA interference (RNAi) is a natural cellular mechanism whereby gene expression is reduced at the posttranscriptional level. Double-stranded RNA (dsRNA) is bound by the endonuclease dicer, which cleaves the dsRNA into small fragments. These small dsRNA fragments, usually 21–25 nucleotides in length, are called small interfering RNA (siRNA). The ribonucleoprotein RNA-induced silencing complex (RISC) binds to the siRNA, which guides the complex to the target mRNA in a sequence-specific manner. This complex subsequently cleaves and degrades the target mRNA, thereby achieving a reduction of gene expression [1–5].

In the laboratory, we can utilize this endogenous process in vitro or in vivo to achieve gene knockdown through the use of short hairpin RNA (shRNA) or chemically synthesized siRNA. While both approaches rely on the mechanism described

David O. Azorsa, Shilpi Arora (eds.), *High-Throughput RNAi Screening: Methods and Protocols*, Methods in Molecular Biology, vol. 1470, DOI 10.1007/978-1-4939-6337-9_11, © Springer Science+Business Media New York 2016

above, there are advantages and disadvantages to consider for either experimental approach. Utilizing shRNA results in more stable gene knockdown due to its incorporation into the host genome, but it requires the use of viral or bacterial vectors in order to deliver the shRNA into cells. Once incorporated, shRNA are transcribed, exported from the nucleus, and then cleaved by dicer into siRNAs. shRNA can be used to transfect primary cells as well as cell lines that are difficult to transfect. However, the use of shRNA necessitates more stringent safety requirements, and longer assay times (weeks), and presents the difficulty of normalizing the concentration of shRNA across the library. In contrast, chemically synthesized siRNA can be introduced into readily transfectable cells by using lipid-based transfection reagents, but the gene knockdown is transient, lasting 5–7 days [6, 7], due to the rapid degradation of siRNAs in mammalian cells. While the temporary nature of the knockdown may be a drawback for some, the duration of silencing is sufficient to identify genes playing important roles in cellular processes and drug response. siRNA also offers the benefits of normalized concentration throughout the whole library with minimal safety concerns. Both approaches are amenable to high-throughput screening with the use of microplates, specialized equipment, and shRNA or siRNA libraries targeting custom sets of genes all the way up to genome-wide scale.

For the purposes of this discussion, and the methods provided below, we will focus on the use of chemically synthesized siRNA libraries. These libraries can be screened using two different methods: pooled or arrayed. The pooled method combines several siRNA for each target gene, whereas the arrayed method tests each siRNA individually. The pooling method can reduce cost, but also increases the false-positive hit rate. Following the appropriate assay incubation time, a variety of endpoint reagents can be used to assess phenotypic readout including but not limited to proliferation, cell viability, cell death, apoptosis, morphology, and migration. In the following section, we describe the method of performing an in vitro high-throughput RNAi screen using chemically synthesized siRNA (applicable for both the pooled and arrayed method) using CellTiter-Glo® (Promega) to measure cell viability.

The most widely used applications of high-throughput RNAi are essential gene screens, synthetic lethal screens, and drug sensitizer screens. Essential gene screens, also called lethality screens, seek to identify individual genes whose knockdown results in a lethal phenotype in one or more cell lines of the disease of interest. Genes whose knockdown results in more cell death compared to controls are considered necessary for cell survival, and therefore termed essential [8–12].

In contrast, synthetic lethal screens seek to identify nonessential genes that produce lethal phenotypes only when in combination with an existing loss-of-function (LOF) gene mutation in the cells of interest [13]. The loss of or knockdown of each gene individually does not produce a lethal phenotype; however when in combination, their concurrent loss of function results in cell death, making them synthetic lethal. These screens have wide appeal in that they aim to help to identify therapeutic drug targets that would be lethal only to diseased cells with known gene mutations while leaving healthy cells unharmed. More recently, some have expanded the use of the term synthetic lethal to apply to gene-drug interactions as well [14, 15]. We, however, refer to these as drug sensitizers.

Drug sensitizer screens aim to identify genes whose knockdown sensitizes cells to a particular drug of interest [16–26]. The knockdown of these genes causes a change in phenotypic readout, such as increased cell death, less invasion, or specific morphology change, compared to controls treated with the same concentration of drug. When performing the screen in a multiple dose format, the knockdown of these genes results in a decrease of the IC_{50} value, indicating that the cells have been sensitized. In a similar manner, these screens can identify genes that confer resistance as well. Drug sensitizer screens are useful to elucidate important genes and pathways that regulate drug response. These types of screens can shed light on potential combination therapies [27–29], and provide clinicians with valuable predictive biomarkers affecting patient response to drug treatment. While each of these applications of RNAi has a slightly different experimental goal, the protocol provided here contains information applicable to all of them.

2   Materials

1. siRNA Library (Qiagen or other).

2. Barcoded white solid tissue culture-treated 384-well plates.

3. Microplate centrifuge.

4. MicroFill™ or other microplate reagent dispenser with BioStack™ (BioTek).

5. Cytomat™ incubator fitted with plate hotels.

6. Foil seals for microplates.

7. Cell line(s) of interest.

8. Serum-free media (DMEM, RPMI, etc.).

9. 10% Fetal bovine serum (FBS) growth media: 890 ml Media containing l-glutamine (DMEM, RPMI, etc.), 100 ml FBS, 10 ml antibiotic-antimycotic (Life Technologies).

10. 10% FBS assay media: 900 ml Media containing l-glutamine (DMEM, RPMI, etc.), 100 ml FBS.

11. 5% FBS assay media: 950 ml Media containing l-glutamine (DMEM, RPMI, etc.), 50 ml FBS.

12. Transfection reagent.

13. Trypsin.

14. Phosphate-buffered saline (PBS).

15. Cell counter with associated consumables (e.g., Countess® II Automated Cell Counter with slides, Life Technologies).

16. Varying sizes of storage bottles (for dispensing transfection reagent/cells).

17. T225 flasks.

18. Serological pipettes.

19. Pipet boy.

20. Manual pipettes and tips (varying volumes).

21. High-capacity microplate incubator with plate hotels set to 37 °C.

22. Cell Titer-Glo® (Promega) or other endpoint reagent.

23. Aluminum foil (help secure MicroFill™ tubing in reagent being dispensed).

24. Microplate reader fitted with stacker.

25. Drug/compound(s) of interest.

26. DMSO or other vehicle.

27. Dilution reservoirs.

---

3   Methods

Prior to utilizing these methods, great care must be taken to perform an assay development (AD) step in order to optimize many of the assay parameters including, but not limited to, cell seeding density, transfection reagent concentration, assay incubation time, drug incubation time, DMSO toxicity, and endpoint reagent for each cell line to be screened (Table 1).

Since screening with a large siRNA library that targets thousands of genes can involve using hundreds of microplates over multiple days, it is strongly recommended that you first proceed by following the provided protocol using a small siRNA library or custom siRNA set that would involve only 1–10 microplates. This step, called assay validation (AV), when performed with biological replicates serves the purpose of confirming that the optimized assay conditions pass all quality control parameters and the assay is robust and reproducible. Assay validation ensures high-quality data in a larger scale setup over multiple days of screening.

3.1   Essential Gene Screen (or Synthetic Lethal)

Refer to Chapter 1 of this book for detailed protocols on siRNA library plate preparation.

Table 1
Key parameters in HT-RNAi assay development for drug sensitization screens

Assay component	Parameter	Considerations
siRNA	siRNA concentration	Must produce effective silencing and have limited off-target effects
	siRNA sequences	Must have no or minimal off-target effects
	Number of siRNA/gene	Should be determined by scope of the experiment
	Negative control siRNA	Should have no effect on cell growth or drug activity
	Positive control siRNA	Previously identified; cell line specific; proliferation specific; lethal sequences
	Sensitizing positive control siRNA	Provides measure of overall assay function
	Plate format	Medium evaporation, machine readout, barcode
Transfection reagent	Transfection reagent	Should be effective in introducing siRNA and have low toxicity
	Transfection reagent diluent	Should not interfere with drug activity, readout, or transfection efficiency
	Transfection reagent ratio	Toxicity versus efficiency
	Complexing time	Enough time to complex siRNA and transfection reagent; reagent dependent
Cells	Cell line for screening	Transfection efficiency, growth rate, assay sensitivity
	Cell growth media	Should not interfere with drug activity, readout, or transfection efficiency
	Cell volume added	Well-to-well, plate-to-plate variability
	Cell number added	Optimized to give greatest dynamic range at readout
	Incubation time (before drug)	Enough time for siRNA to silence transcripts
	Incubation time (after drug)	Enough time for drug action
Drug	Drug	Should have an effect on the screen cell line
	Drug diluent (vehicle)	Should readily solubilize drug
	DMSO toxicity	Should be minimal
	Drug volume	Should be minimal to allow for addition of readout reagent
	Drug stability	Temperature, half-life, solution, medium
	Final drug concentration	Should have desired effect at selected concentration(s)
Read out	Readout reagent/method	Sensitivity, accuracy, and cost
	Added volume of readout reagent	Should be minimal
	Incubation time for readout reagent	Optimized to give greatest dynamic range at readout

1. Transfer the barcoded siRNA library plates from −80 °C (*see* **Note 1**) to room temperature until the plates are completely thawed and have reached room temperature.

2. Centrifuge all of the thawed plates for 1 min at $200 \times g$ to make sure that all siRNA is on the bottom of the plate.

3. Remove lids and foil seals from plates (*see* **Note 2**).

4. Load plates onto the BioTek MicroFill™ fitted with a BioStack™ (*see* **Notes 3** and **4**).

5. Prepare the appropriate concentration transfection reagent in serum-free media (*see* **Notes 5–7**).

6. Dispense 25 μl per well of the transfection reagent solution using MicroFill™ (*see* **Note 8**) and start a 30-min timer once dispensing begins (*see* **Note 9**).

7. Trypsinize cells, collect them in 10% assay media, and count cells (*see* **Notes 10–12**).

8. Prepare the cell solution in 10% FBS assay media at appropriate concentration to achieve the desired cell density per well in 25 μl (*see* **Notes 13** and **14**).

9. Once the 30-min incubation is complete, dispense 25 μl per well of the prepared cell solution using MicroFill™.

10. Put lids back on plates and move plates to 37 °C Cytomat™ incubator fitted with plate hotels (*see* **Note 15**).

11. Incubate for 96 h at 37 °C (*see* **Note 16**).

12. Prepare a sufficient volume of CellTiter-Glo® luminescent cell viability reagent according to the manufacturer's protocol (*see* **Notes 17** and **18**).

13. Remove plates from incubator, remove lids, and load plates onto the MicroFill™ fitted with a BioStack™.

14. Dispense 25 μl per well of the CellTiter-Glo® solution using the MicroFill™ and start a 1-h timer after the CellTiter-Glo® is dispensed into the first plate (*see* **Note 19**).

15. Incubate plates at room temperature for 1 h (*see* **Note 20**).

16. Load plates onto a microplate reader fitted with a stacker and barcode reader (*see* **Note 21**).

17. Measure luminescence for all plates using a multiple mode plate reader (*see* **Note 22**).

3.2 Drug Sensitizer Screen

For the drug sensitizer screen, **steps 1–11** and **13–19** remain the same as in the essential gene screen assay, with the following exceptions:

(a) The dispense volume of transfection reagent solution and cell solution is 20 μl per well instead of 25 μl (**steps 6, 9,** and **10**) to allow for a 10 µl dispense of drug solution while keeping the final assay volume at a total of 50 µl.

(b) The total number of each siRNA library plate needed will increase depending on the number of drug concentrations used for screening (one plate per drug concentration).

Also, in the essential gene screen, **step 12** is purely an incubation step, whereas in the drug sensitizer screen there are some additional steps to perform as outlined below:

1. Same as in Subheading 3.1

2. Incubate plates overnight (~12–24 h) at 37 °C (*see* **Note 23**).

   (a) Prepare a serial dilution of five concentrations of drug solution targeting between IC_{15} and IC_{75} as well as DMSO vehicle control (6 doses total) in 5 % FBS assay media (*see* **Notes 24–26**).

   (b) Dispense 10 µl of drug per well (one concentration per plate) using MicroFill™ (*see* **Note 27**).

   (c) Incubate plates at 37 °C for 72–96 h post-drug addition (96–120 h total assay time) (*see* **Note 28**).

3. Prepare a sufficient volume of CellTiter-Glo® luminescent cell viability reagent according to the manufacturer's protocol (*see* **Notes 17** and **18**).

4. Remove plates from incubator, remove lids, and load plates onto the MicroFill™ fitted with a BioStack™.

5. Dispense 25 µl per well of the CellTiter-Glo® solution using the MicroFill™.

6. Start a 1-h timer after the CellTiter-Glo® is dispensed into the first plate (*see* **Note 19**).

7. Incubate plates at room temperature for 1 h (*see* **Note 20**).

8. Load plates onto a microplate reader fitted with a stacker and barcode reader (*see* **Note 21**).

9. Measure luminescence for all plates using a multiple mode plate reader (*see* **Note 22**).

3.3 Confirmation and Validation

The primary RNAi screening (essential gene, synthetic lethal, or drug sensitizer screen) will result in a list of priority genes to be screened again to confirm the results. This confirmation step follows the same high throughput screening (HTS) protocol and uses the same cell line, except only the selected genes will be screened. If the primary HTS is performed with two siRNAs per target, we highly recommend testing four siRNAs per target during confirmation step. Multiple biological repeats should be performed. Refer to Chapter 1 in this book for hit picking and preparation of the assay plates containing the genes of interest for confirmation.

After plate preparation, the protocol for confirmation follows all the same steps as in the primary screen. Refer to Subheading 3.1 for essential gene/synthetic lethal confirmation screens or Subheading 3.2 for drug sensitizer confirmation screens. This step will produce a reduced confirmed gene list, which will be further tested in the following validation screen.

For the validation step, the candidate genes will be tested with more cell lines, in addition to the cell line used for the primary screen. These cell lines can be of the same or differing genetic profiles, of the same or different disease types, or cell lines with varying degrees of drug sensitivities. In addition, for the drug sensitizer screens, we can also validate genes with additional drugs of the same target or family, targeting the same or parallel pathways, upstream/downstream of the drug target, etc. Moreover, these confirmed genes should be further verified with gene knockdown by either qPCR or western blot.

4   Notes

1. To facilitate screening efficiency the next day, the barcoded siRNA library plates can also be moved to 4 °C the day before screening.

2. Use extreme caution anytime you are physically handling the plates, especially when unstacking/restacking them, lidding or unlidding them, or removing the foil seals. It is very easy to inadvertently bump and/or knock over plates, which will be especially detrimental after the addition of the reagents. Develop personal handling methods that you find helpful such as avoiding moving the plates from a lower stack to a higher stack directly in front of the lower stack. We have found a triangle setup helpful, with the source stack at the top point of the triangle, the destination stack on the left point, and the plate lids on the right point of the triangle.

3. Other microplate reagent dispensers fitted with a stacker can also be used. Depending on the number of library plates to be screened, more than one dispenser may be needed, or multiple runs on one dispenser may be necessary.

4. We recommend placing 1–2 empty black clear bottom plates, referred to as blanks or dummy plates, before the first siRNA library plate to be dispensed and after the last plate to be dispensed. The purpose of the dummy plates is twofold. First, it allows you to ensure that the MicroFill™ is working properly with no clogged pins or other artifacts that would negatively affect screening plates. Second, it allows the visual monitoring of cell density, the presence of possible contamination, and evaluation of overall assay condition at the beginning and end of the screen.

5. Commonly used transfection reagents include, but are not limited to, Lipofectamine® 2000 (Life Technologies), Lipofectamine® RNAiMax (Life Technologies), Dharmafect™ (Dharmacon™), and siLentFect™ (BioRad).

6. Serum can negatively affect transfection by interfering with the lipid's ability to bind and form complexes with the siRNA. Therefore, the transfection reagent must be prepared in serum-free media.

7. Total assay volume will be 50 μl: 25 μl transfection reagent solution prepared in serum-free media + 25 μl cells prepared in 10 % FBS assay media. The amount of transfection reagent (nl/well or nl/25 μl) in that solution should be optimized for every cell line. In our experience, a range of 40–200 nl/well provides a transfection efficiency of 95 % or greater while maintaining low toxicity for adherent cell lines. Suspension cells are not likely to transfect at such a high rate and 75 % or greater efficiency is considered sufficient. Transfection efficiency is calculated by the formula 1 – (raw signal of positive control/raw signal of negative control).

8. After inserting the MicroFill™ tubing into the reagent bottle containing your solution, the placement of aluminum foil over the mouth of the reagent bottle can be very helpful to secure the tubing in place so that it does not slide out or move to a position that would allow air to get into the tubing. Air in the tubing will disrupt proper dispensing and can lead to empty wells or insufficient volume transfer.

9. It is recommended that the transfection reagent and siRNA incubate at room temperature for a minimum of 30 min in order to form complexes before the cells are added. From our experience, allowing the complex to form for more than 50 min will have a negative effect on transfection efficiency.

10. Assay media contains all the components of growth media except the antibiotics. Antibiotics can negatively affect transfection efficiency. When inactivating the trypsin, be sure to use 10 % FBS assay media and not growth media, so that you do not introduce antibiotics into the assay.

11. Since the transfection reagent is dispensed in serum-free media, the serum concentration of the cell solution needs to be 10 % FBS, 2× the desired final concentration of 5 % FBS. We prefer 5 % FBS as our final concentration since serum can affect transfection and can also affect drugs' activity (when performing a drug sensitizer screen using a drug with serum-binding properties).

12. Be sure to measure the cell viability on the day of screening. If the cell viability is lower than 80%, it would be advised to reschedule screening for another day.

13. For example, when we prepare the cells at a concentration of 40,000 cells/ml, it will give us 1000 cells per well when dispensing 25 μl per well.

14. The concentration, or density of cells per well, needs to be optimized during assay development for each cell line. A range of 50–4000 cells per well is seeded into two separate 384-well plates to be read using CellTiter-Glo® luminescent cell viability reagent at time = 0 h (day of seeding) and time = 96 h post-seeding. More plates can be seeded for additional time points as needed for the assay. To choose the optimal cell density, be sure that T96/T0 is greater than twofold and then choose a density that has not reached signal saturation.

15. If a Cytomat™ incubator or incubator with plate hotels is unavailable, plates can be stacked in a regular incubator. However, care must be taken to avoid uneven evaporation and/or edge effects for the plates on top of the stacks by placing 1–2 dummy plates on top filled with water, PBS, or media. Plate hotels provide the best plate-to-plate consistency in terms of incubation conditions.

16. Incubation time will vary; 72–96 h is standard, but it must be determined by assay development for each of the screening cell lines.

17. Other reagents can be used depending on the endpoint being measured, for example endpoints involving high-content imaging, *see* Henderson-Smith et al. [9].

18. Be extra cautious with plate handling once the CellTiter-Glo® has been dispensed as it can be easy to create froth and or bubbles that are detrimental to the reading mechanisms of microplate readers. If such artifacts are observed, use a kimwipe or paper towel to dab the top of the plate to remove the bubbles. Alternately, you could also centrifuge the plate for 2 min at $200 \times g$.

19. The incubation time for CellTiter-Glo® can range from 30 min to 1 h, but should be optimized for your specific needs.

20. Longer incubation times for CellTiter-Glo® in conjunction with the weight of a stack of plates can lead to the plates sticking together due to the moisture between them. Be advised of this potential artifact and re-lid plates during incubation if necessary.

21. Depending on the endpoint, a multiple mode plate reader that can measure luminescence, fluorescence, or absorbance may be required. Some examples are EnVision® (Perkin Elmer), SpectraMax® Paradigm® (Molecular Devices), or Synergy™ Neo2 (BioTek®). Also, if the endpoint involves imaging, a high-content imager that has an automated camera with autofocus will be needed, such as the ImageXpress (Molecular Devices) or Opera (Perkin Elmer).

22. If applicable on your plate reader, integration time will affect plate read time. Optimize integration time so that read time is similar to MicroFill™ dispense time to give an accurate incubation period for each plate.

23. Note the difference in incubation time due to the drug addition protocol. This incubation time of 12–24 h is to allow the siRNA to be transfected into the cells, and for cells to attach to the bottom of the plate, if applicable.

24. Depending on resources, you can choose to treat with 1–7 concentrations of drug plus DMSO or another vehicle control. We prefer to perform the screen in a drug dose response (DDR) manner [16], while other labs prefer to screen just with one sublethal drug concentration compared with vehicle control [14].

25. For the multiple-dose DDR format, first perform dilution of drug using DMSO (or other vehicle) as diluent. Then transfer an equal volume of each drug preparation in DMSO (or other vehicle) to the appropriate volume of 5% FBS assay media to achieve desired concentrations. For example, determine the amount of 20 mM stock needed to prepare a 50 µM (5× the final concentration of 10 µM) drug solution in 50 ml of 5% FBS assay media:

$$(20 \text{ mM}) (x) = (50 \text{ µM}) (50 \text{ ml})$$
$$x = 125 \text{ µl}$$

In the example above, after performing the serial dilution you would need to add 125 µl of drug preparation to 50 ml of 5% FBS assay media. Vehicle control would be prepared in the same manner by adding 125 µl of DMSO to 50 ml of 5% FBS assay media. This method keeps DMSO/vehicle concentration consistent for all doses. Note that the drug preparation in assay media needs to be 5× the final concentration desired in the assay, due to the 1:5 dilution that occurs when adding the 10 µl of drug solution to the 40 µl of assay already in the plate. For the single-dose format, just prepare a single solution of drug at 5× your final desired assay concentration in 5% FBS assay media.

26. After cells are added to the plate, the concentration of FBS in the assay is 5% (equal parts serum-free media from transfection + 10% FBS assay media with cells). Therefore 5% FBS assay media is used for dosing in order to keep the concentration of FBS consistent at 5%.

27. When dosing with drug or vehicle control, only treat columns 2–24. Leave column 1 untreated to evaluate plate-to-plate variation.

28. Incubation time will vary depending on drug response; 72–96 h is usually used, but the exact time must be determined by assay development.

Acknowledgements

We would like to thank TGen for their support, Mr. Chris Sereduk for editing, and Springer Publishing.

References

1. Agrawal N, Dasaradhi PV et al (2003) RNA interference: biology, mechanism, and applications. Microbiol Mol Biol Rev 67(4):657–685

2. Boutros M, Ahringer J (2008) The art and design of genetic screens: RNA interference. Nat Rev Genet 9(7):554–566

3. Caplen NJ, Parrish S et al (2001) Specific inhibition of gene expression by small double-stranded RNAs in invertebrate and vertebrate systems. Proc Natl Acad Sci U S A 98(17):9742–9747

4. Duxbury MS, Whang EE (2004) RNA interference: a practical approach. J Surg Res 117(2):339–344

5. Elbashir SM, Harborth J et al (2001) Duplexes of 21-nucleotide RNAs mediate RNA interference in cultured mammalian cells. Nature 411(6836):494–498

6. Bartlett DW, Davis ME (2006) Insights into the kinetics of siRNA-mediated gene silencing from live-cell and live-animal bioluminescent imaging. Nucleic Acids Res 34(1):322–333

7. Life Technologies. Duration of siRNA induced silencing: your questions answered. https://www.lifetechnologies.com/us/en/home/references/ambion-tech-support/rnai-sirna/tech-notes/duration-of-sirna-induced-silencing.html. Accessed 30 Jul 2015

8. Ganesan AK, Ho H et al (2008) Genome-wide siRNA-based functional genomics of pigmentation identifies novel genes and pathways that impact melanogenesis in human cells. PLoS Genet 4(12):e1000298

9. Henderson-Smith A, Chow D et al (2013) SMG1 identified as a regulator of Parkinson's disease-associated alpha-synuclein through siRNA screening. PLoS One 8(10):e77711

10. Petrocca F, Altschuler G et al (2013) A genome-wide siRNA screen identifies proteasome addiction as a vulnerability of basal-like triple-negative breast cancer cells. Cancer Cell 24(2):182–196

11. Tiedemann RE, Zhu YX et al (2011) Identification of molecular vulnerabilities in human multiple myeloma cells by RNA interference lethality screening of the druggable genome. Cancer Res 72(3):757–768

12. Tiedemann RE, Zhu YX et al (2010) Kinome-wide RNAi studies in human multiple myeloma identify vulnerable kinase targets, including a lymphoid-restricted kinase, GRK6. Blood 115(8):1594–1604

13. Scholl C, Frohling S et al (2009) Synthetic lethal interaction between oncogenic KRAS dependency and STK33 suppression in human cancer cells. Cell 137(5):821–834

14. Turner NC, Lord CJ et al (2008) A synthetic lethal siRNA screen identifying genes mediating sensitivity to a PARP inhibitor. EMBO J 27(9):1368–1377

15. Whitehurst AW, Bodemann BO et al (2007) Synthetic lethal screen identification of chemosensitizer loci in cancer cells. Nature 446(7137):815–819

16. Harradine KA, Kassner M et al (2011) Functional genomics reveals diverse cellular processes that modulate tumor cell response to oxaliplatin. Mol Cancer Res 9(2):173–182

17. Zhu YX, Tiedemann R et al (2011) RNAi screen of the druggable genome identifies modulators of proteasome inhibitor sensitivity in myeloma including CDK5. Blood 117(14):3847–3857

18. Zhu YX, Yin H et al (2015) RNA interference screening identifies lenalidomide sensitizers in multiple myeloma, including RSK2. Blood 125(3):483–491

19. Xie L, Kassner M et al (2012) Kinome-wide siRNA screening identifies molecular targets mediating the sensitivity of pancreatic cancer cells to Aurora kinase inhibitors. Biochem Pharmacol 83(4):452–461

20. Falkenberg KJ, Gould CM et al (2014) Genome-wide functional genomic and transcriptomic analyses for genes regulating sensitivity to vorinostat. Sci Data 1:140017

21. MacKeigan JP, Murphy LO et al (2005) Sensitized RNAi screen of human kinases and phosphatases identifies new regulators of apoptosis and chemoresistance. Nat Cell Biol 7(6):591–600

22. Bartz SR, Zhang Z et al (2006) Small interfering RNA screens reveal enhanced cisplatin cytotoxicity in tumor cells having both BRCA network and TP53 disruptions. Mol Cell Biol 26(24):9377–9386

23. Giroux V, Iovanna J et al (2006) Probing the human kinome for kinases involved in pancreatic cancer cell survival and gemcitabine resistance. FASEB J 20(12):1982–1991

24. Iorns E, Lord CJ et al (2009) Parallel RNAi and compound screens identify the PDK1 pathway as a target for tamoxifen sensitization. Biochem J 417(1):361–370

25. Lord CJ, McDonald S et al (2008) A high-throughput RNA interference screen for DNA repair determinants of PARP inhibitor sensitivity. DNA Repair (Amst) 7(12):2010–2019

26. Morgan-Lappe S, Woods KW et al (2006) RNAi-based screening of the human kinome identifies Akt-cooperating kinases: a new approach to designing efficacious multitargeted kinase inhibitors. Oncogene 25(9):1340–1348

27. Bogenberger JM, Kornblau SM et al (2014) BCL-2 family proteins as 5-Azacytidine-sensitizing targets and determinants of response in myeloid malignancies. Leukemia 28(8):1657–1665

28. Tibes R, Bogenberger JM et al (2012) RNAi screening of the kinome with cytarabine in leukemias. Blood 119(12):2863–2872

29. Yin H, Kiefer J, Kassner M, Tang N, Mousses S (2010) The application of high-throughput RNAi in pancreatic cancer target discovery and drug development. In: Han H, Grippo P (eds) Drug discovery in pancreatic cancer. Springer Science+Business Media, LLC, New York, pp 153–170

Chapter 12

High-Throughput, Liquid-Based Genome-Wide RNAi Screening in *C. elegans*

Linda P. O'Reilly, Ryan R. Knoerdel, Gary A. Silverman, and Stephen C. Pak

Abstract

RNA interference (RNAi) is a process in which double-stranded RNA (dsRNA) molecules mediate the inhibition of gene expression. RNAi in *C. elegans* can be achieved by simply feeding animals with bacteria expressing dsRNA against the gene of interest. This "feeding" method has made it possible to conduct genome-wide RNAi experiments for the systematic knockdown and subsequent investigation of almost every single gene in the genome. Historically, these genome-scale RNAi screens have been labor and time intensive. However, recent advances in automated, high-throughput methodologies have allowed the development of more rapid and efficient screening protocols. In this report, we describe a fast and efficient, liquid-based method for genome-wide RNAi screening.

Key words RNAi, Genome wide, High-throughput screening, *C. elegans*, Arrayscan

1 Introduction

The ability to specifically knockdown gene expression by RNAi is a powerful tool for investigating gene function. In *C. elegans*, RNAi can be achieved by several different methods: (1) direct injection of dsRNA into the animals, (2) soaking animals in a solution of dsRNA, or (3) feeding animals with bacteria expressing dsRNA. Of the three methods, the "feeding" method is the easiest and the most suitable for large-scale investigations. Currently, two RNAi feeding libraries are available. The Ahringer Library (Geneservice) consists of 16,757 clones and was constructed by inserting genomic fragments (500–2500 bp) into a double T7 promoter vector [1, 2]. The Vidal library (Open Biosystems) consisting of 11,511 clones was generated by inserting full-length open reading frames into double T7 vectors via Gateway cloning [3]. These libraries have paved the way for numerous genome-scale RNAi studies in *C. elegans* [4–6].

David O. Azorsa, Shilpi Arora (eds.), *High-Throughput RNAi Screening: Methods and Protocols*, Methods in Molecular Biology, vol. 1470, DOI 10.1007/978-1-4939-6337-9_12, © Springer Science+Business Media New York 2016

Typically, genome-wide RNAi screens are performed on agar plates and are labor intensive and can take 6–12 months to complete [5, 7]. Adapting the screening to a 96-well liquid format allows the use of high-throughput (HT) liquid handlers that can significantly reduce screening time and labor. However, phenotype assessment is usually performed manually using a microscope and represents the most significant bottleneck in the screening process. Recent advancements in imaging technology and data analysis software have made it possible to automate phenotypic measurements (for example, Multi-Worm Tracker [8] or the automated thrashing assay [9], recently reviewed here [9, 10]).

Previously, our laboratory developed an HT, high-content (HC) protocol for screening drugs that affect the accumulation of a misfolded α1-antitrypsin (ATZ) protein that aggregates in *C. elegans* [11, 12]. We subsequently adapted this protocol to perform a semi-automated, genome-wide RNAi screen for genes that modulate ATZ accumulation [13].

An overview of the screening process is outlined in Fig. 1. In brief, a COPAS™ *BIOSORT* (Union Biometric; heretofore referred

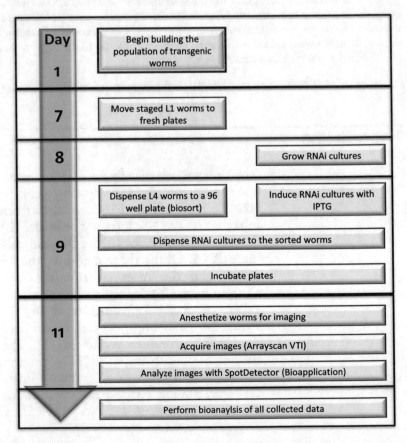

Fig. 1 Schematic of the RNAi screen workflow, detailing the major steps and times (adapted from [13])

to as the "worm sorter") is used to automatically sort 100 L4 stage animals into each well of a 96-well optical bottom assay plate [14]. If a worm sorter is not available, an automated pipetting device like the MultiFlo (BioTek) can be used [15]. Other liquid handling options have recently been reviewed [10]. The worm sorter can precisely sort a predetermined number of animals with desired size and fluorescence properties into each well and thus help reduce assay variability. Individual bacterial clones induced to express dsRNA are then dispensed into the wells utilizing the LIQUIDATOR 96™ (Mettler-Toledo), which allows single-step transfer of liquid into a 96-well plate. After a 48-h incubation on a shaker, an image-based approach is used to monitor the level of GFP transgene accumulation in the intestine of the worm. We utilized the high-speed, HC imager, the ArrayScan V^{TI} (Thermo Fisher Scientific) to automatically acquire images of the animals in the wells. An assortment of built-in BioApplications that convert the image data to numerical values are then used for quantitative assessment of multiple parameters such as fluorescence spot count, intensity, and area. Other options for imaging acquisition and data analysis suitable for *C. elegans* have recently been reviewed [10].

Using this approach, we conducted a genome-wide RNAi screen for modifiers of sGFP::ATZ accumulation in the intestine. However, this approach can be easily adapted for assessing other worm strains expressing fluorescently tagged transgenes such as alpha-synuclein (Parkinson's disease) [16] and polyglutamine repeats (Huntington's disease) [17].

Automation of worm sorting, image acquisition, and data analysis enables RNAi screens to be performed in a HT fashion. Worm sorting times can vary depending on the number of worms being sorted, the degree of synchronization, and gating/sorting parameters. Typically, it takes 30–45 min to sort 100 animals into each well of 96-well plate. Image acquisition can also take 30–45 min per 96-well plate. As such, one can realistically process between 12 and 14 96-well plates (equivalent to 1152–1344 RNAi samples) in a normal workday. While the exact times will vary depending on the assay and phenotype being assessed, one could complete a whole genome RNAi screen in as little as 2 weeks.

2 Materials

2.1 Instruments

1. COPAS™ BIOSORT (Union Biometrica).
2. Arrayscan V^{TI} (Thermo Fisher Scientific).
3. Liquidator™ 96 (Mettler-Toledo).
4. 96-well pinning device (V&P Scientific Inc.).
5. Innova 4300 incubator shaker (New Brunswick Scientific).
6. Orbital plate shaker MP4 (GeneMate, BioExpress).

2.2   Components for Animal Culture

1. Luria Bertani (LB) broth: Weigh out 10 g tryptone, 5 g yeast extract, 10 g NaCl, bring to 1 l with milli-Q water. Prepare 2 l (divided into 2×2 l Erlenmeyer flasks) and 200 ml in a 500 ml screw cap bottle. Autoclave.

2. Phosphate buffered saline (PBS): Prepare a 10× solution by weighing out 2.4 g KH_2PO_4, 80 g NaCl, 14.4 g Na_2HPO_4, 2 g KCl, and bring to 1 l with milli-Q water. Before use dilute to 1× in milli-Q water. Make 2 l and autoclave.

3. 40 % Glycerol: Take 200 ml of glycerol and bring to 500 ml with 1× PBS. Autoclave.

4. Prepare 6×250 ml centrifuge tubes, by wrapping in foil and autoclaving.

5. NGM agar: Weigh out 3 g NaCl, 25 g Difco bacto-agar, 2.5 g bacto-peptone. Make up to 1 l in a 2 l flask and autoclave. Once cooled to 55 °C add 1 ml cholesterol (5 mg/ml in ethanol), 1 ml 1 M $MgSO_4$, 1 ml 1 M $CaCl_2$, 25 ml 1 M KPO_4 pH 6.0. Pour in petri dishes and allow to set (20 ml per 10 cm dish).

2.3   Components for RNAi Bacterial Preparation

1. RNAi clones were obtained from the Ahringer RNAi feeding Library (Geneservice Limited).

2. Sterile 96 well 1 ml deep-well round-bottom plates (BioExpress).

3. LB + Ampicillin: prepare ampicillin aliquots by dissolving 1 g of ampicillin to 10 ml of milli-Q water (100 mg/ml), and filter sterilize. Store at –20 °C in 1 ml aliquots. Add ampicillin to LB broth to a final concentration of 50 μg/ml prior to use.

4. Breathe-EASIER™ film (Diversified Biotech).

2.4   RNAi Assay Procedure

1. IPTG: Make up a 1 M stock in milli-Q water, sterile filter, and store in 1 ml aliquots at –20 °C. Use once and discard.

2. 5-Fluorodeoxyuridine (FuDR): Make up 100 mM stock in milli-Q water, filter sterilize, and store at –80 °C in 1 ml aliquots.

2.5   COPAS BIOSORT Reagents

1. 10 % sodium hypochlorite (Clorox): Dilute 200 ml in milli-Q water, bring to 2 l. Filter sterilize with 1 l Stericup (Millipore) to remove all particulate matter.

2. Sterile H_2O: Autoclave 4 l milli-Q water.

3. 1 l PBS prepared as above and filter sterilize.

4. Sheath fluid: Prepare 3 l PBS and add Triton X-100 to final concentration of 0.01 %. Filter sterilize.

2.6   Image Acquisition

1. Sodium azide (NaN_3): Make a 1 M stock of NaN_3 by dissolving 0.65 g NaN_3 in 10 ml PBS, use within a month. On the day of use dilute the 1 M stock to 0.1 M. Use at a final concentration of 0.05 M.

3 Methods

3.1 Preparation of Animals for RNAi Screening

3.1.1 Preparation of E. coli (OP50) Stock

1. Streak out a culture of OP50 onto a fresh NGM plate. Incubate overnight at 37 °C.

2. Inoculate 2×5 ml LB cultures with a single colony from the NGM plate. Incubate overnight at 37 °C, in an incubator shaker at 250 rpm.

3. The next morning inoculate 2×1 l LB broth with 5 ml of the overnight culture. Place in the 37 °C incubate and shake at 250 rpm. Grow to OD_{600} ~0.5–0.6 (approximately 2 h). Place on ice.

4. Aliquot 200 ml into each of the six centrifuge tubes and centrifuge for 5 min at $4270 \times g$.

5. Discard the supernatant and divide the remaining 2 l of culture equally amongst the tubes (approximately 125 ml each). Centrifuge tubes for 5 min at $4270 \times g$.

6. Discard the supernatant and wash the pellet by resuspending in 130 ml PBS and centrifuge at $4270 \times g$ for 5 min. Discard the supernatant and resuspend the bacterial pellet in a total volume of 400 ml PBS. Add 400 ml of 40 % glycerol and mix by inversion. Divide the solution into 40 ml aliquots in 50 ml falcon tubes and freeze at −80 °C.

7. For working solution, thaw an aliquot of the bacterial stock and pellet by centrifugation at $4270 \times g$ for 20 min. Carefully decant the glycerol solution and resuspend the pellet in 12 ml fresh sterile PBS. Seed each 10 cm prepared NGM plate with 50 μl and incubate overnight at 37 °C. Cool plates to room temperature before use.

3.1.2 Preparation of C. elegans

1. Place 12–15 adult transgenic animals on 5×10 cm NGM/OP50 plates. Maintain all animals at 22 °C on NGM [18], unless otherwise stated. After approximately 7 days incubation, when the population has increased, isolate early-staged larval animals by differential sedimentation, and transfer to 10×10 cm NGM/OP50 plates (see **Note 1**).

2. Incubate the larvae at 22 °C, until the majority of the animals are at the L4 larval stage (approximately 48 h; see **Notes 2** and **3**).

3.2 RNAi Bacterial Preparation and Induction

1. The Ahringer RNAi library was provided in a 384-well plate format. As such, it was necessary to re-array the plates into 96-well plates for screening. For each 384-well plate to be re-arrayed, prepare 4×96-well plates, containing 100 μl LB-Amp. Using a disposable sterile pinning device (V&P Scientific Inc.), inoculate each plate, changing the pin set between each. Seal the plate with Breathe-EASIER™ film, and incubate overnight at 37 °C in an incubator shaker at 250 rpm. Add an equal volume of 40 % glycerol and freeze at −80 °C until use.

2. To grow the RNAi cultures for screening, dispense 400 µl of LB broth into each well of a deep-well 96-well plate using the Liquidator.

3. Using a sterile pinning device inoculate the RNAi clones from the prepared frozen stock plates into the corresponding deep-well 96-well plates.

4. Seal each plate with Breathe-EASIER™ film, and incubate overnight at 37 °C in an incubator shaker at 250 rpm.

5. The next morning thaw and dilute the 1 M IPTG stock to 500 µM with sterile PBS. Add 3.2 µl of the 500 µM IPTG stock solution to each well, with the Liquidator, to bring the final concentration of IPTG to 4 mM. Reseal the plates, and incubate for 1 h with shaking to induce production of dsRNA.

6. Centrifuge the plates at $2205 \times g$ for 5 min to pellet the bacteria. Carefully decant the supernatant, and resuspend the bacterial pellet with 400 µl of fresh LB ampicillin/IPTG.

3.3 Animal Sorting Using the COPAS™ BIOSORT (Worm Sorter)

1. *Worm sorter preparation.* Place the prepared sheath solution in the reservoir, decanting slowly to prevent introducing air bubbles. Turn on pump, laser, and sorter, and allow to warm-up for 1 min. Open the program BioSort 5270, set mixer to 50%, click START, click RUN, click DONE. Check pressure, and click PRESSURE OK. Click AQUIRE to allow sheath solution to flush the system. Use clean function to eliminate air bubbles in the tubing.

2. *Prepare worms for sorting.* Examine worm plates under microscope for any lint or other large debris and remove if present. Wash worms off five 10 cm plates and combine into a 50 ml falcon tube. Allow worms to settle by gravity and remove supernatant. Repeat step twice remove small larvae and debris.

3. Resuspend animals in 50 ml fresh PBS. Check for any particulate matter, and remove with a pipette (*see* **Note 4**).

4. Place worms into the sample cup, and ensure the lid is tightened so that system pressure is maintained. Using the acquire function, acquire data on 500 animals to collect the sample population distribution data. Edit GATE and SORT regions to select the desired population (*see* **Note 5**).

5. Test sort ten worms to five wells. Confirm sorting of correct number and size of worms under a fluorescent stereoscope.

6. Once the sorting parameters have been optimized, 100 L4/young-adult animals were sorted into each well of the 96-well optical bottom plates (Nunc MicroWell 96).

3.4 Addition of RNAi Cultures

1. Using the Liquidator-96 add 40 µl of the induced RNAi culture to each well of a 96-well plate containing 100 L4-stage animals.

2. Add 5-fluorodeoxyuridine (FuDR) to a concentration of 200 μM in each well to prevent eggs from developing and contaminating the plates with young worms. Incubate plates at 22 °C on an orbital plate shaker at 650 rpm for 48 h. To prevent evaporation, place plates into a sealed plastic container, containing moist paper towels.

3.5 Image Acquisition

1. Prior to imaging, the animals are first anesthetized with 50 mM NaN₃. 100 μl of 0.1 M NaN₃ is added to each well with the Liquidator-96, and incubated for 5 min until worm movement was significantly impaired.

2. Acquire images with the ArrayScan V^{TI} HCS Reader (Cellomics, ThermoFisher) fitted with a 5× objective and a 0.63× coupler. Capture the images utilizing a two-channel (Green/Red) assay previously described [11].

3. The ArrayScan V^{TI} is switched on and software booted.

4. In the Protocol Interactive mode, select the plate type and protocol to be used. Load the plate, autofocus, and autoexpose prior to acquiring the well image set. Optimize the SpotDetector BioApplication parameters to identify the transgenes being expressed. Once all the parameters have been optimized, acquire images of each well (*see* **Note 6**).

5. With approximately 10 min left in the plate read, prepare the next plate by adding sodium azide, and begin the next scan immediately upon completion of the first plate. Data is automatically stored on the server and can be accessed at any time after image acquisition.

3.6 Determining the Dynamic Range of the Assay

Before undertaking a full library screen, the dynamic range of the assay must first be determined using control RNAi reagents. In our case we routinely use *Vec*, *GFP*, and *daf-16* RNAis. *Vec(RNAi)* is our negative control. *GFP(RNAi)* and *daf-16(RNAi)* are known to decrease and increase our ATZ transgene, respectively [13]. To accurately assess transgene expression, it is desirable to coexpress another transgene tagged to a different colored reporter, preferably in a different tissue to that of the transgene of interest. We routinely express a red fluorescent protein (RFP or mCherry) in pharynx using the myo-2 promoter. This allows us to efficiently count the number of animals in each well using the SpotDetector BioApplication, and subsequently to normalize our data, by dividing the GFP data by the red head count (Fig. 2 and *see* **Note 7**)

3.7 Identification of Initial Hits

1. For each RNAi sample, a z-score is calculated using the formula: $z = (x - \mu)/\sigma$, where x = sample raw score, μ = mean of the samples on the plate, and σ = the standard deviation of samples on the plate [19]. We arbitrarily selected z-score above or below 2.35 as potential hits for verification as it corresponds to $P < 0.05$ (*see* **Note 7**).

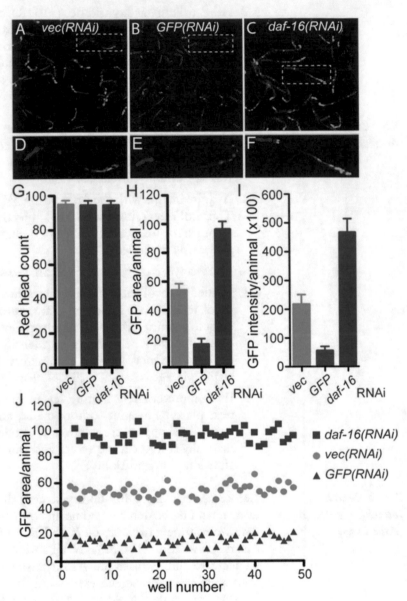

Fig. 2 Arrayscan V^{TI} images of worms treated with *Vec*, *GFP*, and *daf-16* RNAi (A–C) and single animal magnified (D–F). Quantitative data from 48 wells. The GFP transgene expression was normalized by counting the number of red heads (G) and expressed as either GFP area (H) or intensity (I). The dynamic range of the assay (J) shows clear separation between the three RNAi populations. Figure reprinted from [13], O'Reilly LP, Long OS, Cobanoglu MC, et al., (2014) A genome-wide RNAi screen identifies potential drug targets in a *C. elegans* model of alpha1-antitrypsin deficiency. Human Molecular Genetics 23 (19):5123-5132 by permission of Oxford University Press

2. To verify hits, positive RNAi clones are cherry-picked into a new 96-well plate, and the assay repeated 2× to ensure reproducibility of each hit.

3.8 Analysis of Results

In some cases, it may be necessary to take the list of hits and perform pathway analysis to determine which pathways/family of proteins are important to pursue further. However, very few resources are available to perform such bioinformatics directly on *C. elegans* data, therefore it is often necessary to assign human orthologs to *C. elegans* hits.

1. Human orthologs, can be assigned in one of two ways. Firstly, WormBase (http://www.wormbase.org; referential freeze WS236) can be used to query the sequence names of hit genes, and identify the corresponding human orthologs with the highest pBLAST score and/or best predicted human ortholog (based on curated data from TreeFam, Inparanoid, Panther, EnsEMBL-compara ortholog prediction programs). A second more stringent method is to use the OrthoList compiled by Shaye and Greenwald [20], which is now available as an online tool via WormBase. The OrthoList was derived from a meta-analysis of four independent prediction methods, in order to generate a human ortholog list of 7663 *C. elegans* genes.

2. Once human orthologs have been assigned, the data can be analyzed using various bioinformatics programs, listed in Table 1.

3. For pathway analysis, the Database for Annotation, Visualization and Integrated Discovery (DAVID) Bioinformatics Resource v6.7 [21], can be used to generate a functional annotation chart, using a term-centric singular enrichment analysis so that the protein profiles can be investigated. More sophisticated programs such as INGENUITY or MetaCore can also be used to probe specific pathways. However a subscription is needed, whereas DAVID is freely available.

Table 1
List of the various bioinformatics programs available to analyze the RNAi screen hits

Analysis	Software	Website	Access
Pathway	Ingenuity (IPA-Qiagen)	ingenuity.com	Subscription
Pathway	Metacore (Thomson Reuters)	portal.genego.com	Subscription
Drug interaction	STITCH	stitch.embl.de	Free access
Drug interaction	Metadrug (Thomson Reuters)	portal.genego.com	Subscription
Pathway	DAVID	david.abcc.ncifcrf.gov	Free access

4. To probe drug-target interactions the Search Tool for Interactions of Chemicals (STITCH; www.stitch.embl.de) can be queried. STITCH currently contains information on >2 million interactions between more than 300,000 chemicals and 2.6 million proteins from >1100 organisms. STITCH primarily uses keyword mining of the literature and experimental data to predict protein–drug interactions generating a confidence score to indicate the probability that the predicted interaction exists. Another subscription-based software is MetaCore/MetaDrug by Thomson Reuters (http://thomsonreuters.com/products_services/science/science_products/a-z/metacore/). MetaCore is a systems biology platform for pathway analysis and drug discovery, using manually curated literature searches, and links drug-target information to the original references. However, unlike STITCH, no confidence score is provided.

4 Notes

1. The method described was determined specifically for RNAi screening of our sGFP::ATZ transgenic strain. As such, specific parameters and times may vary depending on the worm strain used. Therefore, such parameters should be optimized empirically prior to undertaking the genome-wide RNAi screening. We have found that synchronizing the animal population by bleaching significantly reduced transgene expression. As such, bleaching was avoided in the protocol.

2. We find sorting L4 to work best as older worms tend to contaminate the assay with progeny, which results in starvation, even in the presence on FuDR.

3. Approximately 50,000 transgenic animals are required for each 96-well plate and the sorting time was ~30–45 min/plate. Prepare enough worms for the amount of plates being sorted on that day.

4. The worm sorter is a pressure-driven instrument. As such, any particulate matter present in the sample could impede liquid flow and result in inaccurate worm sorting. Great care must be taken to ensure that the final worm suspension placed into the sample cup is devoid of any debris such as small pieces of agar, bacterial clumps, lint, and/or dust.

5. We routinely choose L4 staged animals expressing moderate levels of the GFP transgene. In some instances, it may be necessary to adjust the worm concentration to achieve the optimum flow rate of 15–20 worms per second.

6. Depending on the algorithm chosen, it takes approximately 30–40 min to read each plate. This limits the number of plates that can be imaged in a given day.

7. To maintain well alignment with the RNAi library, each plate contained 96-samples and no additional RNAi controls. As most RNAi samples are expected to have a minimal effect on fluorescent transgene expression, data from each assay plate served as its own control. This sample-based, rather than a control-based, normalization has been recommended for RNAi screening by Birmingham et al. [19]. However, for each batch of plates run on a single day, we included an additional plate containing GFP(RNAi) and vector(RNAi) as RNAi positive and negative controls, respectively. These controls ensured that the assay was functioning properly (e.g., animals were viable, growth medium was adequate), but this data was not used for normalization, and was not factored into the z-score determinations.

Acknowledgment

This work was supported by a grant from the National Institutes of Health (DK096990) to GAS.

References

1. Fraser AG, Kamath RS, Zipperlen P et al (2000) Functional genomic analysis of C. elegans chromosome I by systematic RNA interference. Nature 408(6810):325–330. doi:10.1038/35042517

2. Kamath RS, Fraser AG, Dong Y et al (2003) Systematic functional analysis of the Caenorhabditis elegans genome using RNAi. Nature 421(6920):231–237. doi:10.1038/nature01278

3. Rual JF, Ceron J, Koreth J et al (2004) Toward improving Caenorhabditis elegans phenome mapping with an ORFeome-based RNAi library. Genome Res 14(10B):2162–2168. doi:10.1101/gr.2505604

4. Hamilton B, Dong Y, Shindo M et al (2005) A systematic RNAi screen for longevity genes in C. elegans. Genes Dev 19(13):1544–1555. doi:10.1101/gad.1308205

5. Lehner B, Tischler J, Fraser AG (2006) RNAi screens in Caenorhabditis elegans in a 96-well liquid format and their application to the systematic identification of genetic interactions. Nat Protoc 1(3):1617–1620. doi:10.1038/nprot.2006.245

6. Lejeune FX, Mesrob L, Parmentier F et al (2012) Large-scale functional RNAi screen in C. elegans identifies genes that regulate the dysfunction of mutant polyglutamine neurons. BMC Genomics 13:91. doi:10.1186/1471-2164-13-91

7. O'Rourke EJ, Conery AL, Moy TI (2009) Whole-animal high-throughput screens: the C. elegans model. Methods Mol Biol 486:57–75. doi:10.1007/978-1-60327-545-3_5

8. Swierczek NA, Giles AC, Rankin CH et al (2011) High-throughput behavioral analysis in C. elegans. Nat Methods 8(7):592–598. doi:10.1038/nmeth.1625

9. Buckingham SD, Sattelle DB (2009) Fast, automated measurement of nematode swimming (thrashing) without morphometry. BMC Neurosci 10:84. doi:10.1186/1471-2202-10-84

10. O'Reilly LP, Luke CJ, Perlmutter DH et al (2014) C. elegans in high-throughput drug discovery. Adv Drug Deliv Rev 69–70:247–253. doi:10.1016/j.addr.2013.12.001

11. Gosai SJ, Kwak JH, Luke CJ et al (2010) Automated high-content live animal drug screening using C. elegans expressing the aggregation prone serpin α1-antitrypsin Z. PLoS One 5(11):e15460. doi:10.1371/journal.pone.0015460

12. Long OS, Gosai SJ, Kwak JH et al (2011) Using Caenorhabditis elegans to study serpinopathies. Methods Enzymol 499:259–281. doi:10.1016/B978-0-12-386471-0.00013-4

13. O'Reilly LP, Long OS, Cobanoglu MC et al (2014) A genome-wide RNAi screen identifies potential drug targets in a C. elegans model of alpha1-antitrypsin deficiency. Hum Mol Genet 23(19):5123–5132. doi:10.1093/hmg/ddu236

14. Benson JA, Cummings EE, O'Reilly LP et al (2014) A high-content assay for identifying small molecules that reprogram C. elegans

germe cell fate. Methods 68(3):529–535. doi:10.1016/j.ymeth.2014.05.011

15. Leung CK, Deonarine A, Strange K et al. High-throughput screening and biosensing with fluorescent *C. elegans* strains. J Vis Exp. 2011;(51). doi:10.3791/2745

16. Hamamichi S, Rivas RN, Knight AL et al (2008) Hypothesis-based RNAi screening identifies neuroprotective genes in a Parkinson's disease model. Proc Natl Acad Sci U S A 105(2):728–733. doi:10.1073/pnas.0711018105

17. Morley JF, Brignull HR, Weyers JJ et al (2002) The threshold for polyglutamine-expansion protein aggregation and cellular toxicity is dynamic and influenced by aging in *Caenorhabditis elegans*. Proc Natl Acad Sci U S A 99(16):10417–10422. doi:10.1073/pnas.152161099

18. Brenner S (1974) The genetics of *Caenorhabditis elegans*. Genetics 77(1):71–94

19. Birmingham A, Selfors LM, Forster T et al (2009) Statistical methods for analysis of high-throughput RNA interference screens. Nat Methods 6(8):569–575, doi:nmeth.1351 [pii] 10.1038/nmeth.1351

20. Shaye DD, Greenwald I (2011) OrthoList: a compendium of *C. elegans* genes with human orthologs. PLoS One 6(5):e20085. doi:10.1371/journal.pone.0020085

21. da Huang W, Sherman BT, Lempicki RA (2009) Systematic and integrative analysis of large gene lists using DAVID bioinformatics resources. Nat Protoc 4(1):44–57. doi:10.1038/nprot.2008.211

Chapter 13

Design and Methods of Large-Scale RNA Interference Screens in *Drosophila*

Jia Zhou and Chao Tong

Abstract

Drosophila is an ideal model system for addressing important questions in biology. The use of RNA interference (RNAi) to knockdown gene expression in fly tissues is both very effective and relatively simple. In the past few decades, genome-wide UAS-RNAi transgenic libraries and thousands of Gal4 strains have been generated and have facilitated large-scale in vivo RNAi screening. Here, we discuss methods for the design and performance of a large-scale in vivo RNAi screen in *Drosophila*. Furthermore, methods for the validation of results and analysis of data will be introduced.

Key words RNA interference, *Drosophila*, UAS-Gal4 system, DAVID, COMPLEAT

1 Introduction

Discoveries in fruit flies (*Drosophila*) have greatly contributed to our understanding of biological questions [1]. Owing to their rapid life cycle, low chromosome number, small genome size, and the wealth of genetic tools available, *Drosophila* has been a first-choice model system for many biologists. In the 1990s, an in vivo ectopic expression system was introduced into flies, which allows for the expression of a specific cDNA sequence followed by UAS, a yeast DNA sequence, under control of the transcriptional activator Gal4, and was so named the UAS-Gal4 system [2]. Since then, thousands of Gal4 lines with different expression patterns have been developed to enable the control of gene expression in a highly versatile and sophisticated manner.

With the subsequent discovery of gene silencing through RNA interference (RNAi) [3], the UAS-Gal4 system has been further applied to express sequence-specific siRNA precursors to trigger the cleavage and destruction of target mRNA in a temporally and spatially specific manner. Genome-wide resources for RNAi in fruit flies have been developed, which have enabled high-throughput gene

David O. Azorsa, Shilpi Arora (eds.), *High-Throughput RNAi Screening: Methods and Protocols*, Methods in Molecular Biology, vol. 1470, DOI 10.1007/978-1-4939-6337-9_13, © Springer Science+Business Media New York 2016

silencing screening at an organism level [4]. Researchers initially generated transgenic fly stock collections for RNAi by introducing long double-stranded hairpin RNAs (dsRNAs) into flies [4]. Recently, new genome-wide RNAi resources have been generated that use short hairpin RNAs (shRNAs) as silencing triggers [5]. The new RNAi collections improved the knockdown efficiency and specificity, and are particularly effective for gene silencing in the female germline. With these powerful tools, many large-scale RNAi screens have been performed, and various gene networks for a wide range of biological processes have been identified [6–9]. Currently, the transgenic RNAi collections are publicly available worldwide. Furthermore, a number of web-based databases have been developed to support data analysis for large-scale RNAi screens.

Here, we discuss how to design and perform a large-scale RNAi screen in *Drosophila*. In addition, we explain the follow-up experiments required to ensure data quality and appropriate methods for analysis of the large dataset (see a flowchart of the screen procedures in Fig. 1).

2   Materials

2.1   Fly Stock Collections

1. RNAi transgenic fly stocks are available in the following stock centers shown in Table 1. Stocks generated by the Drosophila RNAi Screening Center (DRSC) were routinely used in our laboratory.

2. Gal4 lines and UAS-Dicer 2 transgenic flies. Many Gal4 lines and UAS-Dicer 2 transgenic flies are available from the Bloomington Drosophila Stock Center (Indiana University).

2.2   Fly Culture, Dissection, and Phenotype Scoring

1. Fly food recipe: 20 g/l instant dry yeast, 10 g/l concentrated yeast extract powder; 10 g/l tryptone, 15 g/l sucrose, 30 g/l glucose, 0.25 g/l $MgSO_4.7H_2O$, 0.25 g/l $CaCl_2.2H_2O$, 9.5 g/l agar power, 54 g/l corn meal, 9 ml/l propionic acid, 6 ml/l 10% methyl 4-hydroxybenzoate.

2. 25 °C incubators.

3. Stereoscopes.

4. Brushes.

5. Forceps.

2.3   Molecular Biology Reagents

1. Total RNA extraction reagents: Trizol (Life technologies), chloroform, isopropanol, ethanol.

2. Reverse transcription reagents: M-MLV Reverse Transcriptase (Life Technologies).

3. Quantitative reverse transcription-polymerase chain reaction reagents: SYBR® Green PCR master mix.

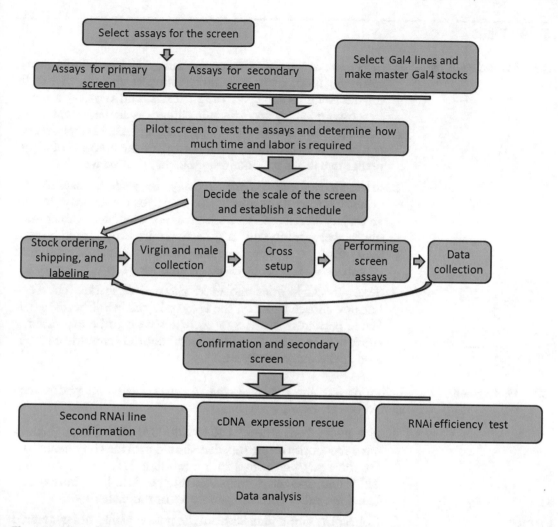

Fig. 1 Work flow for an RNAi screen in *Drosophila*

Table 1 The list of the stock centers that provide RNAi trangenic flies

RNAi Fly resource type/name	URL(s)
Drosophila RNAi Screening Center (DRSC)	http://www.flyrnai.org/
Bloomington Drosophila Stock Center	http://flystocks.bio.indiana.edu/
National Institute of Genetics (NIG)-Japan	http://www.shigen.nig.ac.jp/fly/nigfly/
Vienna Drosophila RNAi Center (VDRC)	http://stockcenter.vdrc.at/control/main
Drosophila Genomics Resource Center (DGRC)	https://dgrc.cgb.indiana.edu/

3 Methods

3.1 Assay Selections

1. Select assays for the primary screening. Many different assays could be used, including: morphological analysis of the fly organs (such as the eyes, wings, testes, and ovaries) under a stereoscope; analyzing the subcellular organelle morphology or the patterns of reporters using imaging-based assays; analyzing protein levels, luciferase intensity, or the amount of a particular metabolic product using biochemical assays.

2. Select assays for secondary screening. In general, assays for the primary screen are relatively easy to perform and assays for the secondary screen are more selective. For example, a direct morphology observation under dissection microscope could be used for a primary screen and immuno-staining of the tissue followed by confocol microscopy could be used for a secondary screen.

3. Select the Gal4 lines and make the master stocks. The Gal4 lines are chosen based on the assays selected in Subheading 3.1. When particular markers or reporters need to be expressed, a stock with both Gal4 and a marker (reporter) should be generated at this stage (*see* **Note 1**).

3.2 Pilot Screen

Before performing the large-scale screen, a small-scale pilot screen should be carried out.

1. Pick males from around 100 to 300 UAS-RNAi lines, including a few positive controls that should provide the phenotypes for the assay performed in Subheading 3.1. For each UAS-RNAi line, 2–3 males are picked and put into fly culture tubes. Label the tubes with the genotypes of the male flies.

2. Collect the virgin females from the master Gal4 lines generated in **step 3** in Subheading 3.1 and put 6–8 virgin females into each of the fly culture tubes containing male flies that were collected in **step 1** in Subheading 3.2.

3. Place the culture tubes into a 25 °C incubator for a few days and dump the adult parents.

4. The resulting progenies from the cross will be analyzed by the selected assay at ideal stages.

5. Data will be collected and analyzed to check the number of positive hits and to ascertain whether the positive control can be isolated by the selected assay (*see* **Note 2**). Calculate how much time and labor is required for this pilot screen.

3.3 Establishment of a Schedule

Before the start of the screening, the total number of RNAi lines to be screened should be determined according to researcher's goal. One can screen the whole collection from the stock centers or screen a group of genes with specific functions, for example, epigenetic factors, kinases, transcriptional factors, etc.

1. Divide the total UAS-RNAi lines that one aimed to screen into groups. The numbers of lines in a group are determined by how complex the assay described in Subheading 3.1 is and how many man-powers are devoted in the screening. Each group can contain as many lines as the screen team can handle. The screen will be performed sequentially from the first group to the last group.

2. Prepare a round-up schedule for fly ordering, shipping, food preparation, virgin collection, cross setting, assay performance, data collection, and stock maintenance. To save time, the screen team members do not have to start the second group after the first group finished. The work can be done simultaneously between different groups and each group has different phase. For example, when they perform assay for group 1 flies, the screen team members can do the virgin collection for group 2 flies and order fly stocks for group 3 flies (*see* **Note 3**).

3.4 Performing the Screen

1. Follow the schedule made in Subheading 3.3 and perform the screen in a similar manner described for the pilot screen.

2. Only keep the RNAi lines for the positive hits to reduce the labor and costs related to fly maintenance.

3.5 Confirmation and Secondary Screening

1. After the whole screen is complete, repeat the assay for the positive hits to confirm the results.

2. An independent assay could be used to further analyze the positive hits obtained from the primary screen. Since the number of the hits is much smaller than the number of lines screened in Subheading 3.4, the assays for the secondary screen could be more sophisticated than those used in the primary screen.

3.6 Quality Control

1. To validate the screened data set, the genes with more than one independent RNAi line are retested by knocking down the gene expression using the second RNAi line and analyzing phenotypes (*see* **Note 4**).

2. The transgenic animals carrying RNAi-resistant versions of cDNA could be used in rescue experiments to exclude the off-target effects (*see* **Note 5**).

3. The efficiency of RNA knockdown can be tested by using quantitative reverse transcription-polymerase chain reaction analysis and antibody staining of desired targets. The knockdown efficiency of 30–50 randomly selected lines should be analyzed.

3.7 Data Analysis

The large-scale RNAi screen will usually produce a large list of hits. The analysis and extraction of the biological meaning of these data could be carried out using several bioinformatics resources such as the Database for Annotation, Visualization and Integrated Discovery (DAVID; http://david.abcc.ncifcrf.gov) [10] and a protein complex enrichment analysis tool (COMPLEAT; http://www.flyrnai.org/compleat) [11] (*see* **Note 6**).

1. For DAVID analysis, a gene list of the hits should be submitted to DAVID, and then the analytic modules could be accessed through the tools menu page. For a given gene list, DAVID analytic modules help users to discover the enriched functionally related gene groups and to identify overrepresented annotation terms. In addition, it helps to visualize genes on BioCarta and KEGG pathway maps and provides gene–disease associations and a list of interacting proteins.

2. COMPLEAT is a protein complex resource that enables the identification and visualization protein complexes generated by high-throughput datasets. For COMPLEAT analysis, an RNAi screen dataset that associated with genes and normalized values or scores can be submitted through a web-based interface (http://www.flyrnai.org/compleat). The results are visualized as an interactive scatter plot using iCanPlot (http://www.icanplot.org/). The enriched complexes could also be saved as a table. The Cytoscape visualizations of selected complexes could be exported as image files.

4   Notes

1. In some cases, the UAS-Dicer2 transgene needs to be incorporated into the Gal4 master stock to enhance the RNAi knockdown efficiency. For RNAi in the female germline, a maternal triple-driver MTD-Gal4 is widely used to produce strong siRNA expression [8].

2. The number of hits obtained from the pilot screen will indicate the quality of the screen design. A good design will produce a reasonable number of hits. If the pilot screen turns out to have too many or too few hits, the screen strategy will need to be changed.

3. If a large-scale screen will be carried out, a detailed schedule needs to be made. Every trivial item needs to be considered, including stock labeling, food preparation, and stock maintenance. If possible, the fly stock should be ordered and shipped in separate bunches with a fixed schedule to avoid fly stock maintenance issues.

4. The newly generated shRNA lines (TRiP lines: shRNA in constructs VALIUM20 and VALIUM22) should have less off-target effects [5].

5. The recently developed clustered regularly interspaced short palindromic repeats (CRISPR)-Cas9 system [12] could also be used to generate gene knockout animals to further confirm the phenotypes.

6. For bioinformatics analysis, many other databases such as BioGrid, IntAct, MINT, DIP, DPiM, and DroID are available to extract more information from the screen.

References

1. Bellen HJ, Tong C, Tsuda H (2010) 100 years of Drosophila research and its impact on vertebrate neuroscience: a history lesson for the future. Nat Rev Neurosci 11:514–522

2. Brand AH, Perrimon N (1993) Targeted gene expression as a means of altering cell fates and generating dominant phenotypes. Development 118:401–415

3. Fire A, Xu S, Montgomery MK, Kostas SA et al (1998) Potent and specific genetic interference by double-stranded RNA in Caenorhabditis elegans. Nature 391:806–811

4. Perrimon N, Ni JQ, Perkins L (2010) In vivo RNAi: today and tomorrow. Cold Spring Harb Perspect Biol 2:a003640

5. Ni JQ, Zhou R, Czech B et al (2011) A genome-scale shRNA resource for transgenic RNAi in Drosophila. Nat Methods 8:405–407

6. Mummery-Widmer JL, Yamazaki M, Stoeger T et al (2009) Genome-wide analysis of Notch signalling in Drosophila by transgenic RNAi. Nature 458:987–992

7. Cronin SJ, Nehme NT, Limmer S et al (2009) Genome-wide RNAi screen identifies genes involved in intestinal pathogenic bacterial infection. Science 325:340–343

8. Yan D, Neumuller RA, Buckner M et al (2014) A regulatory network of Drosophila germline stem cell self-renewal. Dev Cell 28:459–473

9. Neumuller RA, Richter C, Fischer A et al (2011) Genome-wide analysis of self-renewal in Drosophila neural stem cells by transgenic RNAi. Cell Stem Cell 8:580–593

10. da Huang W, Sherman BT, Lempicki RA (2009) Systematic and integrative analysis of large gene lists using DAVID bioinformatics resources. Nat Protoc 4:44–57

11. Vinayagam A, Hu Y, Kulkarni M et al (2013) Protein complex-based analysis framework for high-throughput data sets. Sci Signal 6:rs5

12. Mohr SE, Smith JA, Shamu CE et al (2014) RNAi screening comes of age: improved techniques and complementary approaches. Nat Rev Mol Cell Biol 15:591–600

Chapter 14

Genome-Wide RNAi Screens in *C. elegans* to Identify Genes Influencing Lifespan and Innate Immunity

Amit Sinha and Robbie Rae

Abstract

RNA interference is a rapid, inexpensive, and highly effective tool used to inhibit gene function. In *C. elegans*, whole genome screens have been used to identify genes involved with numerous traits including aging and innate immunity. RNAi in *C. elegans* can be carried out via feeding, soaking, or injection. Here we outline protocols used to maintain, grow, and carry out RNAi via feeding in *C. elegans* and determine whether the inhibited genes are essential for lifespan or innate immunity.

  Key words RNA interference, *Caenorhabditis elegans*, Innate immunity, Ageing, Lifespan

1 Introduction

The model nematode *C. elegans* has been extensively used as a powerful genetic model system to study the cellular and molecular mechanisms of various biological processes such as embryogenesis and development, signaling pathways, sex determination, neurobiology and behavior, ecology and evolution, metabolism, innate immunity and host–pathogen interactions, and genetic basis of longevity regulation [1]. In addition to the standard "forward" genetic screens, the discovery of RNA interference (RNAi) in *C. elegans*, combined with relative ease of inducing RNAi in *C. elegans*, has enabled "reverse genetics" at a genome-wide scale.

RNA interference (RNAi) is an ancient defense mechanism that is present in plants and animals, which is used to regulate gene expression and destroy viral DNA [2–4]. It was originally discovered by researchers investigating flower pigmentation in petunias [5] and was subsequently reported to be also present in animals such as *C. elegans* [2]. Since then, the genetic mechanism of RNAi has been intensely studied [6], and the insights generated from these studies has been utilized in developing RNAi as a reverse genetic tool to understand gene function in various models such as

David O. Azorsa, Shilpi Arora (eds.), *High-Throughput RNAi Screening: Methods and Protocols*, Methods in Molecular Biology, vol. 1470, DOI 10.1007/978-1-4939-6337-9_14, © Springer Science+Business Media New York 2016

C. elegans and *D. melanogaster* and human cells. Essentially, the presence of a double stranded RNA (dsRNA) molecule in a cell cytoplasm induces degradation or translational repression of the mRNA transcripts which harbor a region of sequence complementary to the dsRNA [6]. This results in a reduction of function of the gene whose mRNA was targeted by the dsRNA, and thus provides an alternative to the loss-of-function typically expected from deletion mutants.

RNAi is routinely used in *C. elegans* labs for knockdown of gene function, due to its relative ease and efficiency, as the double stranded RNA corresponding to the gene of interest can be administered by feeding [7], soaking [8], or injection [2]. To obtain the dsRNA for a *C. elegans* gene, a 500–700 base pair fragment of its genomic region or corresponding cDNA is first cloned in a vector such that it is flanked by a T7 RNA polymerase site on either ends, thus facilitating RNA synthesis from both the strands. The transformed bacteria containing this construct (referred to as "dsRNA construct" in the subsequent text) can then be used either directly for feeding to *C. elegans* or the plasmid preparations from these bacteria can be used as a substrate in an in vitro *transcription* reaction for producing dsRNA that can be introduced into *C. elegans* by soaking or injection. The vector L4440 (available from Addgene) is one of the most commonly used vectors to make these dsRNA constructs and is used to transform the *E. coli* strain HT115 which can then be used as food source for *C. elegans*. Genome scale libraries of bacterial strains containing genomic regions of 16,757 *C. elegans* genes [9] and the ORFs of 11,511 genes [10] have already been created and can be obtained from commercial sources (Source Biosciences and Dharmacon, respectively) and used in RNAi-by-feeding screens. Together, these libraries cover about 87% of all *C. elegans* genes and hence it is highly likely to find one's genes of interest in these libraries. Further, high throughput automated systems have been created that can be used to screen the whole genome of *C. elegans* in less than 2 months [11]. Also, there are *C. elegans* mutants available that are more susceptible to RNAi than *C. elegans* wild-type, e.g., *rrf-1*, *eri-1* or *lin-15* [12–14] which are available from the Caenorhabditis Genetic Stock Centre (CGC). These resources have enabled whole genome screens to assess the function of genes in many different physiological and developmental such as fat storage [15] and embryogenesis [16].

Just like for any other biological process of interest, RNAi can be used in *C. elegans* to identify and investigate the genes regulating of lifespan [17, 18] and pathogen resistance [19]. *C. elegans* has been at the forefront of studies in genetic basis of aging as one of the first genes whose mutation leads to increased lifespan was isolated from *C. elegans* [20–22]. The fast developmental time and relatively small lifespan further add to its suitability for longevity studies. *C. elegans* feeds on microbes such as bacteria and fungi and is also useful for study of host-microbe interactions and innate immunity [23]. *C. elegans* has been used to understand the genetic mechanisms involved with tackling pathogenic bacteria and fungi by using transcriptomics, forward and reverse genetics leading to identification of various highly conserved pathways including ERK MAP kinase, p38 MAP kinase, TGF β, JNK-like MAP kinase, the G-protein coupled receptor FSHR-1, bZIP transcription factor *zip-2* and the beta-Catenin/*bar-1* [23]. Together, these pathways regulate various downstream effector genes such as lectins, lysozymes, and antimicrobial peptides in a pathogen-specific manner [24]. Interestingly, some of these pathways and genes that regulate lifespan in *C. elegans* have also been found to affect survival on pathogens. For example, *C. elegans daf-2* mutants that are 60% longer lived than wild-type worms on standard lab food *E. coli* [22] have also been found to be resistant to bacterial pathogens such as *Enterococcus faecalis* [25]. Thus, in order to identify genes involved with both lifespan and innate immunity, survival assays on pathogenic bacteria could be used as a faster alternative to carrying out lengthy lifespan assays [26], although it is best to carry out both experiments [27]. Knockdown of *C. elegans* using the RNAi-by-feeding approach is particularly well suited to study of longevity and innate immunity because of the following key advantages:

1. Survival and lifespan assays need to be carried out on sufficiently large numbers of animals (typically 60–100 animals) for appropriate statistical power to robustly detect any phenotypic differences. Here, RNAi-by-feeding is the method of choice as RNAi-by-injection would be much more time consuming and labor intensive.

2. Mutations in some genes induce early developmental defects or even lethality which can be a confounding factor in survival assays. Use of RNAi-by feeding to knockdown gene function in post-developmental, adult life stages opens up a way to study nondevelopmental function of such genes.

3. Multiple genes, especially redundant genes from a particular gene family might be knocked down simultaneously, e.g., using a common dsRNA targeting the shared, conserved regions of these genes [28]. Genes which do not share sequence similarity can be knocked down simultaneously by combining dsRNA constructs targeting multiple genes in the same vector [29], thus bypassing the need to make double or triple mutants. Similarly, RNAi can be used to test for genetic interactions with a mutant allele quickly by using the mutant strain in the RNAi screen.

4. RNAi is especially useful in quick functional validation of the large number of genes that are typically identified through transcriptomic studies as potential candidates regulating lifespan and or innate immunity can be screened for increased/decreased lifespan or pathogen resistance [26, 27].

5. During RNAi-by-feeding, the animals do need to not be handled or physically manipulated as invasively as in RNAi-by-injection, thus reducing any disturbances which might have adverse effects on survival.

Here we present a protocol for screening a large number of genes for their effect on lifespan and survival on pathogens in *C. elegans* using RNAi-by feeding libraries already available.

2   Materials

There are many protocols on how to maintain a clean, fresh, and lively stock of *C. elegans* (Fig. 1a) [30] but essentially *C. elegans* is maintained on Nematode Growing Media (NGM) agar plates seeded with a lawn of the bacterium *Escherichia coli* strain OP50 as food, and can be stored between 10 and 25 °C. For inducing RNAi-by-feeding, the worms are grown on a modified NGM medium that contains IPTG (Isopropyl β-D-Thiogalactoside), and using the bacterial strains with desired dsRNA constructs as the food source. The IPTG in the medium induces the production of dsRNA in the bacteria, which is then ingested by *C. elegans*.

2.1   NGM Agar Components

1. Weigh 3 g NaCl, 17 g agar, and 2.5 g peptone into 1 L Duran bottle and fill with 1000 ml of H_2O. Autoclave (caution hot!).

2. To prepare 1 M solutions, weigh into separate 100 ml Duran bottles: 11.0 g of $CaCl_2$, 12 g of $MgSO_4$, and 13.6 g of KH_2PO_4. Add 100 ml of water to each, mix, and autoclave. Store at 8 °C.

3. Weigh 500 mg of cholesterol in a 100 ml Duran bottle and add 100 ml Ethanol (5 mg/ml). There is no need to autoclave. Store at 8 °C.

4. 5 cm Petri dishes (Greiner)

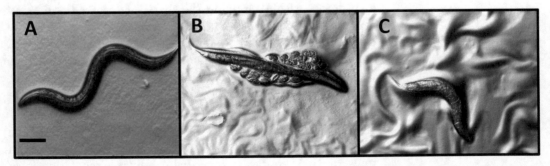

Fig. 1 (a) *C. elegans*. Scale bar represents 100 μm. (b) *C. elegans* after treatment with *unc-22* RNAi. (c) *C. elegans* after treatment with *dpy-9* RNAi

2.2 NGM RNAi Agar Components

1. Weigh 23.8 g of IPTG into 100 ml water to create 1 mM solution. Filter-sterilize with 0.22 μm filter syringe. Store at –20 °C.

2. Weigh 500 mg of ampicillin and add 10 ml of water (50 mg/ml). Filter-sterilize with 0.22 μm filter syringe. Store at –20 °C.

3. Weigh 250 mg of carbenicillin and add 10 ml of water (25 mg/ml). Filter-sterilize with 0.22 μm filter syringe. Store at –20 °C.

2.3 LB Components to Grow E. coli OP50

1. To make LB agar plates, weigh 15 g of agar, 10 g tryptone, 5 g yeast extract, and 10 g NaCl in to 1 l Duran bottle. Add 1000 ml of water, mix, and autoclave. Store at 8 °C.

2. 10 cm Petri dishes.

3. To make LB broth weigh: 10 g tryptone, 5 g yeast extract, and 10 g NaCl in to 1 L Duran bottle. Add 1000 ml of water, mix, and autoclave. Store at 8 °C.

4. *E. coli* strain OP50 which can be purchased from the CGC or obtained from your nearest *C. elegans* lab. Store on LB plates at 8 °C.

2.4 Genome-Wide RNAi Library

Whole genome libraries or sub-libraries can be purchased from Source BioScience (http://www.lifesciences.sourcebioscience.com) and/or GE Dharmacon (http://dharmacon.gelifesciences.com/non-mammalian-cdna-and-orf/c.-elegans-rnai). The methods described below are based on the use of the Ahringer library from Source BioScience.

3 Methods

3.1 Maintenance of C. elegans for Nematode Growing Media (NGM) Agar Plates

1. Once NGM agar has been autoclaved (caution hot!) and cooled then add 1 ml 1 M CaCl₂, 1 ml 5 mg/ml cholesterol in ethanol, 1 ml 1 M MgSO₄ and 25 ml 1 M KH₂PO₄ buffer and mix well.

2. Once the solutions have been added and mixed, 12 ml of NGM can then be poured into 5 cm plastic Petri dishes. If lots of plates are to be made at one time, then a peristaltic pump can be used.

3. *E. coli*, the typical food for *C. elegans*, is maintained as streaked cultures on 10 cm LB plates and usually stored for up to 2 weeks at 8 °C in fridge. To grow a culture of *E. coli* to feed *C. elegans*, a single colony of *E. coli* from the LB plate should be added to 400 ml of LB broth culture in a 500 ml Duran bottle and grown overnight at 37 °C in an incubator. On the following day, add 100–300 μl of *E. coli* to the middle of each plate and let it grow to a lawn overnight at room temperature.

4. *C. elegans* can be added to NGM plates with *E. coli* lawn and stored in an incubator maintained at the assay temperature at

20 °C. If temperature-sensitive mutants such as *glp-1* (*e2141*) are being used, they should be cultured at the appropriate restrictive temperature of 25 °C [31].

3.2 Prepare Working Stocks of the RNAi Library

All steps should be performed in sterile conditions under a laminar flow cabinet.

1. The libraries of bacterial strains containing dsRNA-producing constructs are usually supplied as glycerol stocks in 384-well plates. For the genes to be screened, identify the corresponding clones from the available RNAi libraries and make a note of the location such as the plate number and the well number for each clone. Store the original stocks at –80 °C (*see* **Note 4**).

2. Make working stocks of the clones selected above. Add 1 µl of the glycerol stock to 500 µl of LB broth with 50 µg/ml ampicillin in a 96-well deep-well plate (*see* **Note 4**). Seal the plate with a gas-permeable breathable film and incubate at 37 °C in a shaking incubator overnight. Number the deep-well plates with a permanent marker and make a note of the location of each clone for later reference (*see* **Note 5**).

3. Next day, add equal volume (500 µl) of sterile 50 % glycerol to these cultures. Aliquot about 150 µl from each well to the corresponding well of a 96-well PCR plate. Again, number the plate and keep track of location of each clone. Seal the plates with sealing film and store these working stocks at –20 °C. The PCR plate stocks are faster to thaw when needed. Multiple copies of the same 96-well plate can be kept as backups.

3.3 Performing Feeding RNAi in C. elegans

1. In order to carry out RNAi in *C. elegans*, the NGM substrate is slightly different from the maintenance plates, whereby NGM agar is supplemented with 1 mM Isopropyl β-D-Thiogalactoside (IPTG) which acts as the inducing agent for dsRNA production in the bacteria, and 25 µg/ml carbenicillin which acts as the selection agent for bacteria containing the dsRNA construct.

2. *E. coli* strains containing the correct double stranded RNAi-producing plasmids are grown at 37 °C in LB with 50 µg/ml ampicillin overnight (*see* **Note 1**). For this, thaw the working stocks, the 96-well PCR plates. Add 20–40 µl from each well of the PCR plate to the corresponding well of a deep-well 96-well plate that has 500 µl to 1000 µl of LB with 50 µg/ml ampicillin. Seal with a gas-permeable film and incubate overnight at 37 °C in a shaking incubator. Simultaneously, also grow the control *E. coli* strain HT115 with the empty vector L4440, and other positive control strains such as the cloned carrying *unc-22* and *dpy-7* constructs, in a similar volume and format (*see* **Notes 2,3**).

3. Take the required number of NGM RNAi plates, typically three to five plates per bacterial strain, and place in a laminar flow. Turn them upside down and write on the bottom in permanent marker the ID of the clone and/or the gene of interest that is going to be knocked down via RNAi. Spread 100 µl of bacterial suspension onto each NGM RNAi plate using a sterile metal or plastic spreader. It is important to carry out this step in a laminar flow cabinet to reduce the chances of contamination from other bacteria or fungi. The plates should be left to dry in the cabinet and depending on the age of the plates should take no more than 10 min. The plates should then be placed in a non-airtight box and are allowed to induce overnight at 20 °C (*see* **Note 6**).

4. The next day 2–3 *C. elegans* young adults should be transferred on to three plates per genotype and grown at appropriate temperature, typically 20 °C or 25 °C. Temperature-sensitive mutants such as *glp-1* are first grown and stored at 15 °C to let them be able to lay eggs. Using a worm pick, which consists of a thin piece of metal attached to a glass pipette, L4 or adult *C. elegans* from RNAi plates can be carefully transferred to pathogen plates. It is important to burn the pick in between transferring the worms to avoid contaminating original *E. coli* plates with bacterial pathogen.

5. Once eggs have been laid (1–2 days later), the adults should be removed from the plates so that only eggs collected in the first 2-day window are collected. In case of *glp-1* mutants, the restrictive temperature plates are shifted to the restrictive temperature 25 °C to induce germline depletion in these progeny (*see* **Notes 7,8**).

6. After about 2.5 days, 60–100 young-adult nematodes are then picked onto three to five plates containing *Xenorhabdus nematophila* (our pathogen of choice) and their survival be monitored daily (see immunity assays below). We usually carry out experiments at both 20 °C or 25 °C as the efficacy of RNAi has been shown to be affected by temperature [32].

7. For longevity assays the young adult worms continued to be reared on the respective RNAi clone bearing bacteria on NGM RNAi plates.

8. We also use two positive RNAi controls against *unc-22* (Fig. 1b) and *dpy-9* (Fig. 1c), to ensure that RNAi was efficient. Inhibition of gene function of *unc-22*, which produces the TWITCHIN protein and controls muscle development is easily observable due to worms that "twitch." Also, RNAi against *dpy-9* produces small, "dumpy" like worms that are easy to observe. It is also important to include an empty vector control in the experiment to make sure the plasmid without double stranded RNAi does not affect worm survival.

9. For immunity assays worm survival needs to be monitored daily till all animals are dead, usually between 5 and 7 days, depending on the pathogen. But the lifespan assay can easily take about 30 days (*see* **Notes 9,10**). If *C. elegans* wild-type strain is used then offspring will be produced regularly for the first 4 days which can then crowd the plate and make it difficult to observe the original worms. It is therefore recommended that every 2 days the worms are transferred on to fresh plates to remove the adults from their brood.

3.4 Assessing the Lifespan and Innate Immunity of C. elegans After RNAi Treatment

C. elegans is susceptible to bacterial pathogens including the opportunistic human pathogens *Pseudomonas aeruginosa* and *Staphylococcus aureus* and *Serratia marcescens*, and insect pathogens such as *X. nematophila* and *Photorhabdus luminescens* [33]. Previously we have exposed *C. elegans* and another distantly related nematode (*Pristionchus pacificus*) to hundreds of naturally isolated bacteria by using a rapid NGM agar based assay [33, 34]. We have also used RNAi against over 100 genes in *C. elegans* to determine if they were involved in both lifespan and immunity in germline deficient and *C. elegans* WT [26].

1. To assess the survival of *C. elegans* exposed to bacterial pathogens, standard 5 cm NGM agar plates are made as described above (without addition of IPTG) and left to dry at room temperature for 3 days. For the pathogen assays, one needs three to five plates per RNAi clones being screened. In addition, the same number of plates should be prepared for the no-pathogen controls.

2. On the second day, subculture the bacterial pathogen of choice, taking a single colony from an LB plate and streaking out onto a fresh LB plate. Incubate at 30 °C overnight (or at optimum pathogen growth conditions).

3. On the third day, a 200 ml conical flask should be filled with 50 ml LB broth and inoculated with a single colony of the bacterial pathogen. The flask should be placed on a shaking incubator (200 rpm) overnight at 30 °C (or at optimum pathogen growth conditions). It is also important to simultaneously grow a culture of *E. coli* OP50 from streaked cultures stored at 8 °C, which will serve as the no-pathogen control and should always run in parallel with the infection assays.

4. The next day 50 µl of the bacterial pathogen should be added to each NGM plate and spread evenly across the surface and allowed to dry in a laminar hood. Also spread 50 µl of *E. coli* OP50 on the control plates. Plates should then be stored at 30 °C overnight in a non-airtight box.

5. The next day a solid bacterial lawn should be visible and worms that have undergone RNAi treatment by feeding (**step 5**, above section) can now be transferred to these plates and

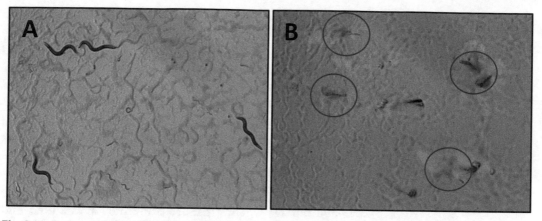

Fig. 2 (a) *C. elegans* fed on *E. coli* OP50. (b) *C. elegans* fed on pathogenic *Serratia marcescens*

tested for survival. For each RNAi clone, we usually place twenty adult *C. elegans* onto a single pathogen plate, with three to five pathogen plates and 20 adult *C. elegans* each onto three to five *E. coli* OP50 control plates for each bacterium to run in parallel. Once worms have been transferred onto NGM pathogen plates they can be placed into a non-airtight box and stored at 20 °C or 25 °C.

6. Each day the number of alive nematodes (Fig. 2a) on each plate is counted daily by using a dissecting microscope at 40× magnification, until all worms have died (Fig. 2b). Any nematodes that look poorly but not dead should be tested with a gentle touch with the worm pick to the head or tail for any signs of slow or sluggish movement which would indicate that the animal is still alive. An animal is considered dead only if it completely fails to respond to the head touch by worm pick, as moribund worms which can barely move and hardly show any pharyngeal pumping can be miscounted as dead. Dead worms can have offspring growing in the body of the hermaphrodite mother and their motion should not be mistaken for the motion of the parent. Similarly, the *E. coli* control should also be monitored in parallel (*see* **Notes 11,12**).

4   Notes

1. It is highly advisable to first do a pilot run of the screen with a smaller number of candidate genes (e.g., 10–20) including all the appropriate controls. This will help not only in fine tuning the procedure for optimum results but also in estimating and planning of time and other resources required for the full scale screen.

2. Always use the bacterial strain with the empty vector as the food source on the control plates, as slight differences in bacterial strains can affect physiology and survival. It is also not uncommon

to use bacteria harboring a non-specific dsRNA construct such as for GFP to be used as a control for RNAi vector.

3. Make sure to include appropriate positive controls in every run to verify that RNAi is working as expected. Common choices are RNAi against *unc-22*, *dpy-7* and/or genes such as *pmk-1* that directly affect innate immunity and survival.

4. RNAi feeding libraries are usually supplied as glycerol stocks in 384 well plates, with small volumes in each well. Make sure not to spill and mix the contents of the wells, especially when taking off or putting back the sealing tape on top of the plate.

5. Store these library stocks at −80 °C. Make working stocks of the 200–300 candidate genes that are being used at one time, and store them in 96 well PCR plates −20 °C. Label the plates with a good permanent marker. Keep track of the identity of clones in each well, preferably in print as well as digitally. If larger volumes of working stocks are desired, one might use deep-well plates but since they take much longer to thaw out, it might be more efficient to make multiple copies of 96-well PCR plates.

6. Use incubators to keep constant temperatures, as temperature affects lifespan as well as the efficiency of RNAi. Carry out experiments at multiple temperatures if possible.

5. The NGM and NGM + IPTG plates used for maintenance or RNAi of *C. elegans* should not be too old or dry as it affects the osmolarity of the medium which can affect the physiology and survival of the worms.

6. The worms should be maintained in constantly fed conditions and not allowed to starve, and also be kept free of bacterial or fungal contaminants to avoid any potential trans-generational effects on survival and resistance to pathogens. In case of accidental starvation or contamination, it is a good practice to let the worms grow for two generations in good conditions.

7. Since the final statistical analysis and plotting of the survival curves needs to be done on a computer, it is advisable to transfer all the survival data from the lab notebook to the computer daily or at the earliest available opportunities. The transfer of data accumulated in notebooks over 3–4 weeks of survival assays becomes a tedious and error-prone task if done in one go.

8. Many good statistical programs and software packages are available for the analysis of survival data such as the calculation of Kaplan-Meier's statistics. We found the online program OASIS convenient and comprehensive for these analyses [35].

9. Once the genes whose RNAi knockdown gives the desired phenotype (e.g., reduced lifespan or survival on pathogen), the correctness of the corresponding RNAi clone should be tested by sequencing. Correct targets and clones of the gene of interest can be identified using the program "Clone mapper" [36].

10. Other variations to the protocol described here exist and should be used if better suited to the research question under consideration. For example, animals might be put on RNAi plates only after the completion of their development to the adult stage to separate the developmental function of gene from that in adult stage. Some *C. elegans* strains and some tissues such as neurons and pharynx are less sensitive to RNAi [2], but can be rendered more sensitive by the use of strains mutant for genes such as *eri-1*, *rrf-3* or *lin-15* [12, 14, 37] or by expression of *sid-1* [38]. For tissue specific screens, it is also possible to restrict RNAi to a particular tissue only, for example by using a RNAi defective strain such as *sid-1* mutant, while rescuing the mutation only in the tissue of interest [39]. Lastly, since *E. coli* itself has been found to be slightly pathogenic to *C. elegans* especially in later stages, one might want to avoid using it as the food source altogether, and use *Bacillus* as a more natural food source, which can also be transformed to carry plasmids harboring dsRNA-producing constructs [40].

References

1. Corsi AK, Wightman B, Chalfie M (2015) A transparent window into biology: a primer on Caenorhabditis elegans. Genetics 200:387–407

2. Fire A, Xu S, Montgomery MK et al (1998) Potent and specific genetic interference by double-stranded RNA in Caenorhabditis elegans. Nature 391:806–811

3. Li H, Li WX, Ding SW (2002) Induction and suppression of RNA silencing by an animal virus. Science 296:1319–1321

4. Ding S-W, Li H, Lu R et al (2004) RNA silencing: a conserved antiviral immunity of plants and animals. Virus Res 102:109–115

5. Napoli C, Lemieux C, Jorgensen R (1990) Introduction of a chimeric chalcone synthase gene into petunia results in reversible co-suppression of homologous genes in trans. Plant Cell 2:279–289

6. Wilson RC, Doudna JA (2013) Molecular mechanisms of RNA interference. Annu Rev Biophys 42:217–239

7. Timmons L, Fire A (1998) Specific interference by ingested dsRNA. Nature 395:854

8. Tabara H, Grishok A, Mello CC (1998) RNAi in C. elegans: soaking in the genome sequence. Science 282:430–431

9. Kamath RS, Fraser AG, Dong Y et al (2003) Systematic functional analysis of the Caenorhabditis elegans genome using RNAi. Nature 421:231–237

10. Rual J-F, Ceron J, Koreth J et al (2004) Toward improving Caenorhabditis elegans phenome mapping with an ORFeome-based RNAi library. Genome Res 14:2162–2168

11. Squiban B, Belougne J, Ewbank J, Zugasti O (2012) Quantitative and automated high-throughput genome-wide RNAi screens in C. elegans. J Vis Exp. doi: 10.3791/3448

12. Simmer F, Tijsterman M, Parrish S et al (2002) Loss of the putative RNA-directed RNA polymerase RRF-3 makes C. elegans hypersensitive to RNAi. Curr Biol 12:1317–1319

13. Kennedy S, Wang D, Ruvkun G (2004) A conserved siRNA-degrading RNase negatively regulates RNA interference in C. elegans. Nature 427:645–649

14. Lehner B, Calixto A, Crombie C et al (2006) Loss of LIN-35, the Caenorhabditis elegans ortholog of the tumor suppressor p105Rb, results in enhanced RNA interference. Genome Biol 7:R4. doi:10.1186/gb-2006-7-1-r4

15. Ashrafi K, Chang FY, Watts JL et al (2003) Genome-wide RNAi analysis of Caenorhabditis elegans fat regulatory genes. Nature 421:268–272

16. Sönnichsen B, Koski LB, Walsh A et al (2005) Full-genome RNAi profiling of early embryogenesis in Caenorhabditis elegans. Nature 434:462–469

17. Lee SS, Lee RYN, Fraser AG et al (2003) A systematic RNAi screen identifies a critical role for mitochondria in C. elegans longevity. Nat Genet 33:40–48

18. Murphy CT, McCarroll SA, Bargmann CI et al (2003) Genes that act downstream of DAF-16

to influence the lifespan of Caenorhabditis elegans. Nature 424:277–283

19. Cronin SJF, Nehme NT, Limmer S et al (2009) Genome-wide RNAi screen identifies genes involved in intestinal pathogenic bacterial infection. Science 325:340–343

20. Klass MR (1983) A method for the isolation of longevity mutants in the nematode Caenorhabditis elegans and initial results. Mech Ageing Dev 22:279–286

21. Friedman DB, Johnson TE (1988) A mutation in the age-1 gene in Caenorhabditis elegans lengthens life and reduces hermaphrodite fertility. Genetics 118:75–86

22. Kenyon C, Chang J, Gensch E et al (1993) A C. elegans mutant that lives twice as long as wild type. Nature 366:461–464

23. Ewbank JJ (2006) Signaling in the immune response. In: The C. elegans Research Community (ed) WormBook. doi: 10.1895/wormbook.1.83.1

24. Sinha A, Rae R, Iatsenko I, Sommer RJ (2012) System wide analysis of the evolution of innate immunity in the nematode model species Caenorhabditis elegans and Pristionchus pacificus. PLoS One 7, e44255. doi:10.1371/journal.pone.0044255

25. Garsin DA, Villanueva JM, Begun J et al (2003) Long-lived C. elegans daf-2 mutants are resistant to bacterial pathogens. Science 300:1921

26. Sinha A, Rae R (2014) A functional genomic screen for evolutionarily conserved genes required for lifespan and immunity in germline-deficient C. elegans. PLoS One 9:e101970. doi:10.1371/journal.pone.0101970

27. Iatsenko I, Sinha A, Rödelsperger C, Sommer RJ (2013) New role for DCR-1/Dicer in Caenorhabditis elegans innate immunity against the highly virulent bacterium Bacillus thuringiensis DB27. Infect Immun 81:3942–3957

28. Grishok A, Pasquinelli AE, Conte D et al (2001) Genes and mechanisms related to RNA interference regulate expression of the small temporal RNAs that control C. elegans developmental timing. Cell 106:23–34

29. Min K, Kang J, Lee J (2010) A modified feeding RNAi method for simultaneous knockdown of more than one gene in Caenorhabditis elegans. Biotechniques 48:229–232

30. Stiernagle T (2006) Maintenance of C. elegans. In: The C. elegans Research Community (ed) WormBook. doi: 10.1895/wormbook.1.101.1

31. Kimble JE, White JG (1981) On the control of germ cell development in Caenorhabditis elegans. Dev Biol 81:208–219

32. Maine EM (2001) RNAi As a tool for understanding germline development in Caenorhabditis elegans: uses and cautions. Dev Biol 239:177–189

33. Rae R, Riebesell M, Dinkelacker I et al (2008) Isolation of naturally associated bacteria of necromenic Pristionchus nematodes and fitness consequences. J Exp Biol 211:1927–36

34. Rae R, Iatsenko I, Witte H, Sommer RJ (2010) A subset of naturally isolated Bacillus strains show extreme virulence to the free-living nematodes Caenorhabditis elegans and Pristionchus pacificus. Environ Microbiol 12:3007–3021

35. Yang J-S, Nam H-J, Seo M et al (2011) OASIS: online application for the survival analysis of lifespan assays performed in aging research. PLoS One 6, e23525. doi:10.1371/journal.pone.0023525

36. Thakur N, Pujol N, Tichit L, Ewbank JJ (2014) Clone mapper: an online suite of tools for RNAi experiments in Caenorhabditis elegans. G3 (Bethesda) 4:2137–2145

37. Schmitz C, Kinge P, Hutter H (2007) Axon guidance genes identified in a large-scale RNAi screen using the RNAi-hypersensitive Caenorhabditis elegans strain nre-1(hd20) lin-15b(hd126). Proc Natl Acad Sci U S A 104:834–839

38. Calixto A, Chelur D, Topalidou I et al (2010) Enhanced neuronal RNAi in C. elegans using SID-1. Nat Methods 7:554–559

39. Firnhaber C, Hammarlund M (2013) Neuron-specific feeding RNAi in C. elegans and its use in a screen for essential genes required for GABA neuron function. PLoS Genet 9(11):e1003921. doi:10.1371/journal.pgen.1003921

40. Lezzerini M, van de Ven K, Veerman M et al (2015) Specific RNA interference in Caenorhabditis elegans by ingested dsRNA expressed in Bacillus subtilis. PLoS One 10, e0124508. doi:10.1371/journal.pone.0124508

Chapter 15

RNAi-Assisted Genome Evolution (RAGE) in *Saccharomyces cerevisiae*

Tong Si and Huimin Zhao

Abstract

RNA interference (RNAi)-assisted genome evolution (RAGE) applies directed evolution principles to engineer *Saccharomyces cerevisiae* genomes. Here, we use acetic acid tolerance as a target trait to describe the key steps of RAGE. Briefly, iterative cycles of RNAi screening are performed to accumulate multiplex knockdown modifications, enabling directed evolution of the yeast genome and continuous improvement of a target phenotype. Detailed protocols are provided on the reconstitution of RNAi machinery, creation of genome-wide RNAi libraries, identification and integration of beneficial knockdown cassettes, and repeated RAGE cycles.

Key words RNA interference, High-throughput screening, *Saccharomyces cerevisiae*, Directed evolution, Genome engineering, Synthetic biology, Inhibitor tolerance

1 Introduction

Successful metabolic engineering practice often requires identification and modulation of multiple gene targets [1]. Whereas recombination-based genetic engineering (recombineering) is able to create combinatorial genetic diversity on a genome scale, such method is mainly limited to bacterial cells [2, 3]. *S. cerevisiae* is both a prominent eukaryotic model and a widely used microbial cell factory for industrial production of chemicals and fuels [4, 5]. To identify relevant genes of a target phenotype, nonessential genes have been individually deleted in *S. cerevisiae* to construct strain libraries for functional screening [6, 7]. Although strain libraries have been invaluable to understand relationship between genotype and phenotype of numerous important biological processes [8], the current procedure to introduce genome-wide perturbations on a wild type or mutated genome is expensive and time consuming. As a result, preconstructed gene-knockout libraries are only available for certain laboratory strains of the *S. cerevisiae* species [9], which is inadequate as different strains often exhibit

David O. Azorsa, Shilpi Arora (eds.), *High-Throughput RNAi Screening: Methods and Protocols*, Methods in Molecular Biology, vol. 1470, DOI 10.1007/978-1-4939-6337-9_15, © Springer Science+Business Media New York 2016

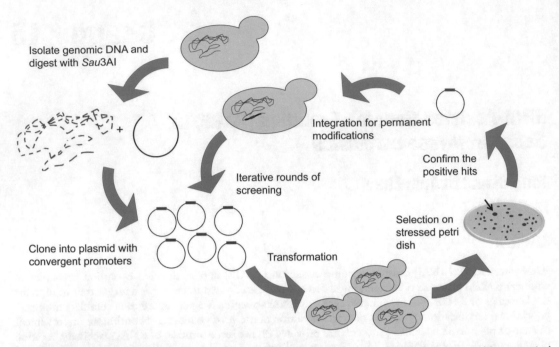

Fig. 1 Scheme of RAGE. The ease of RNAi library construction using a pooled RNAi library enables repeated rounds of screening in an evolving genetic background, which accumulates beneficial modifications identified from the previous rounds of screening by integration. Adapted with permission from [12]. Copyright 2015 American Chemical Society

dramatic differences in phenotypes [10]. In addition, it is difficult to create genetic libraries containing multiple gene deletions in each single strain. The synthetic genetic array (SGA) method has been developed to assay genetic interactions, whereby a query strain with a modified genetic background is crossed with a gene-deletion library to create an ordered array of haploid double-mutant strains [11]. Again, the prohibitively tedious procedure prevents the large scale use of SGA. Together, new tools for rapid and effective introduction of multiplex genome-wide modifications in customized genetic backgrounds are highly desirable for genome engineering in yeast.

To tackle such challenges, we developed the RNAi-*a*ssisted *g*enome *e*volution (RAGE) method in *S. cerevisiae* (Fig. 1) [12]. RNAi is a ubiquitous gene-silencing mechanism in eukaryotic organisms, whereby messenger RNAs (mRNAs) are targeted by homologous double-stranded RNAs (dsRNAs) for degradation [13, 14]. Without allelic modifications, RNAi screening achieves genome-wide knockdown perturbations and is widely used in eukaryotic systems [15, 16]. Although all known *S. cerevisiae* strains lack native RNAi machinery, a heterologous RNAi pathway from *Saccharomyces castelli* was functionally reconstituted in *S. cerevisiae* [17]. To enable RNAi screening in *S. cerevisiae*, we first created a pooled long-dsRNA library by adapting a convergent-promoter design, whereby dsRNA molecules are transcribed from yeast genomic DNA fragments inserted between two promoters that are placed in reverse directions [18]. In this way, genome-wide reduction of function modifications was introduced via a single step of transformation [12, 19]. We then applied a directed evolution strategy to yeast genome engineering through iterative RNAi screening, enabling continuous improvement of a target trait by accumulating beneficial knockdown modifications [12]. In particular, we successfully identified single and multiplex gene-silencing targets to improved acetic acid (HAc) tolerance, which is highly desirable for commercial production of lignocellulosic ethanol by *S. cerevisiae* [20, 21]. RAGE should be generally applicable to engineering other phenotypes in any *S. cerevisiae* strain provided that appropriate screening methods and basic genetic tools are available.

2   Materials

All chemicals were purchased through Sigma-Aldrich or Fisher Scientific unless indicated otherwise. Ultrapure water is prepared by Milli-Q Integral System to prepare cell media and solutions.

2.1   RNAi Plasmid Library Construction

1. pRS416 plasmid (New England Biolabs).

2. *Sau*3AI, *Xho*I, *Kpn*I-HF, *Sac*I-HF restriction enzymes (New England Biolabs).

3. pRS416-TTrc (available upon request): pRS416-GPDtrc-TEF1p-*Xho*I-TPI1prc-PGK1t, created in this study to synthesize long dsRNAs from a pair of convergent promoters P_{TEF1} and P_{TPI1}. Terminators T_{GPD} and T_{PGK1} are placed outside the promoter regions to signal the end of the RNA synthesis. An *Xho*I site is engineered between the two promoters to facilitate the insertion of genomic DNA fragments generated by *Sau*3AI digestion (Fig. 2a).

4. PCR thermal cycler.

5. TAE electrophoresis buffer: Dilute the 50× TAE electrophoresis buffer with Milli-Q water to a 1× working concentration of 40 mM Tris, 20 mM acetic acid, and 1 mM EDTA.

6. 0.7% agarose gel in 1× TAE buffer: Completely dissolve 0.7 g of agarose into 100 mL of 1× TAE buffer by microwaving. Cool the solution to approximately 70–80 °C. Add 5 μL of ethidium bromide into the solution and mix well. Pour 50 mL of solution onto an agarose gel rack with appropriate 2- or 8-well combs. For 1.0% and 1.5% agarose gel, add 1.0 g and 1.5 g of agarose into 100 mL of 1× TAE buffer.

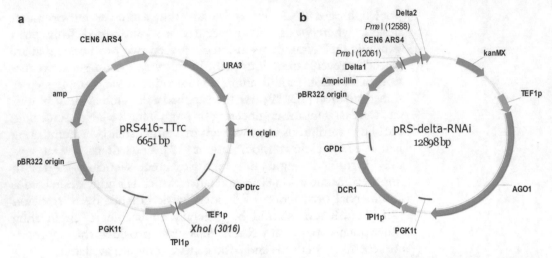

Fig. 2 The vector map of (**a**) pRS416-TTrc and (**b**) pRS-delta-RNAi. CEN6 ARS4: yeast centromere/automatic replication sequence, URA3; kanMX: selection marker in *S. cerevisiae*; amp: selection marker in *E. coli*; pBR322 origin: *E. coli* origin of replication; Delta1/Delta2: homologous sequences of delta sites for integration; TEF1p, TPI1p: yeast promoter; PGK1t, GPDt: yeast terminator; AGO1, DCR1: *S. castelli* RNAi genes. The promoters in pRS416-TTrc are in convergent configuration to synthesize long dsDNA for gene silencing

7. Horizontal electrophoresis system: Mini-Sub Cell GT cells and PowerPac Basic 300 V Power Supply (Bio-Rad).

8. Molecular Imager Gel Doc system.

9. QIAquick PCR Purification and Gel Extraction Kit.

10. QIAprep Miniprep Kit.

11. Wizard Genomic DNA Purification Kit.

12. NanoDrop2000c (Thermo Scientific): measure DNA concentrations.

13. Benchtop centrifuges.

14. T4 DNA ligase.

15. DNA Polymerase I, Large (Klenow) Fragment.

16. 100 mM dATP, dGTP, dCTP, and dTTP.

17. 16 °C water bath.

18. NEB 5α Electrocompetent *E. coli* (New England Biolabs).

19. Zymo 5α Z-competent *E. coli* (Zymo Research).

20. Gene Pulser II and Pulse Controller Plus (Bio-Rad).

21. *N*-butanol.

22. 70 % (v/v) ethanol.

23. 30 % (v/v) glycerol solution: mix 30 mL glycerol with 60 mL ddH$_2$O and bring the total volume to 100 mL using ddH$_2$O. Filter through 0. 22 μm filter.

24. 2 mL cryogenic tube.

25. Q5 High-Fidelity DNA Polymerase.

26. Gibson Assembly Cloning Kit.

27. Luria broth (LB) medium: dissolve 12 g of LB Broth into 600 mL Milli-Q water. Autoclave at 121 °C for 20 min.

28. 1000× ampicillin (Amp) stock: dissolve 1 g of ampicillin sodium salt into 10 mL Milli-Q water and filter through 0.22 μm filter. Aliquot is stored at –20 °C. For LB + Amp medium, dilute ampicillin stock 1000-fold to a working concentration of 100 μg/mL.

29. Bacto Agar: Supplement 20 g/L agar into proper liquid medium before autoclave. Pour 20 mL of autoclaved medium into each 100 × 10 mm Petri dish after being cooled down to 50–60 °C.

2.2 Yeast RNAi Library Construction

1. *S. cerevisiae* strain CEN.PK2-1c (*MATa ura3-52 trp1-289 leu2-3,112 his3Δ1 MAL2-8C SUC2*) (EUROSCARF, Frankfurt, Germany).

2. *S. castellii* strain NRRL number Y-12630 (ARS culture collection).

3. pRS-delta-RNAi (available upon request): pRS-delta-KanMX-LoxP-TEF1p-AGO1-PGK1t-TPI1p-DCR1-GPD1t created in this study to integrate the *S. castelli* RNAi pathway into *S. cerevisiae* genome through delta integration (Fig. 2b).

4. *Pme*I restriction enzyme.

5. *S. cerevisiae* strain CAD: CEN.PK2-1c strain integrated with the *S. castelli* RNAi pathway.

6. YPAD medium: dissolve 6 g of yeast extract, 12 g of peptone, 12 g of dextrose, and 60 mg of adenine hemisulfate in 600 mL of Milli-Q water. Autoclave at 121 °C for 20 min.

7. Synthetic complete dropout medium lacking uracil (SC-Ura): dissolve 3 g of ammonium sulfate, 1.02 g of Difco Yeast Nitrogen Base without Amino Acids and Ammonium Sulfate, 0.50 g of CSM-Ura, 60 mg of adenine hemisulfate, and 12 g of dextrose in 600 mL of deionized water, and adjust pH to 5.6 or 4.5 by 10% (w/v) NaOH. Autoclave at 121 °C for 20 min. For SC, SC-His and SC-His-Trp, use CSM, CSM-His, and CSM-Trp instead of CSM-Ura, respectively.

8. 42 °C water bath.

9. 1.0 M Lithium acetate (1.0 M LiAc): dissolve 10.2 g of lithium acetate dihydrate in 100 mL of ddH$_2$O. Autoclave at 121 °C for 20 min.

10. 0.1 M LiAc: mix 5 mL 1.0 M LiAc with 30 mL sterile ddH$_2$O. Bring the final volume to 50 mL with sterile ddH$_2$O.

11. 50% (w/v) PEG 3350: use a magnetic stirrer hot plate to heat 30 mL of ddH$_2$O to around 80 °C in a 150 mL beaker with a stir bar. Gradually add 50 g of PEG 3350 until all PEG dissolves. Autoclave at 121 °C for 20 min. The bottle should be tightly capped to prevent evaporation. Prepare fresh PEG 3350 solution every 2 months to maintain high transformation efficiency.

12. Tris–EDTA (TE) buffer solution (10 mM Tris–HCl, 1 mM Na$_2$EDTA, pH 8.0).

13. Single-stranded carrier DNA (ssDNA) (2.0 mg/mL): dissolve 200 mg of salmon sperm DNA in 100 mL of sterile TE buffer in a 150 mL beaker at 4 °C overnight, with the help of a magnetic stirrer plate. Store the aliquot in −20 °C.

14. 100× G418 solution (20 g/L): dissolve 0.2 g of G418 disulfate salt into 10 mL of Milli-Q water and filter through 0.22 μm filter. Aliquot is stored at −20 °C. For YPAD + G418 medium, dilute G418 stock 100-fold to a working concentration of 0.2 g/L in the YPAD medium.

2.3 RNAi Screening for Acetic Acid Tolerance

1. 10% (v/v) acetic acid stock: mix 10 mL glacial acetic acid with 80 mL Milli-Q water. Adjust pH to 4.5 with 10% (w/v) NaOH. Adjust the total volume to 100 mL. Filter through 0.22 μm filter.

2. 0.5% (v/v) acetic acid SC-Ura solid medium: autoclave 600 mL SC-Ura medium (pH = 4.5) containing 12 g agar at 121 °C for 20 min and then cooled to 50–60 °C. Add 31.6 mL of 10% (v/v) acetic acid to the medium and mixed well. Pour 40 mL of the medium into each 150×15 mm Petri dish. For 0.6% and 0.7% (v/v) acetic acid SC-Ura solid medium, add 38.2 and 45.2 mL of 10% (v/v) acetic acid to 600 mL medium.

3. Zymoprep II yeast plasmid isolation kit.

2.4 Further Rounds of RAGE

1. pRS403, pRS404 plasmids (New England Biolabs).

2. *XhoI*, *SacI*, *KpnI* restriction enzymes.

---

3 Methods

3.1 RNAi Plasmid Library Construction

1. Isolation of *S. cerevisiae* genomic DNA. Inoculate a single colony of the CEN.PK2-1c strain into 3 mL YPAD medium and grow overnight at 37 °C and 250 rpm (*see* **Note 1**). Isolate the genomic DNA from 3 mL cell culture using Wizard Genomic DNA Purification Kit in six separate reactions. Measure the concentrations using NanoDrop.

2. Digest yeast genomic DNA at 37 °C for 15 min in a 50 μL reaction containing 1 μL of *Sau*3AI (5 U/μL), 5 μL of 10× CutSmart Buffer, and 50 μg of yeast genomic DNA (Fig. 1).

Purify the digestion products using QIAquick PCR Purification Kit and elute DNA in 86 μL ddH$_2$O.

3. Fill in the *Sau*3AI overhangs with dATP and dGTP using Klenow fragment. Reaction conditions: 86 μL of digested yeast genomic DNA, 10 μL of 10× NEBuffer 2, 3 μL of Klenow fragment, 0.5 μL of 5 mM dATP, 0.5 μL of 5 mM dGTP. Incubate at 30 °C for 30 min in a thermocycler. Purify the fill-in products using QIAquick PCR Purification Kit. Measure the concentrations using NanoDrop (*see* **Note 2**).

4. Digest pRS416-TTrc at 37 °C for 6 h in a thermocycler (Fig. 2a). Reaction condition: 2 μL of *Xho*I, 5 μL of 10× CutSmart buffer, and 10 μg of pRS416-TTrc. Add ddH$_2$O to a final volume of 100 μL. Purify the digestion products using QIAquick PCR Purification Kit and elute DNA in 86 μL ddH$_2$O.

5. Fill in the digested pRS416-TTrc overhangs with dCTP and dTTP by Klenow fragment. Reaction conditions: 86 μL of digested pRS416-TTrc, 10 μL of 10× NEBuffer 2, 3 μL of Klenow fragment, 0.5 μL of 5 mM dCTP, 0.5 μL of 5 mM dTTP. Incubate at 30 °C for 30 min in a thermocycler. Purify the fill-in products using QIAquick PCR Purification Kit into 30 μL ddH$_2$O.

6. Remove digested pRS416-TTrc that is not filled-in by ligation at 16 °C overnight. Reaction conditions: 30 μL of purified fill-in pRS416-TTrc products, 5 μL of 10× T4 DNA ligase buffer, 2 μL of T4 DNA ligase, 13 μL of ddH$_2$O. Load the ligation products onto 0.7 % agarose gels and perform electrophoresis at 120 V for 20 min. Cut the gel slice containing the linear DNA (~6.6 kb). Purify using QIAquick Gel Extraction Kit, and measure the concentrations of purified products (*see* **Note 3**).

7. Assembly of the RNAi plasmid library by ligation at 16 °C overnight (Fig. 1). Reaction conditions: 300 ng of genomic DNA fragments, 100 ng of pRS416-TTrc, 2 μL of 10× T4 DNA ligase buffer, 1 μL of T4 DNA ligase. Add ddH$_2$O to a final volume of 20 μL. A control experiment is also performed where genomic DNA fragments are omitted.

8. The ligation product is precipitated by addition of *n*-butanol. Add 200 μL *n*-butanol and vortex for 20 s. Centrifuge at 16,100×*g* for 5 min. Remove the supernatant, add 200 μL 70 % ethanol, and vortex for 20 s. Centrifuge at 16,100×*g* for 5 min. Remove the supernatant and air dry the pellet until no liquid is visible. Resuspend in 10 μL of ddH$_2$O.

9. Transform 10 μL of ligation products into 100 μL of NEB 5α electrocompetent *E. coli* by electroporation. Conditions: 1.7 kV, 200 Omega and 25 μF in a 1 mm electroporation cuvettes. The typical time constant is 4.8–5.1 ms.

10. The *E. coli* cells are immediately transferred into 1 mL of SOC medium and incubated at 37 °C for 1 h. Cells are then used to inoculate 25 mL of LB + Amp medium in a 125 mL baffled Erlenmeyer flask and allowed to grow overnight at 37 °C and 250 rpm. One hundredth of the cells were plated on an LB + Amp plate to grow overnight at 37 °C to estimate the transformation efficiency (*see* **Note 4**).

3.2 Quality Estimation of the RNAi Plasmid Library

1. Inoculate 20 colonies randomly from the library plates into 3 mL of LB + Amp liquid medium and grow overnight at 37 °C and 250 rpm.

2. Isolate the plasmids from overnight culture using QIAprep Miniprep Kit.

3. Amplify the inserts from the isolated plasmids by PCR. PCR reaction conditions: 4 μL of 5× Q5 Reaction Buffer, 0.4 μL of 10 mM dNTPs, 1 μL of 10 μM "S TEF1p For" primer (Table 1), 1 μL of 10 μM "S TPI1p For" primer (Table 1), 1 ng of plasmid, 0.2 μL of Q5 DNA Polymerase. Add ddH₂O to a final volume of 20 μL. PCR thermocycling condition: initial denaturation at 98 °C for 30 s, followed by 25 cycles of 98 °C for 10 s, 50 °C for 30 s, and 72 °C for 30 s, with a final extension at 72 °C for 2 min. A control PCR reaction with the empty pRS416-TTrc as the template will also be performed.

4. Load PCR products onto 1.5 % agarose gel and perform electrophoresis at 120 V for 20 min. The insert size of the library plasmids can be estimated by comparing the sizes of PCR products with that of the empty plasmid (130 bp) (*see* **Note 5**).

5. If the plasmid library is of satisfactory quality, use 1 mL library cell culture to make frozen stocks for long-term storage as follows: mix 1 mL cell culture with 1 mL 30 % (v/v) glycerol solution in 2 mL cryogenic tubes, and store at –80 °C. Miniprep the rest 20 mL cell culture using QIAprep Miniprep Kit and measure the concentrations using NanoDrop.

Table 1
The primers used in this chapter

Name	Sequence (5′ → 3′)
S TEF1p For	TTTTACTTCTTGCTCATTAG
S TPI1p For	TTTTTGTTTGTATTCTTTTC
pRS-GPDtrc For	TTGGGTACCGGGCCCGGAATCTGTGTATATTACTGC
PGK1t-pRS Rev	GGAGCTCCACCGCGGCAGGAAGAATACACTATAC
TPI1p-DCR1 For	CATAAACTAAAAATGAATAGAG
DCR1-GPD1t Rev	TTCACACTAGTTCACAGATTGTTGC

**3.3 Integration
of the RNAi Pathway**

1. Linearization of the integration plasmid pRS-delta-RNAi (Fig. 2b). Digestion condition: 5 µL of *Pme*I, 5 µL of 10× CutSmart buffer, and 10 µg of pRS-delta-RNAi. Add ddH$_2$O to a final volume of 50 µL. Incubate at 37 °C for 6 h in a PCR thermocycler. Load the digestion products onto 0.7 % agarose gels and perform electrophoresis at 120 V for 20 min. Gel purify the digestion products using QIAquick Gel Extraction Kit (*see* **Note 6**).

2. Inoculate a single colony of the CEN.PK2-1c strain into 3 mL of YPAD medium and grow for 16 h at 30 °C and 250 rpm.

3. Add 0.15 mL of overnight culture into 5 mL of YPAD medium in a 125 mL baffled flask to grow for 4 h at 30 °C and 250 rpm (*see* **Note 7**).

4. Boil a 1.0 mL sample of carrier ssDNA in water bath for 5 min and chill immediately on ice.

5. Harvest the cells by centrifugation at 3220×g for 5 min. Resuspend the cell pellet in 20 mL of sterile ddH$_2$O and centrifuge at 3220×g for 5 min at room temperature. Repeat the wash step once. Resuspend pellet in 1 mL of 0.1 M LiAc.

6. Transfer the cell suspension to a 1.5 mL Eppendorf microcentrifuge tube. Centrifuge at 7500×g for 30 s and remove the supernatant.

7. Add 240 µL of 50 % (w/v) PEG 3350, 36 µL of 1 M LiAc, 50 µL of carrier ssDNA, and 1 µg of linearized integration plasmid DNA to the cell pellet. Add ddH$_2$O to a final volume of 360 µL. Mix vigorously on a vortex mixer for 1 min (*see* **Note 8**).

8. Incubate the tube in a 42 °C water bath for 1 h (*see* **Note 9**).

9. Centrifuge the tubes at 16,100×g for 1 min and remove the supernatant completely. Resuspend the cell pellet in 1 mL of YPAD medium. Transfer the cell suspension to a 14 mL round-bottom Falcon tube. Incubate at 30 °C and 250 rpm for 1 h (*see* **Note 10**).

10. Centrifuge the tube at 3220×g for 5 min. Remove 900 µL of the supernatant. Resuspend the cell pellet in the remaining YPAD medium and spread onto an YPAD + 0.2 g/L G418 plate (*see* **Note 11**).

11. Incubate the plates at 30 °C for 2–3 days until colonies appear

12. Inoculate six colonies into 3 mL YPAD + G418 medium Isolate the genomic DNA as described above.

13. Perform diagnostic PCR using the genomic DNA as template. PCR reaction condition: 4 µL of 5× Q5 Reaction Buffer, 0.4 µL of 10 mM dNTPs, 1 µL of 10 µM "TPI1p-DCR1 For" primer (Table 1), 1 µL of 10 µM "DCR-GPD1t Rev" primer (Table 1), 100 ng of genomic DNA, 0.2 µL of Q5 DNA

Polymerase. Add ddH$_2$O to a final volume of 20 μL. PCR thermocycling condition: initial denaturation at 98 °C for 30 s, followed by 30 cycles of 98 °C for 10 s, 55 °C for 30 s, and 72 °C for 1 min, with a final extension at 72 °C for 2 min.

14. Load the PCR products onto 0.7 % agarose gels and perform electrophoresis at 120 V for 20 min. A ~1.8 kb PCR band indicates correct integration (*see* **Note 12**).

3.4 Creation of Yeast RNAi Strain Library

1. Transform 20 μg of the RNAi plasmid library DNA into the CAD strain (*see* **Note 13**) using the heat shock protocol described above with the following modifications: add 2 μg of the library DNA in each transformation reaction; scale-up by performing ten transformation reactions in parallel; following heat shock, resuspend the cell pellet in 1 mL SC-Ura medium for each reaction, and combine ten reactions into a 125 mL baffled flask to incubate at 30 °C and 250 rpm for 4 h (*see* **Note 14**).

2. Spread 10 μL of cell culture onto SC-Ura (pH = 5.6) plates to estimate the transformation efficiency.

3. Centrifuge the cell culture at 3220 × *g* for 5 min in 15 mL conical tubes. Resuspend the cell pellet in 2 mL of sterile ddH$_2$O.

4. For the control plasmid, employ a similar protocol as in "Transformation of the RNAi plasmid library" except that only one transformation reaction is performed with 2 μg of pRS416-TTrc and finally resuspend the cell pellet in 200 μL of sterile ddH$_2$O.

5. Screening for acetic acid tolerant mutants. Spread 200 μL cell suspension onto each 150 × 15 mm SC-Ura with 0.5 % (v/v) acetic acid plate (*see* **Note 15**). For the control strain and the RNAi library, use one and ten plates, respectively. Incubate the plates at 30 °C for 3–4 days (*see* **Note 16**).

3.5 First Round of Screening of the RAGE Library

1. From the library plates, inoculate the colonies of sizes that are substantially larger than the colonies on the control plate into 3 mL of SC-Ura medium (pH 4.5). Also inoculate three colonies of average sizes from the control plate into 3 mL of SC-Ura medium. Incubate at 30 °C for 16 h until saturation.

2. Re-inoculate 50 μL of saturated culture into 3 mL fresh SC-Ura medium to synchronize the growth phase at 30 °C for 20 h (*see* **Note 17**). Measure the cell density OD$_{600}$ using NanoDrop.

3. For each strain, start new cell culture by transferring stationary-phase cells into 4 mL of SC-Ura medium (pH 4.5) containing 0.5 % (v/v) HAc with an initial OD$_{600}$ value of 0.2.

4. Incubate at 30 °C and 250 rpm. Monitor the cell density using NanoDrop at 4, 8, 12, 16, and 24 h.

5. Strains that accumulate substantially more biomass than the control strain at 12 h are considered to exhibit improved acetic acid tolerance (*see* **Note 18**).

6. Confirmation of tolerance improvement by retransformation (*see* **Note 19**). For mutant strains with improved acetic acid tolerance, re-inoculate into 3 mL of SC-Ura medium (pH 5.6) to grow at 30 °C and 250 rpm for 16 h.

7. Isolate the yeast plasmids using Zymoprep II Yeast Plasmid Isolation Kit from 1 mL of yeast cell culture

8. Transform 5 µL of the yeast plasmids into Zymo 5α Z-competent *E. coli* following the manufacturer's instruction. Select *E. coli* colonies on LB + Amp plates

9. Inoculate a single *E. coli* colony for each mutant strain into 3 mL of LB + Amp medium to grow at 37 °C and 250 rpm for 16 h.

10. Miniprep the plasmid using QIAprep Miniprep Kit and measure the concentrations using NanoDrop.

11. Transform 100 ng of the plasmid into the CAD strain using the heat shock protocol described above with the following modifications: after heat shock and removal of supernatant, resuspend the cell pellet in 1 mL of SC-Ura medium and spread 100 µL of cell suspension onto 100×10 mm SC-Ura plates. Incubate at 30 °C for 2–3 days.

12. Inoculate three colonies for each re-transformed mutants into 3 mL of SC-Ura medium. Also inoculate three colonies from the control plates. Compare the acetic acid tolerance using the protocol described above. Mutants that accumulate significantly more biomass ($p < 0.05$) than the control strain at 12 h are confirmed with improved acetic acid tolerance.

13. Identification of knockdown mutations. For confirmed mutants, sequence the inserts of their *E. coli* plasmids using the primers "S TEF1p For" and "S TPI1p For" (Table 1) using commercial DNA sequencing services. Use BLAST search to map the sources of the genomic fragments (*see* **Note 20**).

3.6 Further Rounds of RAGE

1. Creation of the parent strains for the second round of RAGE (Fig. 3a). Amplify the long-dsRNA expression cassettes from the mutant *E. coli* plasmids using PCR. PCR reaction condition: 10 µL of 5× Q5 Reaction Buffer, 1 µL of 10 mM dNTPs, 2.5 µL of 10 µM "pRS-GPDtrc For" primer (Table 1), 2.5 µL of 10 µM "PGK1t-pRS Rev" primer (Table 1), 1 ng of mutant *E. coli* plasmid, 0.5 µL of Q5 DNA Polymerase. Add ddH₂O to a final volume of 50 µL. PCR thermocycling condition: initial denaturation at 98 °C for 30 s, followed by 25 cycles of 98 °C for 10 s, 55 °C for 30 s, and 72 °C for 2 min, with a final extension at 72 °C for 2 min. Gel purify the PCR products as described above.

2. Digestion of integration plasmid pRS403. Digestion condition: 2 µL of *Xho*I, 2 µL of *Sac*I, 5 µL of 10× CutSmart buffer, and 3 µg of pRS403. Add ddH₂O to a final volume of 50 µL. Incubate at 37 °C for 3 h in a PCR thermocycler. Gel purify the digestion products as described above.

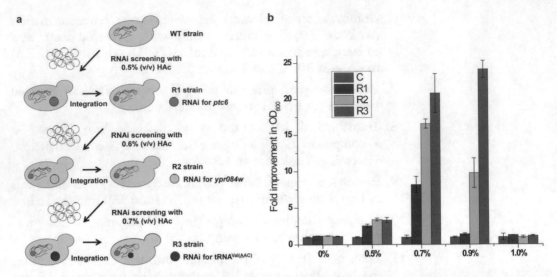

Fig. 3 Engineered yeast strains with improved acetic acid tolerance. (**a**) Scheme of iterative RAGE rounds to accumulate knockdown modifications in a yeast genome. (**b**) Continuous improvement in acetic acid tolerance. Adapted with permission from [12]. Copyright 2015 American Chemical Society

3. Mix 100 ng of the linearized pRS403 plasmid with 100 ng of the amplified RNAi cassette with 10 μL of 2× Gibson Assembly Master Mix. Add ddH$_2$O to a final volume of 20 μL. Incubate the mixture at 50 °C for 1 h in a thermocycler.

4. Transform 5 μL of Gibson Assembly products into the competent cells included in the Gibson Assembly Cloning Kit following the manufacturer's instructions. Spread all the *E. coli* transformant mix onto LB + Amp plates. Incubate at 37 °C for 16–20 h.

5. Inoculate three *E. coli* colonies into 3 mL of LB + Amp medium to grow at 37 °C and 250 rpm for 16–20 h. Isolate the plasmids from overnight culture using QIAprep Miniprep Kit.

6. Confirm the successful insertion of RNAi cassettes into pRS403-RNAi using the protocol described above in "Quality estimation of the RNAi plasmid library."

7. For a confirmed integration plasmid, linearize the plasmid at a unique restriction site within the *HIS3* gene by digestion (*see* **Note 21**). Digestion condition: 2 μL of a chosen enzyme, 5 μL of 10× CutSmart buffer, and 3 μg of pRS403-RNAi plasmid. Add ddH$_2$O to a final volume of 50 μL. Incubate at 37 °C for 3 h in a PCR thermocycler. Purify the digestion products using QIAquick PCR Purification Kit and elute in 34 μL ddH$_2$O.

8. Transform 34 μL of linearized pRS403-RNAi plasmid into the CAD strain using the heat shock protocol described above with the following modifications: after heat shock and removal of the supernatant, resuspend the cell pellet in 1 mL of SC-His

medium and spread 100 µL of cell suspension onto 100 × 10 mm SC-His plates. Incubate at 30 °C for 2–3 days.

9. Compare the acetic acid tolerance between the integrated mutants and the CAD strain using the protocol described above except that SC medium is used instead of SC-Ura medium. Mutants that accumulate significantly more biomass ($p < 0.05$) than the control strain at 12 h are confirmed with improved acetic acid tolerance. The mutant exhibited the highest acetic acid tolerance is used as the parent strain for the second round of RAGE (see **Note 22**).

10. The second round of RAGE (Fig. 3a). Using the newly constructed integration mutant, perform the RNAi screening as described in "Yeast RNAi library construction" with the following modifications: use SC-Ura with 0.6% (v/v) HAc as the liquid and solid media for screening and comparison of acetic acid tolerance (see **Note 23**); use the new parent strains for the second round of RAGE with the empty pRS416-TTrc as the control strains (the R1 strain).

11. Creation of the parent strains for the third round of RAGE (Fig. 3a). The same procedure is performed as in "Creation of the parent strains for the second round of RAGE" with the following modifications: use pRS404 as the integration vector; *Kpn*I and *Sac*I are used to linearize the pRS404 plasmid; the pRS404-RNAi plasmids are linearized at a unique restriction site within the *TRP1* gene (see **Note 21**); integration transformants are selected on SC-His-Trp plates.

12. The third round of RAGE (Fig. 3a). The similar procedure is performed in "The second round of RAGE" with the following modifications: use SC-Ura with 0.7% (v/v) HAc as the liquid and solid media for screening and comparison of acetic acid tolerance (see **Note 23**); use the new parent strains for the third round of RAGE transformed with the empty pRS416-TTrc as the control strains (the R2 strain). After confirmation by retransformation, the best mutant from the third round of RAGE is named the R3 strain.

13. Comparison of acetic acid tolerance of the engineered strains and the control strain (Fig. 3b). The similar protocol in "Growth assay to measure acetic acid tolerance" is used with the following modifications: SC-Ura media (pH = 4.5) containing 0, 0.5, 0.7, 0.9, and 1.0% (v/v) HAc is used to examine biomass accumulation; initial OD_{600} is adjusted to 0.01; cell density is monitored at 24, 48, and 72 h. Fold improvements in biomass accumulation are compared to the CAD strain containing the control plasmid (the C strain). A typical result can be found in Fig. 3b, indicating stepwise and continuous improvement of acetic acid tolerance.

4   Notes

1. This rotation speed (250 rpm) can be used for most incubator shakers with orbit diameters ranging from 0.5 to 2 in. (1.27–5.1 cm).

2. In the original report, a *Bam*HI site was used to linearize the pRS416-TTrc plasmid to create compatible sticky ends with genomic DNA fragments generated by *Sau*3AI. However, in some RNAi plasmids, the inserts contained more than one fragment that were resulted from ligation between genomic DNA fragments. To prevent self-ligation between different genomic fragments, a fill-in reaction of the overhangs in genomic fragments may be performed by Klenow fragment. To be compatible after the fill-in reaction, the *Bam*HI site in pRS416-TTrc plasmid is changed to an *Xho*I site.

3. This fill-in step of the plasmid can greatly reduce the background of plasmid self-ligation, in addition to creation of compatible overhangs with the filled-in genomic fragments.

4. Typically, a library size of more than 4×10^5 should be obtained to achieve a satisfying coverage of the yeast genome. The transformation efficiency of the control experiment should be at least 50 times lower than the library.

5. The PCR product from the control plasmid should be run adjacent to the PCR products from the library plasmids for better comparison. Also, no more than 1 out of the 20 isolated plasmids from the library should be empty.

6. Complete digestion and gel purification is essential for this step. As the pRS-delta-RNAi plasmid contains a CEN/ARS replication origin, the undigested circular plasmid can also support colony growth on YPAD + G418 plates.

7. This empirical inoculation ratio should be adequate for high-efficiency transformation in most laboratory yeast strains. However, for custom strains, the recommended cell density before the 4 h incubation is around 5×10^6 cells/ mL. Also, adjust the incubation time to allow at least two generations of cell replication (4 h is recommended for typical laboratory *S. cerevisiae* strains with a doubling time of 2 h).

8. For delta integration, up to 20 μg of linear integration plasmid DNA may be used to improve transformation efficiency if necessary.

9. Different *S. cerevisiae* strains may have different optimal heat shock time.

10. This recovery step in YPAD medium is essential for yeast cells to develop G418 resistance. The incubation time may be prolonged up to 4 h to improve transformation efficiency.

11. Different *S. cerevisiae* strains may have different selection concentrations of G418.

12. For such a long RNAi pathway, only one copy of integration will typically be achieved. Moreover, as the integration location will affect the expression of the RNAi pathway, an optional gene-silencing assay is recommended to screen for strains with higher RNAi activity. For example, silencing of a GFP reporter by a full-length antisense RNA construct may be used to estimate the RNAi activity.

13. This amount of RNAi plasmid DNA is used to achieve at least 4×10^5 independent clones in the library. Use more DNA for the transformation if necessary.

14. This recovery step is required before screening with acetic acid containing medium.

15. The amount of cells to be spread on each 150×15 mm petri dish should be adjusted to form about 10^4 colonies in the normal SC-Ura medium. The concentration of acetic acid for screening should be adjusted so that about 10^3 colonies will form on each 150×15 mm stressed plate (a tenfold reduction relative to the normal medium). These parameters are chosen to facilitate screening based on colony size. For other tolerance phenotypes, the inhibitor concentration for screening should be optimized to match these parameters.

16. The optimal time window for colony-based screening should be determined empirically.

17. This re-inoculation step is essential as the growth phases greatly affect the tolerance phenotype.

18. For other tolerance phenotypes, the time point where the maximal differences in biomass accumulation should be determined individually.

19. Retransformation is required to rule out the possibility of host adaptation in isolation of a specific mutant.

20. An optional step to estimate gene knockdown efficiency can be performed using GFP as a carboxy-terminal fusion reporter [12, 22] or semiquantitative RT-PCR [12, 17].

21. The insertion of the RNAi cassette may affect the unique restriction sites in an integration plasmid. So the choice of restriction enzyme should be determined individually.

22. The confirmation of phenotype improvement of integration mutants is essential, as integration of knockdown cassettes may affect gene-silencing efficiency and therefore the tolerance trait.

23. Generally, a higher screening stress will be used in a later round of RAGE compared with that in a previous round. The new stress level should be determined according to **Note 15**.

References

1. Si T, Xiao H, Zhao H (2014) Rapid prototyping of microbial cell factories via genome-scale engineering. Biotechnol Adv. doi:10.1016/j.biotechadv.2014.11.007

2. Wang HH, Isaacs FJ, Carr PA, Sun ZZ, Xu G, Forest CR, Church GM (2009) Programming cells by multiplex genome engineering and accelerated evolution. Nature 460:894–898

3. Warner JR, Reeder PJ, Karimpour-Fard A, Woodruff LBA, Gill RT (2010) Rapid profiling of a microbial genome using mixtures of barcoded oligonucleotides. Nat Biotechnol 28:856–862

4. Nevoigt E (2008) Progress in metabolic engineering of *Saccharomyces cerevisiae*. Microbiol Mol Biol Rev 72:379–412

5. Hong K-K, Nielsen J (2012) Metabolic engineering of *Saccharomyces cerevisiae*: a key cell factory platform for future biorefineries. Cell Mol Life Sci 69:2671–2690

6. Winzeler EA, Shoemaker DD, Astromoff A, Liang H, Anderson K, Andre B, Bangham R, Benito R, Boeke JD, Bussey H, Chu AM, Connelly C, Davis K, Dietrich F, Dow SW, El Bakkoury M, Foury F, Friend SH, Gentalen E, Giaever G, Hegemann JH, Jones T, Laub M, Liao H, Liebundguth N, Lockhart DJ, Lucau-Danila A, Lussier M, M'Rabet N, Menard P, Mittmann M, Pai C, Rebischung C, Revuelta JL, Riles L, Roberts CJ, Ross-MacDonald P, Scherens B, Snyder M, Sookhai-Mahadeo S, Storms RK, Véronneau S, Voet M, Volckaert G, Ward TR, Wysocki R, Yen GS, Yu K, Zimmermann K, Philippsen P, Johnston M, Davis RW (1999) Functional characterization of the *S. cerevisiae* genome by gene deletion and parallel analysis. Science 285:901–906

7. Giaever G, Chu AM, Ni L, Connelly C, Riles L, Veronneau S, Dow S, Lucau-Danila A, Anderson K, Andre B, Arkin AP, Astromoff A, El Bakkoury M, Bangham R, Benito R, Brachat S, Campanaro S, Curtiss M, Davis K, Deutschbauer A, Entian K-D, Flaherty P, Foury F, Garfinkel DJ, Gerstein M, Gotte D, Guldener U, Hegemann JH, Hempel S, Herman Z, Jaramillo DF, Kelly DE, Kelly SL, Kotter P, LaBonte D, Lamb DC, Lan N, Liang H, Liao H, Liu L, Luo C, Lussier M, Mao R, Menard P, Ooi SL, Revuelta JL, Roberts CJ, Rose M, Ross-Macdonald P, Scherens B, Schimmack G, Shafer B, Shoemaker DD, Sookhai-Mahadeo S, Storms RK, Strathern JN, Valle G, Voet M, Volckaert G, Wang C-y, Ward TR, Wilhelmy J, Winzeler EA, Yang Y, Yen G, Youngman E, Yu K, Bussey H, Boeke JD, Snyder M, Philippsen P, Davis RW, Johnston M (2002) Functional profiling of the *Saccharomyces cerevisiae* genome. Nature 418:387–391

8. Forsburg SL (2001) The art and design of genetic screens: yeast. Nat Rev Genet 2:659–668

9. Scherens B, Goffeau A (2004) The uses of genome-wide yeast mutant collections. Genome Biol 5(7)

10. van Dijken JP, Bauer J, Brambilla L, Duboc P, Francois JM, Gancedo C, Giuseppin MLF, Heijnen JJ, Hoare M, Lange HC, Madden EA, Niederberger P, Nielsen J, Parrou JL, Petit T, Porro D, Reuss M, van Riel N, Rizzi M, Steensma HY, Verrips CT, Vindeløv J, Pronk JT (2000) An interlaboratory comparison of physiological and genetic properties of four *Saccharomyces cerevisiae* strains. Enzyme Microb Technol 26:706–714

11. Tong AHY, Evangelista M, Parsons AB, Xu H, Bader GD, Pagé N, Robinson M, Raghibizadeh S, Hogue CWV, Bussey H, Andrews B, Tyers M, Boone C (2001) Systematic genetic analysis with ordered arrays of yeast deletion mutants. Science 294:2364–2368

12. Si T, Luo Y, Bao Z, Zhao H (2015) RNAi-assisted genome evolution in *Saccharomyces cerevisiae* for complex phenotype engineering. ACS Synth Biol 4:283–291

13. Fire A, Xu SQ, Montgomery MK, Kostas SA, Driver SE, Mello CC (1998) Potent and specific genetic interference by double-stranded RNA in *Caenorhabditis elegans*. Nature 391:806–811

14. Hannon GJ (2002) RNA interference. Nature 418:244–251

15. Echeverri CJ, Perrimon N (2006) High-throughput RNAi screening in cultured cells: a user's guide. Nat Rev Genet 7:373–384

16. Boutros M, Ahringer J (2008) The art and design of genetic screens: RNA interference. Nat Rev Genet 9:554–566

17. Drinnenberg IA, Weinberg DE, Xie KT, Mower JP, Wolfe KH, Fink GR, Bartel DP (2009) RNAi in budding yeast. Science 326:544–550

18. Cheng X, Jian R (2010) Construction and application of random dsRNA interference library for functional genetic screens in embryonic stem cells. Methods Mol Biol 650:65–74

19. Xiao H, Zhao H (2014) Genome-wide RNAi screen reveals the E3 SUMO-protein ligase gene *SIZ1* as a novel determinant of furfural tolerance in *Saccharomyces cerevisiae*. Biotechnol Biofuels 7:78

20. Olsson L, HahnHagerdal B (1996) Fermentation of lignocellulosic hydrolysates for ethanol production. Enzyme Microb Technol 18:312–331

21. Mira NP, Teixeira MC, Sa-Correia I (2010) Adaptive response and tolerance to weak acids in *Saccharomyces cerevisiae*: a genome-wide view. OMICS 14:525–540

22. Huh WK, Falvo JV, Gerke LC, Carroll AS, Howson RW, Weissman JS, O'Shea EK (2003) Global analysis of protein localization in budding yeast. Nature 425:686–691

Chapter 16

RNAi Screening in *Spodoptera frugiperda*

Subhanita Ghosh, Gatikrushna Singh, Bindiya Sachdev, Ajit Kumar, Pawan Malhotra*, Sunil K. Mukherjee*, and Raj K. Bhatnagar*

Abstract

RNA interference is a potent and precise reverse genetic approach to carryout large-scale functional genomic studies in a given organism. During the past decade, RNAi has also emerged as an important investigative tool to understand the process of viral pathogenesis. Our laboratory has successfully generated transgenic reporter and RNAi sensor line of *Spodoptera frugiperda* (Sf21) cells and developed a reversal of silencing assay via siRNA or shRNA guided screening to investigate RNAi factors or viral pathogenic factors with extraordinary fidelity. Here we describe empirical approaches and conceptual understanding to execute successful RNAi screening in *Spodoptera frugiperda* 21-cell line.

Key words RNA interference, RNAi screening, Sf21 cells, Insect RNAi, *Spodoptera frugiperda*, siRNA screening

1 Introduction

1.1 RNA Interference Basic Biology

RNA interference and its related processes have emerged as leading mechanisms that suppress unwanted genetic elements and transcripts, thereby acting as gene-regulatory mechanisms for host defense. These processes thus play a variety of biological functions such as antiviral defense, epigenetic regulation, DNA elimination, and heterochromatin formation [1, 2]. RNAi/miRNA regulation is a two-step process; the first step involves cleavage of long dsRNA or pre-miRNA into ~21–25 nts long small interfering RNA (siRNAs) or miRNA by RNAseIII class of proteins called Dicer(s) and other cognate RNA-binding proteins such as R2D2, TRBP, and PACT. The second step, which is also referred to as the splicing step, is the main mRNA degradation step where siRNA/miRNA joins multinuclease complex to degrade or transcriptionally suppress miRNAs [3]. It has been reported that besides conserved proteins,

---

* Author contributed equally with all other contributors.

David O. Azorsa, Shilpi Arora (eds.), *High-Throughput RNAi Screening: Methods and Protocols*, Methods in Molecular Biology, vol. 1470, DOI 10.1007/978-1-4939-6337-9_16, © Springer Science+Business Media New York 2016

Dicer as well as Argonautes involved in various RNAi pathways, a number of auxiliary proteins also participate in these processes and these proteins stabilize various RNAi-related multiprotein complexes and bring specificity to the reactions [4–6]. Genome-wide RNAi screens have identified variable numbers of RNAi-related proteins in different organisms [7, 8]. Since RNAi is a conserved mechanism in invertebrates and vertebrates, many invertebrate species are being widely exploited to study the endogenous biological pathway of eukaryotes. In insect science, RNAi has revolutionized the notion of sequence-specific loss of function gene expression in high-throughput format especially to explore genetic basis, insecticidal management, and reduce disease pathogens [9]. Additionally, the increasing availability of NGS data and rapidly evolving bioinformatics tools have aided significantly in the functional genomic research in cell-based RNAi screen in insects. We have been earlier involved in understanding ligand-receptor interactions and elucidating the mechanisms of action of known insecticides like *Bacillus thuringiensis* (BT) toxin using *Spodoptera frugiperda* cells [10, 11]. Further, we have developed RNAi silenced lines to identify animal virus suppressor proteins. Additionally, we have assembled draft genome and transcriptome data from *Spodoptera frugiperda* cells that has allowed us to comprehend comparative genomics studies and develop small RNA-based approaches [12–15]. RNAi allied functional studies are being carried out efficiently in *Spodoptera* system either as dsRNA/siRNA-induced inhibition to modulate baculovirus-mediated expression of heterologous gene [16] or to study mechanisms of action of known insecticides like *Bacillus thuringiensis* (BT) toxin [10, 11]. However, the empirical exercise of the technology is species specific, which makes *Spodoptera frugiperda* one of the prime candidates to study regulatory genetic network within different insect groups. Application of RNAi screening is indeed robust and cell line-based approaches made this approach conceivable to carry out efficiently.

1.2 Origin and Application of Spodoptera frugiperda Cells

From primary explants of the pupal tissue of *Spodoptera frugiperda*, two cell lines were developed [17]; Sf21 cells, a cell line made from ovarian cells isolated from *Spodoptera frugiperda*, and Sf9 cells, a clonal isolate derived from the parental Sf21 cell which is sometimes favored for their relatively faster growth rate and higher cell densities than Sf21. These cell lines are commercially available and may be sourced from different vendors (such as Invitrogen and ATCC). Both Sf21 and Sf9 cells are spherical in shape with somewhat unequal sizes and granular appearance. The advantage of using *Spodoptera* cell line is that they adhere firmly to surfaces, permitting expansion as monolayer in stationary systems for transfection or plaque assay applications and can easily be maintained in suspension culture. The Sf21 cell line is highly susceptible to infection with *Autographa californica* nuclear polyhedrosis virus (AcNPV baculovirus), and thus is widely used as a suitable host for the rapid propagation of baculovirus stocks, and production of recombinant proteins using baculovirus expression vectors (BEVs). Sf21-based Baculo system proved to be uniquely beneficial as it generates high levels of expression of homologous and heterologous proteins under the control of the strong polyhedrin or p10 promoter. The expression system supports post-translation modifications including phosphorylation, glycosylation, authentic peptide cleavage, and simultaneous expression of multiple genes, with unlimited protein size in functional form using most simplistic manner. Sf21 cells are preferred expression vehicles as compared to Sf9 cell lines in certain conditions. However, latest technological breakthroughs using next-generation sequencing reveal differential expression of either host microRNAs (miRNAs) or virus-encoded mRNAs upon Baculovirus expression using Sf21 or Sf9 systems, thus unraveling a new window for host pathogen interactive aspect of *Spodoptera* small RNA biology [15, 18]. Earlier studies have shown that the Sf21 cellular system possesses full complement of RNAi factors [11] and efficacy of RNAi screening in *Spodoptera frugiperda* is influenced strongly by the mode of delivery that triggers cell-autonomous RNAi. A handful of parameters are always in consideration for successful RNAi screens involving concentration of siRNA/dsRNA, accurate nucleotide sequence, length of the siRNA/dsRNA fragment, library design, persistence of the suppression effect, life cycle of the target organism [19] etc. We have successfully carried out genome-wide screening of components of RNA silencing machinery of *Spodoptera frugiperda* using indigenously developed Sf21 transgenic line. Protocols and technologies optimized in our laboratory over several years are described here.

1.3 siRNA-Mediated Genome-Wide Screening in Sf21 Cell Line

Our laboratory performed NGS and transcriptome studies on the Sf21 cell line and bioinformatically analyzed the genome sequence data of Sf21 cells to identify various putative RNAi factors. Such analysis allowed us to narrow down to a data set of 80 putative RNAi factors. These factors were later validated by siRNA screening using transgenic Sf21 insect cell line expressing GFP (green fluorescent protein) reporter [13, 20]. At least two siRNAs (three to five in some cases) were designed for each putative gene. Inactivation of endogenously expressed GFP transcript along with putative RNAi factor mRNA were simultaneously targeted with GFP-siRNA and gene-specific individual siRNAs to monitor the altered expression of the reporter. The putative siRNAs that were able to reverse the GFP-siRNA-mediated loss of GFP fluorescence during siRNA library screening in the transiently silenced cell line were identified; and the target gene(s) required for RNAi pathway were considered as the true RNAi factor in *Spodoptera frugiperda* system (Fig. 1) [13]. In total, 42 candidate RNAi factors were confirmed from a pool of potential candidates, which showed significant GFP reversion in the Sf21 functional assay. In Sf21 cell line-based assay system, transient silencing of the targeted gene

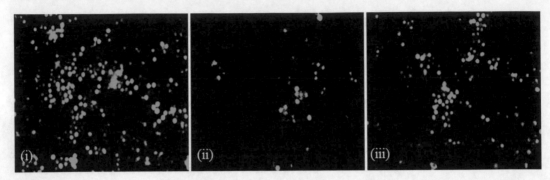

Fig. 1 Fluorescence imaging of siRNA-mediated screening approach for Sf21 RNAi factor. (i) Sf21/GFP reporter cell line (ii) Sf21/GFP reporter cell line transfected with GFP siRNA (iii) Sf21/GFP reporter cell line co-transfected with putative RNAi factor Sf-Dicer-2 specific siRNA and GFP siRNA. Adapted from reference [12] with permission

makes the siRNA approach suitable for rapid analysis of knock-down phenotypes, which may be adapted for high-throughput screening platform.

1.4 Screening in Sf21 Cells Harboring GFP Along with GFP-shRNA for Viral RNAi Suppressor via Reversion Assay of Reporter

We employed the RNAi pathway of Sf21 cells to develop a shRNA-guided sensor line that regain expression of the silent GFP reporter gene due to suppression of RNAi machinery caused by viral-encoded suppressor protein(s). The assay uses the ability of the pathogenic viruses to counteract the host RNAi response by encoding specific RSS (RNA silencing suppressor) elements. Utilizing the underlying suppression mechanism of RNAi setup by GFP-shRNA, we have identified the functionality of Flock House virus B2 (FHVB2) protein that suppresses the insect's anti-viral RNA-induced silencing response [20]. The Sf21 RNAi sensor line is essentially a GFP-silenced line in which GFP expression levels are reduced to the minimum by constitutive expression of GFP reporter and short hairpin RNA (shRNA) of GFP under the control of the same promoter (Fig. 2). This pre-established GFP silencing was suppressed due to transient expression of FHVB2 leading to elevated level of GFP transcript. It has been established by Singh et al. that FHVB2-Dicer interaction leads to a reduction of siRNA biogenesis. To test the RNAi suppressor activity, similar approaches were studied for NS4B protein of Dengue virus which also showed reverted level in GFP expression [21]. It is significant to note that Sf21 cell line is particularly useful as it lacks the immunological response and thus is an excellent system in discriminating between the interferon response and the RNAi pathway. Furthermore, functionality of HBV (Hepatitis B virus) encoded suppressor protein HBx was also assessed using Sf21 heterologous RNAi sensor system [22]. Reversion of silencing assay indeed set up a novel platform to characterize RSSs of different animal viruses expending the RNAi mechanism of *Spodoptera frugiperda*. The principle for developing such shRNA-guided sensor line is that its

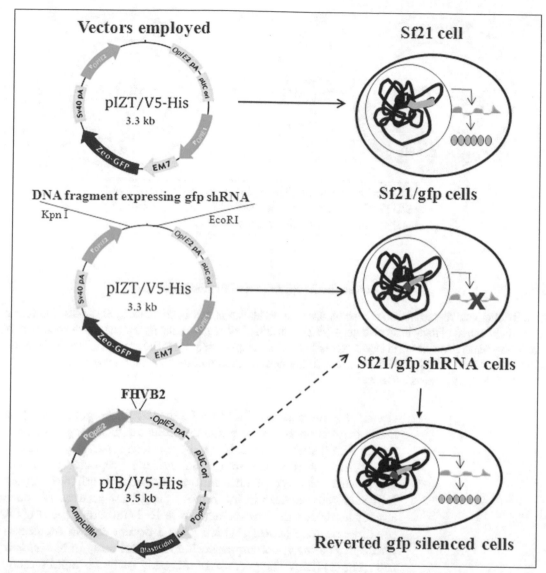

Fig. 2 Generation of Sf21 transgenic cell line and RNAi screening for viral suppressor. Schematic representation of plasmid constructs used for the generation of the Sf21/GFP reporter line, Sf21/GFP shRNA RNAi sensor line, and GFP reverted in Sf21/GFP shRNA line that overexpressed viral RNAi suppressor (FHVB2). Adapted from reference [20] with permission

use would expose the RNAi factors that act in Sf21 cells and allow for a significant comparison to be made between the RNAi machinery of *Spodoptera* and its close relative.

1.5 Reporter Assay for Validation of miRNA Target Using Sf21 Cells

An effective strategy to validate annotated miRNA/3′UTR target interactions has been pursued by using phenotypic expression optimized assay in Sf21 cells. We have studied the potential interaction of gene-specific miRNA by conducting luciferase assays in Sf21 cell-based system. For the assay, 3′UTR of targeted gene was

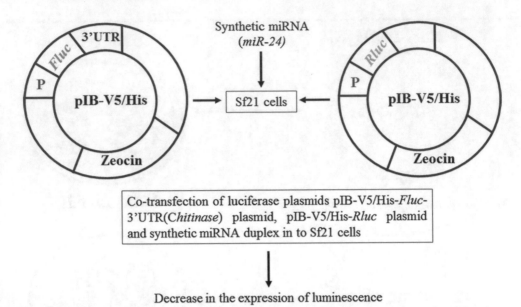

Co-transfection of luciferase plasmids pIB-V5/His-*Fluc*-3'UTR(*Chitinase*) plasmid, pIB-V5/His-*Rluc* plasmid and synthetic miRNA duplex in to Sf21 cells

Decrease in the expression of luminescence

Fig. 3 Schematic representation of reporter assay for validation of miRNA target using Sf21 cells. The vector constructs contain Firefly luciferase gene (*Fluc*) with 3'UTR of targeted chitinase gene (*hachi*) and Renilla luciferase (*Rluc*) gene cloned in insect expression vector independently. Plasmids are transfected in the presence of synthetic miRNA (*miR-24*) resulting in the downregulation of reporter expression expending Sf21-based miRNA target validation assay

cloned downstream to 3'end of Firefly luciferase gene (*Fluc*) in insect expression vector to generate firefly luciferase reporter construct. Renilla luciferase (*Rluc*) gene was also separately cloned in the vector. Co-transfection of the luciferase reporter construct along with *Rluc* vector and annotated synthetic miRNA duplex into Sf21 cells resulted in inhibition of luciferase activity. We have already identified the involvement of *miR-24* targeting the 3'UTR of chitinase gene (*hachi*), which plays a potent role in metamorphosis in *Helicoverpa armigera* using luciferase assay in *Spodoptera* cells (Fig. 3) [23]. The premise of this assay facilitates rapid screening of insect derived tentatively identified microRNAs to execute direct binding of 3'UTR of targeted gene leading to reduction in luminescence using Sf21 as a support platform.

1.6 Baculovirus-Encoded miRNA Profiling Using Sf21 Cells

Differential expression profiling of *Spodoptera litura* nucleopolyhedrovirus (SpltNPV) encoded miRNAs has been validated using Sf21 cells. We have identified and characterized baculoviral miRNAs and have established their roles during viral pathogenesis at dynamic stages of infection. The virus responsive miRNAs can impact signaling pathways, and translation and metabolic processes [15]. Expression pattern of baculovirus-encoded small RNAs could be analyzed at different stages of viral infection in Sf21 cells as well as in mid-gut and fat-body tissue samples to determine their potential roles in host pathogen interactions, adopting the next-generation sequencing technology. As Sf21 is permissive of multiple virus infection, it is ideal to use *Spodoptera* as a useful model system scaffolding to screen and study temporal expression of insect-specific viral RNomics.

2   Materials

1. TNM-FH Insect Medium with serum: Supplemented form of Grace's Insect Medium known as TNM-FH (*Trichoplusia ni* Medium-Formulation Hink) with trace metals, lactalbumin hydrolysate, yeastolate, and 10% heat inactivated fetal bovine serum (pH of 6.2) (BD BaculoGold™ TNM-FH Insect Medium).

2. Serum-Free Insect Media: Media without any supplementation or the addition of serum (BD BaculoGold™ Max-XP Serum-Free Insect Cell Medium).

3. 75 cm² flasks.

4. Cellfectin® II Reagent (Invitrogen).

5. InsectSelect™ Glow System (pIZT-V5/His) (Invitrogen).

6. pIB/V5-His TOPO (Invitrogen).

7. Zeocin (Invitrogen).

8. Dual Luciferase assay kit (Promega).

3   Methods

Sf9 and Sf21 cells may be grown in both adherent and suspension culture. In adherent culture cells are grown in monolayer. In suspension, cells are maintained in spinner culture for rapid expansion of cell stocks, propagation of baculovirus stocks, or production of recombinant proteins. Here we describe the protocols for Sf21 cells in adherent culture.

3.1   Maintenance of Sf21 Cell Line

1. Incubate Sf21 cells with complete insect medium with serum at optimum conditions of 27 °C in a non-humidified environment for adherent culture. After 24 h, suspend the cells with 10 ml fresh complete media and transfer to new flasks in 1:2 or 1:3 dilutions as per requirement (*see* **Note 1**).

2. Inoculate new 25 cm² flasks with $1.5–2.0 \times 10^6$ cells in 5 ml of complete medium or $3.5–4.5 \times 10^6$ cells in 10–15 ml of medium for 75 cm² flasks.

3. Passage cells when the flask is close to fully confluent to maintain growth of the cells as a monolayer (*see* **Notes 2 and 3**).

3.2 Generation of Transgenic Cell Line for RNAi Screening in Spodoptera frugiperda (Sf21 Cells)

1. To explore the RNA silencing mechanism in *Spodoptera frugiperda*, generate stable Sf21 transgenic cell lines.

   (a) Sf21/GFP line: The reporter line that constitutively expresses fluorescence due to transfection-mediated integration of GFP gene into Sf21 genome using commercial vector InsectSelect™ Glow System (pIZT-V5/His) [20].

   (b) Sf21/GFP shRNA line: RNAi sensor line with suppressed GFP expression developed via genomic integration of pIZT-V5/His+GFP shRNA construct in Sf21 cells which target the GFP mRNA to inhibit fluorescence expression in the transgenic line [20] (*see* **Note 4**). A schematic representation of Sf21/GFP RNAi sensor lines is shown in Fig. 1.

2. Select and maintain isolated colonies in complete insect medium with gradual increment of antibiotic pressure up to final concentration 300 µg/ml of zeocin.

3. Monitor the GFP expression using Immunofluorescence microscopy.

4. Quantify different patterns of fluorescence using flow cytometric analysis (FACS).

3.3 siRNA-Mediated Screening in Sf21 Cell Line

3.3.1 Dispersion of Sf21 Cells

1. Before transfection slough Sf21 and Sf21/GFP cells (70–80% confluent) individually with 5 ml of fresh TNM-FH Insect Medium. Check viability of the cells with an assay for trypan blue exclusion. Cell viability should be at least 90–95% for healthy log phase cultures.

2. Seed the cells uniformly in each well of a multi-well culture plate with serum containing medium according to Table 1. Rock the plate slowly forward and backward and sideways to allow even distribution of cells over the entire surface to avoid asymmetric monolayer.

Table 1
Transfection parameters for Sf21 cells

Culture vessel	Number of cells/well	Total DNA/ well (µg)	Total RNA/ well (nM/ pmoles)	Transfection reagent (µl) (Cellfectin II) (Invitrogen)	Volume of serum-free medium during transfection/ well (µl)	Volume of serum containing medium after transfection/well (ml)
6-well	$0.5–1.0 \times 10^6$	4–6	16–30/ 10–20	10	600	2
12-well	$0.25–0.5 \times 10^6$	2–3	1–15/5–10	5	300	1
24-well	$0.1–0.25 \times 10^6$	1–1.5	4–8/3–5	2.5	150	0.5

3. Allow cells to attach for at least 1 h. Cell seeding density should be within 50–60% confluence at the time of transfection.

3.3.2 siRNA Transfection in Sf21 Cells

1. For siRNA-mediated knock down assay transfect Sf21/GFP cells with 2.5 pmoles GFP siRNA (*see* **Note 5**) in a 24-well plate. Follow Table 1 to determine the protocols for 6-well and 12-well formats [13].

2. To identify factors involved in *Spodoptera frugiperda* RNA interference pathway, co-transfect Sf21/GFP reporter cells with 2.5 pmoles GFP siRNA and 5 pmoles RNAi factor specific test siRNA along with 2.5 μl Cellfectin II reagent/well.

3. Use 5 pmoles scrambled siRNA with 2.5 pmoles GFP siRNA to transfect Sf21/GFP cells as negative control.

4. For transfection control separately incubate Sf21 and Sf21/GFP reporter cells only with serum-free medium devoid of any siRNA.

5. Prepare all transfection mixture individually with siRNAs in 200 μl serum-free medium with 2.5 μl Cellfectin II reagent and incubate for 20 min at room temperature (*see* **Note 6**).

6. Prior to the addition of transfection mix, wash the cells settled in the plate three times with serum-free insect cell medium.

7. Add 200 μl of reaction mixture dropwise to each well of 24-well plates (*see* **Note 7**).

8. Keep the plate for transfection at 27 °C for 4 h (*see* **Note 8**).

9. Four hours post-transfection, add 500 μl serum plus medium to all the cells and keep the culture plate stationary at 27 °C for 48 h.

10. Quantify the GFP fluorescence of the assay with FACS analysis.

11. Wash Sf21 cells with 400 μl FACS-grade phosphate buffered saline.

12. From the FACS data, determine the following quantitative parameters:

    (a) The number of Sf21/GFP expressing cells co-transfected with test siRNA and GFP siRNA.

    (b) The number of Sf21/GFP expressing cells transfected only with GFP siRNA.

    (c) Sf21/GFP expressing cells.

13. Calculate the % of GFP reversion for putative RNAi candidate as

$$\{(a-b)/(c-b)\}\times 100$$

3.4 shRNA-Guided Screening in Sf21 for Viral Suppresser

3.4.1 Generation of Viral RSS Expressing Plasmids

1. Amplify the putative viral RSS gene using adequate primers and ligate into the pIB-V5/His-TOPO vector and transform into *E. coli* DH5α and plate on LB agar medium following standard protocol.

2. Analyze the transformants by restriction analysis, PCR, and plasmid DNA sequencing.

3.4.2 Maintenance and Dispersion of Sf21 and Sf21/GFP shRNA Cell Line

1. Dispense cells as mentioned in Subheadings 3.1 and 3.3.1.

2. Propagate Sf21/GFP shRNA line in the presence of 300 μg/ml of antibiotic zeocin in complete media. Do not use zeocin while transfecting cells.

3.4.3 Transfection of Viral Suppressor in Sf21/GFP shRNA Cells

1. An hour before transfection, slough Sf21 and Sf21/GFP shRNA cells separately (60–70 % confluent) and seed approximately $0.5–1.0 \times 10^6$ cells/well into 6-well plates.

2. In 600 μl serum-free medium mix 1 μg of pIB-V5/His-TOPO RSS plasmid construct using 10 μl Cellfectin II reagent and incubate for 20 min.

3. Prior to transfection, wash the cells three times with serum-free insect cell medium.

4. Transfect Sf21/GFP shRNA cells with viral suppressor by adding transfection mixture.

5. After 4 h, add 2 ml serum medium and allow cells to transiently overexpress RNAi suppressor protein.

6. Transfect empty vector pIB-V5/His-TOPO independently to serve as a control.

7. Incubate Sf21/GFP shRNA cells with transfection mixture without any plasmid as negative control.

8. Use Sf21 cells as cell control for FACS analysis.

9. 48 h post-infection resuspend the cells with 400 μl of FACS-grade PBS and quantify reversion of GFP expression in suppressor transfected Sf21/GFP shRNA RNAi sensor line in comparison to Sf21 line and control Sf21/shRNA GFP line by flow cytometric analysis.

10. Calculate the reverted % of GFP expression using the formula:

$$\{(X - Y / Y)\} \times 100$$

where (X) is the number of Sf21/shRNA GFP expressing cells transfected with viral suppressor

(Y) is the number of Sf21/shRNA expressing cells

3.5 Luciferase Assay for miRNA Target Validation in Sf21 Cells

3.5.1 Cloning of Luciferase and 3′ UTR of Target Gene

1. Amplify and clone full-length Firefly luciferase (*Fluc*) and Renilla luciferase (*Rluc*) cDNAs in an insect expression vector (pIB/V5-His TOPO), referred as "pIB-*Fluc* control vector" and "pIB-*Rluc* control vector," respectively.

2. Clone 3′UTR of potential target gene downstream to pIB-*Fluc* after the 3′end of *Fluc* in EcoRV/SacII sites and referred as "recombinant firefly luciferase reporter vector."

3.5.2 Co-transfection of Luciferase Plasmids and miRNA Duplex

1. Disperse Sf21 cells as previously described in Subheading 3.3.1.

2. One hour before transfection, slough Sf21 cells (60–70 % confluent) and seed approximately 0.5–1.0×10^6 cells/well into 6-well plates.

3. In an eppendorf mix pIB-*Fluc* plasmid (1 μg), pIB-*Rluc* plasmid (1 μg), and synthetic miRNA duplex with varying concentrations (10–200 nM) in 600 μl serum-free media using 10 μl Cellfectin II reagent and incubate for 20 min.

4. Carefully wash the cells settled in the plate three times with serum-free insect cell medium.

5. Add 600 μl of reaction mixture dropwise to each well of 6-well plates to co-transfect the cells.

6. Set up the following controls:

   First control: Only Sf21 cells

   Second control: Sf21 cells transfected with empty pIB vector

   Third control: Sf21 cells co-transfected with pIB-*Fluc* vector and pIB-Rluc vector without 3′UTR of target gene (*see* **Note 9**).

7. Four hours post-transfection, add 2 ml serum plus TNM-FH medium to the cells and hold the culture plate stationary at 27 °C for 48 h.

8. After 48 h, measure Firefly and Renilla luciferase activity sequentially using Dual Luciferase assay kit as directed by the manufacturer.

9. Normalize luminescence from the test samples against the ratio of *Fluc/Rluc* obtained from the third control [23].

3.6 Baculovirus-Encoded miRNA Profiling Using Sf21 Cells

1. Maintain neonate *S. frugiperda* larvae with a semisynthetic diet at 25 °C with a 16 h light/8 h dark photoperiod.

2. Administer third instar larvae with ~10^5 NPV occlusion bodies that had been partially purified using deionized water.

3. Extract Hemolymph from infected fifth-instar larvae on ice and dilute in a 1:2 ratio with ice-cold PBS containing 20 mM reduced glutathione to prevent melanization.

4. Maintain Sf21 cells as a monolayer in serum-free TNM-FH insect medium at 27 °C as mentioned earlier.

5. Pass the diluted hemolymph through a 0.22 mm Millipore filter and infect Sf21 cells for 1 h. Replace serum containing TNM-FH medium after infection.

6. Monitor cells for signs of infection after 48 h and collect the supernatant from infected cells to titrate the virus by the plaque assay method.

7. Sf21 cells infected at m.o.i. 2 can be used for subsequent studies.

4 Notes

1. Suspend cells pipetting the medium across the monolayer with a sterile glass pasteur pipette to minimize mechanical pressure.

2. Passage Sf21 cells only when confluency is reached, as cells will be easy to dislodge and it shows better viability too. It is better to passage the cells in log phase; log phase growth can be maintained by splitting cells in 1:3 or 1:5 dilutions.

3. While maintaining the cells, avoid overgrowth of Sf21 cells as it may result in reduced viability.

4. The GFP shRNA contains two identical 19 nt sequence motifs in an inverted orientation and separated by 9 nt spacer of non-homologous sequence and two thymidine nucleotide overhang; Forward strand (5′GGT TAT GTA CAG GAA CGC ATT CAA GAG ATG CGT TCC TGT ACA TAA CCT T 3′) and Reverse strand (5′AAG GTT ATG TAC AGG AAC GCA TCT CTT GAA TGC GTT CCT GTA CAT AAC C 3′). Introduce amplified GFP shRNA sequence into the pIZT-V5/ His vector under the control of baculovirus immediate early OpIE2 promoter.

5. GFP siRNA sequence: GGU UAU GUA CAG GAA CGC AUU.

6. Do not add antibiotics to media during transfection.

7. Vortex briefly before adding the transfection mixture to the cells.

8. To obtain the highest transfection efficiency and minimize nonspecific effects, optimize transfection conditions by varying cell density, DNA and Cellfectin® II concentrations, and transfection incubation time.

9. Transfect Sf21 cells individually with pIB-*Fluc* vector/pIB-*Rluc* vector (without 3′UTR of target gene) to optimize transfection regimen.

Acknowledgements

We gratefully acknowledge Late Dr. Neema Agrawal for making substantial contribution in conceptualizing RNAi application in initial experimentation. This work was supported by a financial grant (BT/PR10673/AGR/36/579/2008) from Department of Biotechnology, NFBSFARA (National Fund for Basic, Strategic and Frontier Application Research in Agriculture), ICAR (Indian Council for Agricultural Research), India [Grant no. RNAi-2012]. Reproduction of Figs. 1 and 2 is duly acknowledged from BMC Genomics [13] and FASEB [20] journal respectively.

References

1. Djupedal I, Ekwall K (2009) Epigenetics: heterochromatin meets RNAi. Cell Res 19(3):282–295. doi:10.1038/cr.2009.13

2. Wilkins C, Dishongh R, Moore SC, Whitt MA, Chow M, Machaca K (2005) RNA interference is an antiviral defence mechanism in Caenorhabditis elegans. Nature 436(7053):1044–1047. doi:10.1038/nature03957

3. Agrawal N, Dasaradhi PV, Mohmmed A, Malhotra P, Bhatnagar RK, Mukherjee SK (2003) RNA interference: biology, mechanism, and applications. Microbiol Mol Biol Rev 67(4):657–685

4. Bernstein E, Caudy AA, Hammond SM, Hannon GJ (2001) Role for a bidentate ribonuclease in the initiation step of RNA interference. Nature 409(6818):363–366. doi:10.1038/35053110

5. Elbashir SM, Lendeckel W, Tuschl T (2001) RNA interference is mediated by 21- and 22-nucleotide RNAs. Genes Dev 15(2):188–200

6. Liu Q, Rand TA, Kalidas S, Du F, Kim HE, Smith DP, Wang X (2003) R2D2, a bridge between the initiation and effector steps of the Drosophila RNAi pathway. Science 301(5641):1921–1925. doi:10.1126/science.1088710

7. Kim JK, Gabel HW, Kamath RS, Tewari M, Pasquinelli A, Rual JF, Kennedy S, Dybbs M, Bertin N, Kaplan JM, Vidal M, Ruvkun G (2005) Functional genomic analysis of RNA interference in C. elegans. Science 308(5725):1164–1167. doi:10.1126/science.1109267

8. Tomoyasu Y, Miller SC, Tomita S, Schoppmeier M, Grossmann D, Bucher G (2008) Exploring systemic RNA interference in insects: a genome-wide survey for RNAi genes in Tribolium. Genome Biol 9(1):R10. doi:10.1186/gb-2008-9-1-r10

9. Zhang H, Li HC, Miao XX (2013) Feasibility, limitation and possible solutions of RNAi-based technology for insect pest control. Insect Sci 20(1):15–30. doi:10.1111/j.1744-7917.2012.01513.x

10. Agrawal N, Malhotra P, Bhatnagar RK (2002) Interaction of gene-cloned and insect cell-expressed aminopeptidase N of Spodoptera litura with insecticidal crystal protein Cry1C. Appl Environ Microbiol 68(9):4583–4592

11. Sivakumar S, Rajagopal R, Venkatesh GR, Srivastava A, Bhatnagar RK (2007) Knockdown of aminopeptidase-N from Helicoverpa armigera larvae and in transfected Sf21 cells by RNA interference reveals its functional interaction with Bacillus thuringiensis insecticidal protein Cry1Ac. J Biol Chem 282(10):7312–7319. doi:10.1074/jbc.M607442200

12. Kakumani PK, Malhotra P, Mukherjee SK, Bhatnagar RK (2014) A draft genome assembly of the army worm, Spodoptera frugiperda. Genomics. doi:10.1016/j.ygeno.2014.06.005

13. Ghosh S, Kakumani PK, Kumar A, Malhotra P, Mukherjee SK, Bhatnagar RK (2014) Genome wide screening of RNAi factors of Sf21 cells reveal several novel pathway associated proteins. BMC Genomics 15:775. doi:10.1186/1471-2164-15-775

14. Kakumani PK, Chinnappan M, Singh AK, Malhotra P, Mukherjee SK, Bhatnagar RK (2015) Identification and characteristics of microRNAs from army worm, Spodoptera frugiperda cell line Sf21. PLoS One 10(2), e0116988. doi:10.1371/journal.pone.0116988

15. Kharbanda N, Jalali SK, Ojha R, Bhatnagar RK (2015) Temporal expression profiling of novel Spodoptera litura nucleopolyhedrovirus-encoded microRNAs upon infection of Sf21 cells. J Gen Virol 96(Pt 3):688–700. doi:10.1099/jgv.0.000008

16. Agrawal N, Malhotra P, Bhatnagar RK (2004) siRNA-directed silencing of transgene expressed in cultured insect cells. Biochem Biophys Res Commun 320(2):428–434. doi:10.1016/j.bbrc.2004.05.184

17. Vaughn JL, Goodwin RH, Tompkins GJ, McCawley P (1977) The establishment of two cell lines from the insect Spodoptera frugiperda (Lepidoptera; Noctuidae). In Vitro 13(4):213–217

18. Mehrabadi M, Hussain M, Asgari S (2013) MicroRNAome of Spodoptera frugiperda cells (Sf9) and its alteration following baculovirus

infection. J Gen Virol 94(Pt 6):1385–1397. doi:10.1099/vir.0.051060-0

19. Huvenne H, Smagghe G (2010) Mechanisms of dsRNA uptake in insects and potential of RNAi for pest control: a review. J Insect Physiol 56(3):227–235. doi:10.1016/j.jinsphys.2009.10.004

20. Singh G, Popli S, Hari Y, Malhotra P, Mukherjee S, Bhatnagar RK (2009) Suppression of RNA silencing by Flock house virus B2 protein is mediated through its interaction with the PAZ domain of Dicer. FASEB J 23(6):1845–1857. doi:10.1096/fj.08-125120

21. Kakumani PK, Ponia SS, S RK, Sood V, Chinnappan M, Banerjea AC, Medigeshi GR, Malhotra P, Mukherjee SK, Bhatnagar RK (2013) Role of RNA interference (RNAi) in den-gue virus replication and identification of NS4B as an RNAi suppressor. J Virol 87(16):8870–8883. doi:10.1128/JVI.02774-12

22. Chinnappan M, Singh AK, Kakumani PK, Kumar G, Rooge SB, Kumari A, Varshney A, Rastogi A, Sarin SK, Malhotra P, Mukherjee SK, Bhatnagar RK (2014) Key elements of the RNAi pathway are regulated by hepatitis B virus replication and HBx acts as a viral suppressor of RNA silencing. Biochem J 462(2):347–358. doi:10.1042/BJ20140316

23. Agrawal N, Sachdev B, Rodrigues J, Sree KS, Bhatnagar RK (2013) Development associated profiling of chitinase and microRNA of Helicoverpa armigera identified chitinase repressive microRNA. Sci Rep 3:2292. doi:10.1038/srep02292

Chapter 17

Morphology and Gene Expression Screening with Morpholinos in Zebrafish Embryos

Li-Chuan Tseng, Chih-Hao Tang, and Yun-Jin Jiang

Abstract

High-throughput screening with a loss-of-function strategy is a logical and efficient way to identify novel genes involved in biological processes of interest. In zebrafish, morpholinos have been developed as a convenient tool to knock down gene expression. Here, we describe procedures for systematic screening using morpholinos in zebrafish to identify novel deubiquitylases involved in convergent extension during gastrulation. In this example, we examine candidates based on embryonic morphology and molecular signals of whole mount in situ hybridization assay.

Key words Zebrafish, Morpholinos, In situ hybridization, Knockdown, RNA probe

1 Introduction

A well-designed high-throughput functional screen allows for the investigation of novel and important candidate genes. Many high-throughput functional screens are performed in bacteria, yeast, cell lines, worms, and flies due to their ease of manipulation and low cost. The findings obtained in invertebrate screens are sometimes artificial and inapplicable to higher order organisms (e.g., mice and humans). Additionally, conducting a high-throughput screen in mouse models retains excessive cost. The zebrafish (*Danio rerio*) is a small vertebrate and can be a model organism for functional screens. The raising and breeding of thousands of zebrafish is much cheaper and easier than that of mice. Results from whole genome sequencing indicate a high level of conservation between the zebrafish and human genomes as 71.4% of human genes have at least one orthologous gene in zebrafish, including 2601 disease-associated genes [1]. Since both loss-of-function and gain-of-function studies have been conducted in zebrafish, the zebrafish has become a popular animal model to study embryonic development and human diseases.

David O. Azorsa, Shilpi Arora (eds.), *High-Throughput RNAi Screening: Methods and Protocols*, Methods in Molecular Biology, vol. 1470, DOI 10.1007/978-1-4939-6337-9_17, © Springer Science+Business Media New York 2016

In zebrafish, gene knockdown can be easily performed by microinjection of morpholinos into embryos. Morpholinos are DNA analogues with nucleic acid bases that are bound to morpholine rings, in replacement of deoxyribose rings, and linked through neutral-charged phosphorodiamidate groups instead of phosphates. Because of the neutral charge, morpholinos do not bind to proteins, which make it less toxic and more resistant to nuclease degradation. Antisense morpholinos bind to RNA specifically following Watson-Crick base-pairing rule. Instead of RNase H dependent action of RNAi, morpholinos result in gene knockdown by blocking protein translation or disrupting the mRNA splicing process. In addition to zebrafish, morpholinos have also been used for efficient gene knockdown in *Xenopus*, chicken, sea urchin, and *Drosophila* [2, 3].

In this chapter, we describe a high-throughput screening method using morpholinos to identify novel deubiquitylases involved in the convergent extension. In zebrafish, there are about 90 deubiquitylases identified so far belonging to the following categories: ubiquitin-specific proteases (USP), ovarian tumor proteases (OTU), ubiquitin C-terminal hydrolases (UCH), Machado-Joseph disease proteases (MJD), JAMM/MPN+ metalloproteases (JAMM), and permuted papain fold peptidases of dsRNA viruses and eukaryotes (PPPDE) [4]. The protease activity of deubiquitylases removes ubiquitin from target proteins to reverse ubiquitylation. Convergent extension is an action of collective cell movement and cell intercalation that narrows and extends body axis of zebrafish at late gastrulation [5]. The defects in convergent extension cause phenotypes like shorter body, wider somites, and thicker notochord [6, 7]. In the following procedure, morpholinos are injected into zebrafish embryos to knock down the expression of deubiquitylases. Through observation of live phenotypes of morphants (embryos injected with morpholinos) or gene expression patterns by whole mount in situ hybridization assay, deubiquitylases participating in convergent extension are identified and selected for further studies.

2   Materials

2.1   Microinjection of Morpholinos

1. Morpholinos: anti-sense oligomers with 25 bases are customized from Gene Tools Inc. To confirm the function of genes, at least two different morpholinos for each gene are required.

2. Zebrafish: 6 months to 1 year old.

3. Small tank for fish setting: a small tank with a meshed bottom to separate fish from eggs (Fig. 1a).

4. Tea strainer for egg collection.

5. Plastic Petri dish.

6. Dropper.

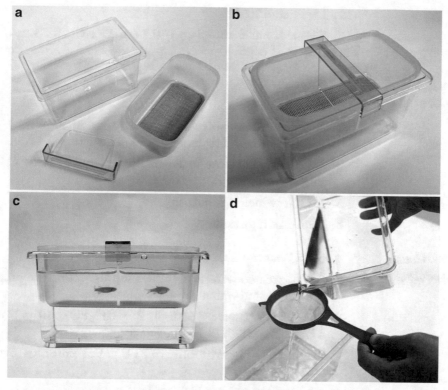

Fig. 1 Devices for fish setting and egg collection. (**a**) A small tank for fish setting includes an outer container, an inner container with meshed bottom, and a separator. (**b**) Assembly of fish setting devices. (**c**) Fish setting with a pair of fish in a small tank filled with water to 70 % full. (**d**) Eggs are collected by pouring the tank water over a tea strainer

7. P-97 Flaming/Brown micropipette puller.

8. Glass capillary: 3.5-in. long, outside diameter 0.044 in., inside diameter 0.02 in.

9. Small glass tip: it can be prepared by flaming a glass capillary in the middle until it becomes soft. Pulling it quickly to make a very thin tube. Cut it from the middle and fuse the tiny opening by flame.

10. Mineral oil.

11. Microinjector.

12. Dissecting microscope.

13. Injection dish: you can make one by pouring liquid 2 % agarose into a plastic Petri dish and float a mould to create ditches for egg sitting. If the mould is not available, float several capillaries (1–1.5 mm) in the liquid agarose. Remove the mould or capillaries when agarose solidifies.

14. 1% Phenol Red.

15. E3 medium: 5 mM NaCl, 0.17 mM KCl, 0.33 mM $CaCl_2$, 0.33 mM $MgSO_4$.

2.2 Phenotype Observation of Live Embryos

1. Forceps.

2. 1 mg/ml Pronase.

3. 23× Tricaine: dissolve 400 mg Tricaine in 97.9 ml H_2O and add 2.1 ml 1 M Tris base (pH 9), adjust to pH 7.

4. 3% Methyl cellulose in E3 medium: store at –20 °C in small aliquots.

5. 1.5% low melting agarose.

6. Depression glass slide.

2.3 Whole Mount In Situ Hybridization

1. 68 °C water bath.

2. DEPC treated water: All buffers in this section are prepared in DEPC treated water.

3. 10× PBS: Dissolve 2 g KCl, 2 g KH_2PO_4, 80 g NaCl, and 11.5 g Na_2HPO_4 in H_2O to final 1 L.

4. 0.4 mM N-phenylthiourea (PTU): For embryos over 24 h post-fertilization.

5. 4% (w/v) paraformaldehyde in PBS.

6. PBST: PBS with 0.1% (v/v) Tween 20.

7. Methanol.

8. H_2O_2.

9. 0.5 mg/ml Protease K stock solution.

10. Probes prepared by MEGAscript Kit (Ambion).

11. 20× SSC: Dissolve 175.3 g NaCl and 88.2 g Sodium citrate in H_2O to final 1 L.

12. HYB⁻: 50% formamide, 5× SSC and 0.1% (v/v) Tween 20, adjust to pH 5.5 with citric acid.

13. HYB⁺: HYB⁻ supplemented with 50 mg/ml Heparin and 500 mg/ml yeast tRNA.

14. Maleic acid buffer: 100 mM Maleic acid, 150 mM NaCl, 0.1% Tween 20, adjust to pH 7.5 with NaOH.

15. Blocking buffer: 1% (w/v) blocking reagent (Roche) in Maleic acid buffer.

16. Anti-digoxigenin alkaline-phosphatase conjugated antibody (Roche, 1:5000 dilution in blocking buffer).

17. NTMT: freshly prepare 0.1 M NaCl, 0.1% Tween 20, 50 mM $MgCl_2$, 0.1 M Tris–HCl (pH 9.5).

18. NBT (nitroblue tetrazolium)/BCIP (5-bromo-4-chloro-3-indolyl phosphate).

19. 100% glycerol.

3   Methods

3.1   Microinjection of Morpholinos

3.1.1   Sequence Design and Working Dose of Morpholinos

A morpholino is usually an anti-sense oligomer with 25 bases. It is able to knock down gene expression by blocking translation or splicing process. To block translation, select a target sequence in a region of mature mRNA from the 5′ cap to 25 bases upstream of the AUG translation start site. The binding of a morpholino in this region disrupts the formation of the translation initiation complex. For blocking splicing processes, choose a sequence located at an exon/intron or an intron/exon boundary of pre-mRNA. The blocking of splicing process leads to a deletion or insertion of mRNA, which often accompanies a nonsense mutation to generate a nonfunctional protein. Effective morpholino sequences should contain the following: (a) 40–60% GC content, (b) little or no significant self-complementarity, (c) less than nine total guanines (<36% G), and (d) no more than three contiguous guanines. For convenience, Gene Tools Inc. provides free services in designing morpholinos according to these rules. Request for design can be made at their website (http://www.gene-tools.com/). In addition, many morpholinos have been used and published in the literature. Published and validated morpholino sequences can be found in the ZFIN database (http://zfin.org/).

For targeting a gene of interest, there are at least three types of morpholinos that one can choose: (1) morpholinos targeting the AUG start site, (2) morpholinos targeting the 5′ untranslated region, and (3) morpholinos disrupting the splicing process. Testing all three kinds of morpholinos is the best way to understand the effects of the particular morpholino on gene knockdown. Since the efficacy of each morpholino subtype can vary depending on the target, empirically assessing each subtype can be time and cost consuming; thus, we recommend selecting morpholinos targeting the AUG start site first and secondly, choosing morpholinos specific for splicing disruption. Since genome sequences for a noncoding region are often not confirmed as seriously as a coding region, the inefficacy of a morpholino may be due to sequence errors in a noncoding region. Additionally, it is easy to determine the efficacy of morpholinos that disrupt the splicing process by RT-PCR.

Obtaining the optimal working dose is also very important. Different morpholinos may have different optimal working doses. We routinely evaluate 2 ng, 4 ng, and 8 ng per embryo for an untested morpholino. An adjustment of the dose is done to obtain the optimal condition and avoid high doses that may result in off-target effects.

3.1.2   Fish Setting and Egg Collection

1. Net a pair of male and female zebrafish into a small tank, and divide them using a separator in the afternoon (Fig. 1b). It is

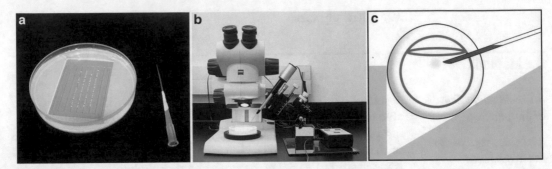

Fig. 2 Devices for microinjection. (**a**) Alignment of eggs on an injection dish (*left*) with a small glass tip (*right*). (**b**) Microinjection setting is composed of a dissecting microscope (*left*) and an oil-driven microinjector with a needle (*right*). Aligned eggs on the injection dish are ready for microinjection under the microscope. (**c**) Illustration of a suitable position for injection with morpholinos in yolk

better to net fish at least 30 min after feeding to allow fish to consume the food.

2. The next morning, after light turns on, remove the partition. Fish will mate and lay eggs (Fig. 1c).

3. After 10–15 min, bring the fish to a new tank and collect eggs with a tea strainer (Fig. 1d).

4. Rinse eggs gently with E3 medium and transfer them to a Petri dish containing the E3 medium.

5. Remove debris or dead eggs (white eggs) with a dropper.

6. Before microinjection, put eggs on an injection dish and line up with a small glass tip (Fig. 2a).

7. Remove excess water from the injection dish without letting the eggs dry up. At the same time, retain about 30 eggs that are not injected as a quality control measure.

3.1.3 Microinjection of Morpholinos

1. Morpholino preparation: dissolve morpholinos in sterilized ddH$_2$O to 3 mM as a stock solution. Aliquot into several small volumes and store at −20 °C. For injection, morpholino stocks are heated at 65 °C on a heat block for 5–10 min, and then placed on ice immediately to completely dissolve precipitated morpholinos and to avoid any secondary structure. Mix morpholinos with sterilized water and phenol red, to a final working concentration of about 0.05–0.1%, and keep it at room temperature.

2. Needle preparation: pull glass capillary by Flaming/Brown micropipette puller. A program that we usually use has the following parameters:

Heat: 607

Pull strength: 180

Velocity: 150

Delay: 100

Pressure: 500

Ramp: 587

3. Cut a needle with a razor blade or forceps to create an oblique opening on the micropipette.

4. Microinjector setup: fill a needle with mineral oil avoiding bubbles. Set the needle on an oil-driven microinjector (Fig. 2b). Drop morpholino working solution on a piece of parafilm and fill the needle by aspirating up slowly. Then, inject the working solution into an oil droplet on a piece of parafilm several times to make sure that each injecting volume is equal. The injection volume should be less than 1/10 volume of eggs (about 1 nl).

5. Microinjection: microinjection can be conducted into cells or yolk. Injections into cells deliver materials directly, but it sometimes causes cell damage and usually takes more time. Thus, for small molecules such as morpholinos, it is recommended to inject into the yolk to avoid unpredictable cell damage and save time. Penetrate the needle across the chorion and then into yolk. Inject the morpholino mix near the boundary of yolk and cell (Fig. 2c). After injection, transfer the eggs back to a dish containing E3 medium and incubate them at 28.5 °C. It is recommended to inject about 60–80 eggs for each morpholino.

6. About 2 h later, remove any unfertilized, damaged, or unsuccessfully injected eggs. Only successfully injected eggs showing the pink color of phenol red should be kept.

7. It is recommended to change with fresh E3 medium and clean any dead embryos again in the late afternoon.

3.2 Observation and Image Acquisition

Phenotype observation under a microscope is a basic and convenient way to understand effects of morpholinos on embryonic development. For example, embryos with defects in convergent extension exhibit wider somites at an early stage and a shorter body at a later stage. Therefore, based on somite width at 9–10 somite stage and body length at 24 h post-fertilization, candidate genes that participate in convergent extension can be identified easily. For quick screening, observation can be carried out directly in Petri dishes with E3 medium using a dissecting microscope. However, to acquire more detailed images, mounting is an essential step. Methyl cellulose and low melting agarose are usually used for mounting live embryos.

3.2.1 Mounting with Methyl Cellulose

1. Dechorionate manually with forceps to tear chorion or chemically with 1 mg/ml pronase incubating at room temperature for 10 min. Gently shake embryos during incubation until chorion is digested by pronase. Wash embryos with 2–3 ml E3 medium several times to remove pronase.

2. At 24 h post-fertilization (hpf), embryos can move quickly. Thus, they should be immersed in 23× Tricaine for 1–2 s to anesthetize them. For embryos at early stages like the 9-somite stage, this step is not necessary.

3. Smear 3 % methyl cellulose on a depression glass slide.

4. Transfer embryos onto the methyl cellulose containing slide with a dropper. Remove excess E3 medium with tissue paper but do not let embryos completely dry up. Since E3 medium is also taken up quickly by methyl cellulose, it can make the embryos too dry to be manipulated.

5. Orientate embryos to proper pose for image acquisition with a small glass tip.

3.3 Mounting with Low Melting Agarose

1. Heat agarose at 60 °C on a heat block until completely melted.

2. Wait for cooling to about 40 °C.

3. Put a drop of agarose on a slide and immerse an embryo into the agarose.

4. Using a small glass tip, orientate the embryo and maintain its orientation for image acquisition until the agarose hardens.

3.4 Whole Mount In Situ Hybridization

Whole mount in situ hybridization detects mRNA expression levels and patterns. With tissue-specific probes, it is possible to label tissues and organs. Here, we perform a whole mount in situ hybridization with *dlx3*, *hgg1*, and *ntl* probes to label neural plate (np), polster (pl), and notochord (nt), respectively. The relative position and shape of neural plate, polster, and notochord are indicators of convergent extension of zebrafish at tail bud stage (Fig. 3). Through observation using a microscope, the results of whole mount in situ hybridization can show the effects of each morpholino on convergent extension.

1. Transfer embryos at tail bud stage into microcentrifuge tubes and add 1 ml 4 % paraformaldehyde to fix embryos at 4 °C for at least 1 day. Fixation can be extended up to 7 days.

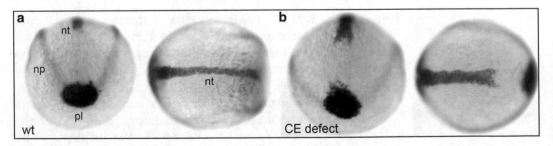

Fig. 3 Whole mount in situ hybridization assay probed for *ntl*, *hgg1*, and *dlx3*. (**a**) Normal wild-type (wt) embryos and (**b**) embryos with convergent extension defects (CE defect) at tail bud stage. Neural plate (np), polster (pl), and notochord (nt) were labeled by *dlx3*, *hgg1*, and *ntl* probes, respectively

2. Wash with 1 ml PBS, and dechorionate manually with forceps.

3. Dehydrate embryos gradually by PBST/methanol gradient using following steps:

   (a) Wash twice with 1 ml PBST for 5 min,

   (b) Wash with 1 ml 75 % PBST + 25 % methanol for 5 min,

   (c) Wash with 1 ml 50 % PBST + 50 % methanol for 5 min,

   (d) Wash with 1 ml 25 % PBST + 75 % methanol for 5 min,

   (e) Wash with 1 ml 100 % methanol for 5 min and

   (f) Store embryos in 100 % methanol at –20 °C overnight.

4. Rehydrate embryos gradually by using a methanol/PBST gradient as follows:

   (a) Wash with 1 ml methanol for 5 min,

   (b) Wash with 1 ml methanol + 2 % H2O2 for 20 min,

   (c) Wash with 1 ml 75 % methanol + 25 % PBST for 5 min,

   (d) Wash with 1 ml 50 % methanol + 50 % PBST for 5 min,

   (e) Wash with 1 ml 25 % methanol + 75 % PBST for 5 min and

   (f) Wash twice with 1 ml PBST for 5 min.

5. Protease K treatment: Embryos older than 24 hpf (hour post-fertilization) should be treated with protease K. For embryos under 24 hpf, protease K treatment is not required. Proceed to **step 6** directly. Protease K treatment is as follows:

   (a) Wash with 1 ml PBS for 5 min, 4 times,

   (b) For 24 hpf embryos, treat with 10 mg/ml protease K for 15 min; for 48 hpf embryos, treat with 25 mg/ml protease K for 25 min; for 72 hpf embryos, treat with 50 mg/ml protease K for 25 min,

   (c) Wash with 1 ml PBS for 5 min, twice,

   (d) Fix embryos again with 4 % paraformaldehyde for 20 min at room temperature and

   (e) Wash with 1 ml PBST for 5 min, 3 times.

6. Hybridization with RNA probes.

   (a) Prehybridize embryos with 1 ml HYB+ at 68 °C for 2.5 h,

   (b) Probe preparation: add RNA probes (1250 ng/ml dlx3, 250 ng/ml hgg1, and 250 ng/ml ntl probes) synthesized using the MEGAscript Kit into 0.5 ml HYB+, heat probes at 80 °C for 10 min, then quickly place on ice at least for 2 min,

   (c) Prewarm probes at 68 °C before hybridization,

   (d) Hybridize embryos with probes at 68 °C overnight.

7. Wash embryos with a HYB⁻/SSC gradient at 68 °C as follows:

(a) Collect probe into a new tube (it can be reused for next experiments),

(b) Wash with 1 ml 75 % HYB– + 25 % 2×SSC for 10 min,

(c) Wash with 1 ml 50 % HYB– + 50 % 2×SSC for 10 min,

(d) Wash with 1 ml 25 % HYB– + 75 % 2×SSC for 10 min,

(e) Wash with 1 ml 2× SSC for 10 min and

(f) Wash with 1 ml 0.2× SSC for 30 min, three times.

8. Detection with an antibody can be done at room temperature as follows:

(a) Wash with 1 ml maleic acid buffer for 5 min,

(b) Block samples with 1 ml 1× blocking buffer for 1.5 h,

(c) Add 0.5 ml antibody for 2 h at room temperature or over-night at 4 °C on a shaker with a gentle speed (based on the labeling of the probes, choose the appropriate antibodies; anti-digoxigenin (DIG) and anti-fluorescein antibodies conjugated with alkaline-phosphatase are routinely used at a dilution of 1:5000 in 1× blocking buffer),

(d) Wash with 1 ml maleic acid buffer for 30 min at least 4 times on a shaker,

(e) Wash with 1 ml NTMT for 5 min, 3 times on a shaker,

(f) Stain with 1 ml NBT/BCIP solution at 28.5 °C; check regularly until signal appears (needs to be kept in dark dur-ing coloring reaction),

(g) Wash with 1 ml PBST pH 5.5 for 5 min on a shaker, twice,

(h) Wash with 1 ml methanol for 5 min, several times, to remove background,

(i) Wash with 1 ml PBST pH 5.5 for 5 min on a shake, twice and

(j) Fix with 4 % paraformaldehyde and store at 4 °C.

9. Observing whole embryos under a microscope:

(a) Replace 4 % paraformaldehyde with 1 ml PBST pH 5.5.

(b) Place embryos onto a glass dish and observe the patterns of dlx3, hgg1, and ntl. Compare the differences between wild-type embryos and morphants.

(c) For image acquisition, mount embryos with glycerol or with low melting agarose as previously described. For mounting with glycerol, add a drop 100 % glycerol onto a slide and place embryos onto the droplet. Be careful to avoid dropping extra PBST on a slide with embryos, which will dilute the glycerol.

(d) Orientate embryos with a glass tip and acquire images.

4   Notes

1. Although several morpholinos have been demonstrated to knock down gene expression and phenocopy mutant zebrafish successfully, some cases indicate that the phenotypes of the morphants were not a result of gene knockdown by morpholinos [8]. The misleading phenotypes may be due to an off-target effect. Therefore, candidate genes identified in a high-throughput screen using morpholinos should be further examined and validated with caution. It is recommended to try two additional and different morpholinos targeting the same gene in order to confirm the phenotypes. Rescue experiments using a coinjection of mRNA and morpholinos are an approach that can be used to validate the phenotypes [3]. Alternatively, other ways of disrupting the functions of interested genes can be applied simultaneously to verify the function of morpholinos. For example, CRISPR interference technology [9, 10] or injection of dominant-negative mRNA. Furthermore, using TALEN or CRISPR systems to generate gene knockout zebrafish mutants can also result in the desired phenotype and could avoid the off-target effects exhibited by morpholinos. Notably, there is a case showing that the inconsistency between knockout mutants and knockdown morphants is due to gene compensation induced by deleterious mutations but not morpholino knockdown [10]. A recent perspective article on the use of morpholinos provides an in-depth discussion in comparison of this method to other engineered knockouts and on the advantages and unique applications associated with morpholinos [11].

2. Obtaining good quality eggs is key to producing a robust high-throughput morpholino screen in zebrafish. The egg quality of older fish is diminished when compared to those of younger fish. Thus, choosing young fish between 6 and 12 months is best for these experiments. Additionally, it is recommended that the fish mate and lay eggs once per 1/2 weeks to avoid aged eggs in the fish. The fish should also be fed nutritional sustenance to maintain good health and egg quality. Furthermore, during experiments, eggs that have not been injected should be retained to evaluate egg quality. If a large number of dead eggs or abnormal development is seen in the control eggs, the injected eggs should be discarded.

3. Because yolk of zebrafish, especially at the early stage, is very fragile and easily sticks on a plastic dish, it is preferred to use a glass slide for dechorionation.

4. Methyl cellulose is not easily dissolved and it is recommended to make smaller aliquots. Once dissolved, store the solution at –20 °C in small aliquots. If bubbles are present in the methyl cellulose solution, centrifuge it briefly before use.

5. Melanophores appear gradually after 24 hpf. It obstructs the observation of gene expression by in situ hybridization assay. To avoid pigmentation, treat embryos with N-phenylthiourea (PTU) on the first evening. Since PTU blocks all tyrosinase-dependent steps, it is used to inhibit pigmentation. Additionally, overexposure with PTU is toxic for embryos. Thus, it is best to treat the embryos with PTU as late as possible but before pigmentation.

6. Fixation with paraformaldehyde is important to maintain the integrity of embryos in whole mount in situ hybridization assays. Occasionally, the yolk can become loose, especially after protease K treatment. Increasing fixation time can improve this.

7. Different probes can work at varying hybridization temperatures and concentrations. A temperature of 68 °C is acceptable for the most probes. If the signal of whole mount in situ hybridization is too weak to be observed, it is recommended to try different hybridization temperatures and concentrations of the probes.

Acknowledgements

The authors are grateful to the Taiwan Zebrafish Core Facility in NHRI for their technical supports and fish maintenance. The deubiquitylase work is funded by the Ministry of Science and Technology, Taiwan, with a grant (MOST 103-2633-B-400-001) awarded to Y.J.J.

References

1. Howe K, Clark MD, Torroja CF et al (2013) The zebrafish reference genome sequence and its relationship to the human genome. Nature 496:498–503

2. Nasevicius A, Ekker SC (2000) Effective targeted gene 'knockdown' in zebrafish. Nat Genet 26:216–220

3. Eisen JS, Smith JC (2008) Controlling morpholino experiments: don't stop making antisense. Development 135:1735–1743

4. Tse WK, Eisenhaber B, Ho SH et al (2009) Genome-wide loss-of-function analysis of deubiquitylating enzymes for zebrafish development. BMC Genomics 10:637

5. Tada M, Heisenberg CP (2012) Convergent extension: using collective cell migration and cell intercalation to shape embryos. Development 139:3897–3904

6. Hammerschmidt M, Pelegri F, Mullins MC et al (1996) Mutations affecting morphogenesis during gastrulation and tail formation in the zebrafish, *Danio rerio*. Development 123:143–151

7. Heisenberg CP, Tada M, Rauch GJ et al (2000) Silberblick/Wnt11 mediates convergent extension movements during zebrafish gastrulation. Nature 405:76–81

8. Kok FO, Shin M, Ni CW et al (2015) Reverse genetic screening reveals poor correlation between morpholino-induced and mutant phenotypes in zebrafish. Dev Cell 32:97–108

9. Larson MH, Gilbert LA, Wang X et al (2013) CRISPR interference (CRISPRi) for sequence-specific control of gene expression. Nat Protoc 8:2180–2196

10. Rossi A, Kontarakis Z, Gerri C et al (2015) Genetic compensation induced by deleterious mutations but not gene knockdowns. Nature 524:230–233

11. Blum M, De Robertis EM, Wallingford JB et al (2015) Morpholinos: antisense and sensibility. Dev Cell 35:145–149

Chapter 18

Live Cell Microscopy-Based RNAi Screening in the Moss *Physcomitrella patens*

Tomohiro Miki*, Yuki Nakaoka*, and Gohta Goshima

Abstract

RNA interference (RNAi) is a powerful technique enabling the identification of the genes involved in a certain cellular process. Here, we discuss protocols for microscopy-based RNAi screening in protonemal cells of the moss *Physcomitrella patens*, an emerging model system for plant cell biology. Our method is characterized by the use of conditional (inducible) RNAi vectors, transgenic moss lines in which the RNAi vector is integrated, and time-lapse fluorescent microscopy. This method allows for effective and efficient screening of >100 genes involved in various cellular processes such as mitotic cell division, organelle distribution, or cell growth.

Key words *Physcomitrella patens*, Inducible RNAi, Kinesin, Protonemal cell, Live cell imaging

1 Introduction

The moss *Physcomitrella patens* is an excellent plant model for cell and developmental biology, partly because of its great suitability for live imaging [1–7]. The availability of the full *P. patens* genome sequence has enabled the use of RNA interference (RNAi) technology to screen for genes involved in certain cellular processes. Two types of RNAi screens are currently available. The first type uses the "transient RNAi" method in which a plasmid expressing double-stranded RNAs (dsRNAs) is transiently introduced into the protoplast, and the effect of RNAi knockdown is monitored throughout the process of protoplast regeneration. This method has been used to screen for genes involved in polarized cell growth of protonemal cells, which identified key regulators of the actin cytoskeleton [8–10]. However, this method is not readily applicable to other intercellular processes such as mitosis or organelle dynamics; mitosis is a rare event during protoplast regeneration and organelle dynamics are more easily tracked at later stages (e.g., in caulonemal cells).

---

*Author contributed equally with all other contributors.

David O. Azorsa, Shilpi Arora (eds.), *High-Throughput RNAi Screening: Methods and Protocols*, Methods in Molecular Biology, vol. 1470, DOI 10.1007/978-1-4939-6337-9_18, © Springer Science+Business Media New York 2016

The second method of RNAi screening is based on transgenic RNAi lines that can be maintained in culture, enabling various cell types to be observed. However, constitutive RNAi prevents viable essential gene RNAi lines from being obtained. To overcome this problem, we recently developed a conditional RNAi system enabling the knockdown of target genes in an inducible manner [5]. Thus, we can create an inducible RNAi transgenic line for any gene of interest, including genes that are essential for organism viability.

By using this methodology, we have screened for >100 genes including kinesin superfamily genes (there are 78 kinesins in *P. patens*) and many possible microtubule regulators [4, 5, 11–14]. Here, we describe RNAi screening protocols combining live cell microscopy with inducible RNAi in *P. patens*.

The detailed protocols for basic moss techniques (e.g., culturing, maintenance, transformation) are described in the PHYSCOmanual, written by the Mitsuyasu Hasebe laboratory at the National Institute for Basic Biology, Okazaki, Japan (http://www.nibb.ac.jp/evodevo/PHYSCOmanual/00Eindex.htm). Moreover, several methodologies were recently summarized by Yamada et al. [15]. In this chapter, we focus on our protocol for RNAi plasmid construction, transgenic line selection, and imaging that were not fully covered in the PHYSCOmanual or by Yamada et al. [15].

2 Materials

2.1 Plasmid Construction for Inducible RNAi

1. RNA extraction kit (e.g., RNeasy Plant Mini Kit, QIAGEN).
2. RNase-free DNase set (QIAGEN).
3. Mortar and pestle.
4. Liquid nitrogen.
5. 1.5 ml Tube.
6. β-Mercaptoethanol.
7. 100% Ethanol.
8. 70% Ethanol (at −20 °C).
9. Benchtop centrifuge.
10. Vortex.
11. cDNA synthesis kit (PrimeScript II first-strand cDNA Synthesis Kit, TAKARA).
12. PCR tubes.
13. PCR machine.
14. pENTR/D-TOPO Cloning Kit (Invitrogen) or a circular plasmid whose backbone is pENTR/D-TOPO (e.g., the plasmid in which a gene is cloned into pENTR/D-TOPO by the TOPO cloning). The latter is preferable.
15. PCR kit (PrimeSTAR HS DNA Polymerase kit, TAKARA).

16. Ligation kit (DNA Ligation Kit <Mighty Mix>, TAKARA).

17. Restriction enzymes: *Not*I, *Asc*I, *Xho*I, *Spe*I, *Kpn*I, *Pme*I, *Eco*RV, *Apa*I, *Hpa*I.

18. DNA Clean & Concentrator (Zymo Research).

19. Gateway LR Clonase II Enzyme mix (Invitrogen).

20. *Escherichia coli* competent cells (e.g., DH5α).

21. Plasmid DNA purification kit (e.g., Invitrogen's Midiprep kit).

22. 3 M Sodium acetate.

2.2 Transformation

All materials necessary for transformation are described in the PHYSCOmanual. This methodology was also recently described in Yamada et al. [15]. Here, we have provided further details of the process in order to create a stand-alone chapter.

1. Parental host cell: We routinely use the GFP-tubulin/histoneh2b-mRFP line to screen for mitosis, microtubule dynamics, and nuclear dynamics [5, 12]. However, any other transgenic line can be used, unless it contains a hygromycin resistance gene (since the RNAi vector used confers hygromycin resistance).

2. 50 ml Conical tubes.

3. 15 ml Conical tubes.

4. 15 ml Round-bottom tubes.

5. 50 ml Round-bottom, glass tubes.

6. 0.22 μm Syringe-driven filter unit and 10 and 20 ml syringes.

7. Funnel with a sheet of 50 μm nylon mesh.

8. 6 cm Petri dish.

9. Cellophane (autoclaved, gift from Futamura Chemical Co., Ltd).

10. 2 g PEG6000 in a 50 ml vial and a small stir bar (autoclaved).

11. Driselase.

12. 8 % Mannitol.

13. 1 M $Ca(NO_3)_2$.

14. 1 M Tris–HCl (pH 8.0).

15. 1 % MES (pH 5.6).

16. 1 M $MgCl_2$.

17. Stock solutions:

    (a) Stock A (0.5 M $Ca(NO_3)_2$, 4.5 mM $FeSO_4$) (do not autoclave).

    (b) Stock B (0.1 M $MgSO_4$).

    (c) Stock C (184 mM KH_2PO_4, pH 6.5).

(d) Stock D (1 M KNO_3, 4.5 mM $FeSO_4$) (do not autoclave).

(e) Alternative TES (0.22 mM $CuSO_4$, 10 mM H_3BO_3, 0.23 mM $CoCl_2$, 0.1 mM Na_2MoO_4, 0.19 mM $ZnSO_4$, 2 mM $MnCl_2$, 0.17 mM KI).

(f) 500 mM Ammonium tartrate.

(g) 50 mM $CaCl_2$.

18. Plating medium:

(a) BCDAT plate (2000 ml).

Stock B/C/D	20 ml each
500 mM Ammonium tartrate	20 ml
50 mM $CaCl_2$	40 ml
Alternative TES	2 ml
Agar	16 g
H_2O	Up to 2000 ml

(b) PRM plate (2000 ml).

Stock B/C/D	20 ml each
500 mM Ammonium tartrate	20 ml
Alternative TES	2 ml
Mannitol	120 g
$CaCl_2$	2.2 g
Agar	16 g
H_2O	Up to 2000 ml

(c) BCD plate (2000 ml).

Stock B/C/D	20 ml each
50 mM $CaCl_2$	40 ml
Alternative TES	2 ml
Agar	16 g
H_2O	Up to 2000 ml

(d) Protoplast liquid medium (100 ml).

Stock A/B	1 ml each
Stock C	0.1 ml
500 mM Ammonium tartrate	54 μl
Mannitol	6.6 g
Glucose	0.5 g
H_2O	Up to 100 ml

(e) PRM/T solution (200 ml).

Stock B/C/D	2 ml each
500 mM Ammonium tartrate	2 ml
Alternative TES	0.2 ml
Mannitol	16 g
$CaCl_2$	0.217 g
Agar (should not have solidified at 45 °C)	1.6 g
H_2O	Up to 200 ml

2.3 Transgenic Line Selection

1. Hygromycin B solution.
2. BCDAT medium supplemented with 30 mg/l hygromycin B.

2.4 Selection of Putative RNAi Lines Based on Histone-RFP Intensity (Optional)

1. 35 mm Glass-bottom dish (Mattek).
2. 6-Well, glass-bottom plate (IWAKI).
3. BCD agar medium (see Subheading 2.2 or PHYSCOmanual).
4. β-Estradiol (1–100 mM in DMSO, stored at –80 °C).
5. DMSO.
6. Microscopy (spinning-disc confocal microscope [100× objective lens, EMCCD camera, 488/561 nm lasers], epifluorescence microscope [10× objective lens, CCD camera, filter cubes (CFP/GFP/mCherry/Cy5)]).

2.5 Rescue Experiment

1. Blasticidin S.
2. Nourseothicin (NTC).
3. BCDAT medium supplemented with 75 mg/l blasticidin S or 75 mg/l nourseothricin.

3   Methods

3.1   Plasmid Construction for the Inducible RNAi System

3.1.1   Inducible RNAi Vector

Two available vectors, pGG624 and pGG626, allow for inducible RNAi (Fig. 1); both vectors confer hygromycin resistance. pGG624 contains an estrogen-inducible promoter and two copies of the Gateway cassette sequences (containing two *ccdB* sequences in opposite directions) with GPA intron sequences inserted in between (Fig. 1a) (*see* **Note 1**). pGG626 contains additional partial RFP sequences, which enable inducible co-knockdown of RFP (or mCherry) and the target gene (Fig. 1b). The backbone of these plasmids is pPGX8 [16], in which the XVE chimeric receptor protein is constitutively expressed [17]. The XVE receptor protein is activated by β-estradiol in the medium, promoting the transcription of the RNAi cassettes that are under the control of LexA operator sequences. Subsequent to *Pme*I digestion and transformation, the RNAi constructs integrate at a high frequency into the *PIG1* genome locus, which is dispensable for moss growth [18].

3.1.2   Primer Design for the RNAi Construct

1. Selection of target sequences
   Target gene sequences are identified by using BLAST and the Phytozome database (select *Physcomitrella patens* in the "species" tab) (http://phytozome.jgi.doe.gov/pz/portal.html). Generally, open reading frame (ORF) sequences 500–700 bp in length are selected (we use cDNA, not genomic DNA, as the dsRNA template; *see* **Note 2**). However, 5′-untranslated region (UTR) sequences can also be selected (e.g., when the ORF size is <500 bp or for rescue experiments utilizing ectopic ORF expression). Since many *P. patens* genes have paralogues, the sequence searches should be performed carefully. If co-knockdown of paralogous genes is desired, the most homologous regions of the paralogues should be selected; since the DNA sequences of paralogous genes in *P. patens* are usually very similar to each other, we have occasionally succeeded in co-knockdown of all paralogues (up to four) with a single RNAi construct [4, 5, 11–13] (*see* **Notes 3** and **4**).

2. PCR primer design
   Prepare ≥2 sets of primers to amplify ≥2 non-overlapping regions of the gene. When an identical phenotype is detected subsequent to RNAi targeting two non-overlapping sequences, the phenotype is most likely due to knockdown of the target gene, not an off-target effect. The primers should be 20–23 nucleotides in length (*see* **Note 5**), with a *Not*I (GCGGCCGC) and *Asc*I (GGCGCGCC) site added to the forward and reverse primer, respectively (*see* **Note 6**).

3.1.3   RNA Extraction

P. patens total RNA is extracted by using the RNeasy Plant Mini Kit (QIAGEN) according to the manufacturer's instructions with some modifications. Here, we summarize the protocol.

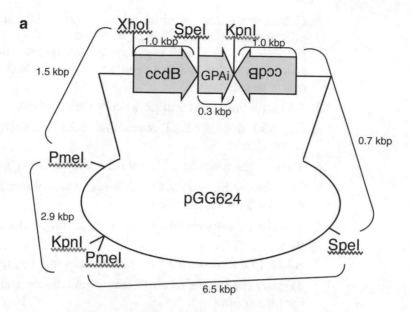

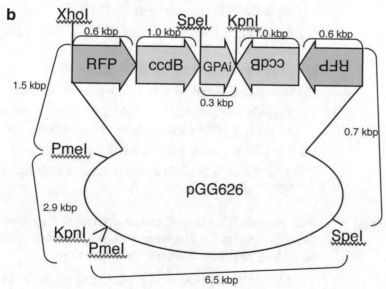

Fig. 1 Inducible RNAi vectors. Schematic diagrams of two inducible RNAi vectors, pGG624 (**a**) and pGG626 (**b**). As described in detail in Nakaoka et al. [5], integration plasmid pGG626 enables the induction of RFP and target gene RNAi. A chimeric transcription activator (XVE) comprised of the DNA-binding domain of the bacterial repressor LexA, the VP16 trans-activating domain, and the regulatory region of the human estrogen receptor is constitutively induced by the *KINID1a* promoter [22] in protonemal cells. β-Estradiol-activated XVE stimulates expression of 300 to 1000 bp partial inverted sequences homologous to the target gene of interest and the *RFP* gene, both of which are controlled by the LexA operator (LexAop) fused to the 35S minimal promoter (m35S pro). A hygromycin resistance cassette (P35S pro, hyg^r, and 35SPA) [22] was also added to the construct for selection of stable transformants. pGG624 was constructed in a similar way, except that the RFP-RNAi cassette is deleted from pGG626 [13]

1. Collect sonicated protonemal cells on a 10 cm diameter cellophane-covered BCDAT plate (day 6 or 7); total tissue should not exceed 100 mg. Gently squeeze out the water by sandwiching the cells between paper towels, and then place cells into the mortar.

2. Add liquid nitrogen and grind cells with a pestle.

3. Add 450 µl Buffer RLT containing 3.5 µl β-mercaptoethanol to the mortar.

4. Transfer the lysate to a 1.5 ml tube and vortex vigorously.

5. Transfer the lysate to a QIAshredder spin column and centrifuge for 2 min at 20,000×g.

6. Transfer the supernatant of the flow-through to a new 1.5 ml tube.

7. Add a 1/2 volume of 100% ethanol and mix by pipetting.

8. Transfer the sample to an RNeasy spin column and centrifuge for 30 s at 9000×g.

9. Wash the spin column with 350 µl Buffer RW1.

10. Add 70 µl Buffer RDD with 10 µl DNase to the column and incubate for 20 min at room temperature.

11. Wash the column with 350 µl Buffer RW1.

12. Wash the column with 500 µl Buffer RPE twice.

13. Transfer the column to a new 2.0 ml tube and centrifuge for 1 min at 20,000×g to remove any remaining buffer.

14. Transfer the column to a new 1.5 ml tube.

15. Add 40 µl RNase-free water and centrifuge for 1 min at 9000×g to elute total RNA.

3.1.4 cDNA Synthesis

First-strand cDNA is synthesised from total *P. patens* RNA by using the PrimeScript II first-strand cDNA Synthesis Kit (TAKARA) according to the manufacturer's instructions.

1. Mix RNA and buffers in a PCR tube on ice as follows:

   1 µl Oligo dT primer (50 µM)

   1 µl dNTP mixture (10 mM each)

   3–5 µg Template total RNA

   RNase-free dH$_2$O up to 10 µl

2. Incubate for 5 min at 65 °C and then rapidly cool on ice.

3. Mix the reaction sample (from **step 1**) as follows:

   10 µl Reaction sample (**step 1**)

   4 µl 5× PrimeScript II Buffer

   0.5 µl RNase inhibitor (40 U/µl)

   1 µl PrimeScript II RTase (200 U/µl)

   RNase-free dH$_2$O up to 20 µl

4. Place the tube in the PCR machine using the following conditions:

   42 °C for 30 or 45 min

   95 °C for 5 min

5. Cool rapidly on ice.

3.1.5 PCR and Ligation

PCR is performed with the PrimeSTAR HS DNA Polymerase kit (TAKARA). The PCR product is then digested with *Not*I/*Asc*I and ligated into the plasmid that has pENTR/D-TOPO backbone by using the Mighty Mix DNA Ligation Kit (TAKARA; *see* **Note 6**). The resulting plasmid constitutes the entry vector for the LR reaction.

3.1.6 LR Reaction

The standard Gateway LR reaction (Invitrogen) was performed with some modifications.

1. Linearize the entry vector constructed in Subheading 3.1.5 (~1520 ng) by *Eco*RV, *Apa*I, or *Hpa*I digestion (an enzyme with a single cutting site should be selected).

2. Purify the reaction solution by using DNA Clean & Concentrator (Zymo Research). Elute with 8 μl distilled water.

3. LR reaction: Mix the plasmid and enzyme as follows:

   0.6 μl Linearized entry vector

   0.2 μl Destination vector pGG624 or pGG626 (100 ng/μl)

   0.2 μl Invitrogen Gateway® LR Clonase® II Enzyme mix

4. Incubate tubes at room temperature for 1 h to overnight.

5. Transform into *E. coli*-competent cells (DH5α) and plate on ampicillin-containing plates.

6. Pick ~8 colonies (at least four colonies) and extract the plasmids by using a standard "miniprep" method.

3.1.7 Plasmid Confirmation

The resulting plasmids should be verified by restriction enzyme digestion. Since the protocol involves two LR reactions, plasmid confirmation is more complex than for conventional DNA ligation or a single Gateway LR reaction.

Following the LR reaction, there is 50% probability that the sequences between the two Gateway cassettes (the 300 bp GPAi sequences in pGG624 and pGG626) are inverted; such plasmids can no longer function as RNAi plasmids. The following procedure outlines how to select for correctly recombined plasmids.

1. Digest the plasmid with *Xho*I/*Spe*I and *Xho*I/*Kpn*I (when the RNAi target sequences do not contain *Spe*I, *Xho*I, and/or *Kpn*I sites). As shown in Fig. 2, the band patterns for correct and incorrect recombination are clearly discernible.

2. If the RNAi target sequences contain *Spe*I, *Xho*I, or *Kpn*I sites, use *Pme*I as an alternative (Fig. 2b); however, the difference

a

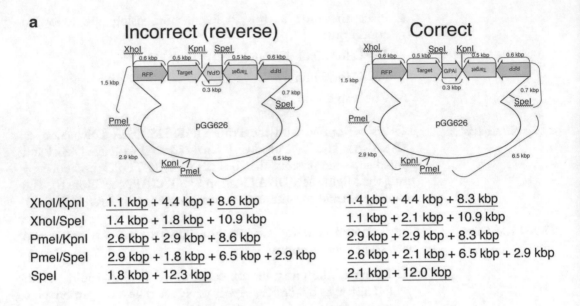

	Incorrect (reverse)	Correct
XhoI/KpnI	1.1 kbp + 4.4 kbp + 8.6 kbp	1.4 kbp + 4.4 kbp + 8.3 kbp
XhoI/SpeI	1.4 kbp + 1.8 kbp + 10.9 kbp	1.1 kbp + 2.1 kbp + 10.9 kbp
PmeI/KpnI	2.6 kbp + 2.9 kbp + 8.6 kbp	2.9 kbp + 2.9 kbp + 8.3 kbp
PmeI/SpeI	2.9 kbp + 1.8 kbp + 6.5 kbp + 2.9 kbp	2.6 kbp + 2.1 kbp + 6.5 kbp + 2.9 kbp
SpeI	1.8 kbp + 12.3 kbp	2.1 kbp + 12.0 kbp

b

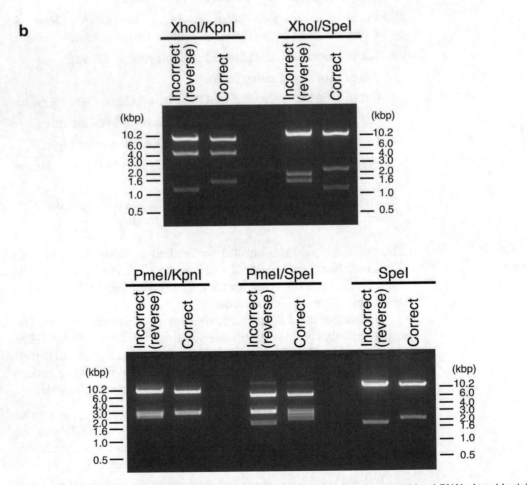

Fig. 2 Plasmid selection method. An example of the selection of correctly recombined RNAi plasmids. (**a**) (*Top panel*) Two Gateway LR reactions result in two plasmid products at equal frequency; the GPAi sequence between

between the band patterns of the correct and incorrect plasmids is more subtle than in Case #1 (*see* **Note 2**).

3.2 Transformation [15]

1. Prepare protonemata of the GFP-tubulin/histoneh2b-mRFP line in ~10 culture dishes (cellophane on top).

2. Prepare the Driselase solution. Add 0.5 g of Driselase to a 50 ml conical tube and add 25 ml of 8% mannitol solution. Mix well for >30 min at room temperature. Centrifuge at $2150 \times g$ for 7 min. Transfer the supernatant to a 20 ml syringe with a 0.22 μm filter unit and filter into a 50 ml centrifuge tube. Discard the pelleted Driselase.

3. Prepare the polyethylene glycol (PEG) solution. Add 1 ml of 1 M $Ca(NO_3)_2$ and 100 μl of 1 M Tris–HCl (pH 8.0) into 9 ml of 8% (w/v) mannitol solution and mix. Filter the solution with a 0.22 μm filter. Add 5 ml of the filtered solution to 2 g autoclaved PEG 6000. Stir for >1 h at room temperature to dissolve the PEG completely.

4. Prepare the MMM solution. Mix 910 mg of mannitol, 150 μl of 1 M $MgCl_2$, 1 ml of 1% MES (pH 5.6), and 8.85 ml of H_2O. Filter the solution by using a 0.22 μm filter.

5. Transfer the propagated, healthy protonemata (collected from ten culture plates) into the Driselase solution with sterile tweezers, and then incubate in the dark at 25 °C for 30 min. Mix gently every 5 min. Healthy protonemata are often obtained 5–6 days following sonication. This amount of protonemata allows for the transformation of ~10 different plasmids.

6. Filter the protonemata through a 50 μm nylon-mesh sheet attached to a funnel.

7. Centrifuge the filtrated protoplasts at $180 \times g$ for 2 min at room temperature, and remove the supernatant with a pipette. Do not discard all of the solution.

8. Rotate the tube very gently by hand and resuspend the centrifuged protoplasts in the remaining 1–2 ml of solution.

9. Resuspend gently in 20 ml of 8% (w/v) mannitol solution. Repeat this washing procedure twice.

10. Count the number of resuspended protoplasts by using a hemocytometer and resuspend to 1.6×10^6 ml^{-1} in MMM solution following centrifugation.

Fig. 2 (continued) the two target-gene sequences is in an opposite orientation in the two products. Only the constructs on the right-hand side are capable of effective RNAi. The target RNAi sequence is 500 bp and pGG626 is used in this example. (*Bottom panel*) The expected band size for each plasmid following restriction enzyme digestion. The underlined values are variable depending on the length of the target RNAi sequence. (**b**) An example of DNA gel electrophoresis following restriction enzyme digestion

11. Add 30 μg of *Pme*I-linearized DNA into a 15 ml round-bottom tube. Then add 300 μl of the protoplast suspension and 300 μl of the PEG solution. Mix gently by tapping the tube 2–3 times.

12. Incubate the tubes containing the transformation mixture in a 45 °C water bath for 5 min, and then in a 20 °C water bath for 10 min.

13. Dilute the transformation mixture by sequentially adding the protoplast liquid medium (300 μl, 500 μl, 700 μl, 1 ml, and 4 ml at 3-min intervals). Upon each addition, mix the solution very gently by tilting the tube.

14. Pour the diluted protoplast solution into a 6 cm Petri dish, seal it with Parafilm, and incubate at 25 °C overnight in the dark.

15. On the next day, prepare the PRM/T solution.

16. Overlay three PRM plates with a sheet of cellophane.

17. Transfer the protoplast suspension into a 15 ml conical tube and centrifuge at $180 \times g$ for 2 min at room temperature.

18. Discard the supernatant and add 9 ml of the PRM/T medium stored at 45 °C. Resuspend the protoplasts gently by pipetting.

19. Pour the protoplast suspension on the cellophane-layered PRM plates ($3 \text{ ml} \times 3$ plates).

20. Seal the Petri dish by using surgical tape. Incubate the plate at 25 °C under continuous white light.

3.3 Line Selection [15]

1. Following 4–6 days of culturing on the PRM plates, the cellophane on which regenerated cells are growing is transferred to a hygromycin-containing BCDAT plate.

2. 3–5 days later, the cellophane is transferred to a drug-free PRM plate. This extra step facilitates the selection of drug-resistant lines in the next step.

3. 4–6 days later, the cellophane is again transferred to a drug-containing BCDAT plate.

4. 3–7 days later, 50–100 colonies are selected and inoculated onto a drug-free BCDAT plate.

5. Colonies are cultured for 10–14 days.

6. A section of moss from each colony is transferred to a drug-containing BCDAT plate.

7. Drug-resistant lines should be identifiable in ~7 days; ≥10 independent transgenic lines are usually obtained.

3.4 Putative RNAi Line Selection Based on Histone-RFP Intensity (Optional; See Note 7)

The RNAi vectors are designed to be integrated into the *PIG1* locus via homologous recombination. However, it is not easy to check the actual integration site and numbers. We therefore skip this step in RNAi screening; it is possible that the selected lines contain multiple copies of the RNAi cassettes at *PIG1* and/or other chromosomal sites. When pGG626 is used as the RNAi vector, putative RNAi transgenic lines are selected on the basis of intensity of histone-RFP, which is constitutively expressed in the parental moss line (*see* **Note** 7).

3.4.1 Preparation of Culture Plates for Imaging [15]

1. Dispense BCD agar medium (15–35 ml) into a 50 ml tube.
2. Melt the BCD agar by using a microwave oven.
3. Add β-estradiol (to a final concentration of 1 μM) and mix well (*see* **Notes** 8 and 9).
4. Pour 3 ml of the BCD β-estradiol agar medium into a 35 mm glass-bottom dish.
5. Cut out the central part of the agar (~1 cm × ~1 cm).
6. Pour ~80 μl of the molten BCD medium (with 1 μM β-estradiol) into the cut area so that a thin agar layer forms on the glass.
7. Inoculate a piece of protonemata from 10 RNAi candidate lines onto five agar dishes prepared as described above (i.e., two lines per dish). Include control lines (parental lines expressing GFP-tubulin and histone-RFP, and if available an RNAi knockdown-confirmed line).
8. Culture for 5 days.

3.4.2 Imaging and Quantification of Histone-RFP Signals

1. By using a fluorescence wide-field microscope with a 10× objective lens, take images of histone-RFP in protonemal tip cells. We typically select four image sites per transgenic line, in which >150 cells can be identified including protonemal tip cells (*see* **Note** 10).
2. Quantify RFP intensities by using ImageJ or other image analysis software.
3. Select five lines with the lowest RFP signal intensities. If essential genes have been knocked down, cells may become very sick by day 5. In such cases, RFP intensity measurements should be performed at earlier time points or the RFP quantification step should be skipped altogether.

3.5   Live Imaging

We usually observe protonemal tissue, in which the actively dividing caulonemal apical cell is the major target (cell cycle duration is ~6 h) [15]. Long-term imaging, such as when image acquisition is conducted every 3 min for ~12 h, is often used for phenotypic screening. For example, an RNAi screen of ~60 kinesin genes involved in nuclear positioning or cell division was performed by using this microscopy [12, 13]. For long-term wide-field imaging, we use 6-well, glass-bottom plates to observe >2 transgenic lines simultaneously (e.g., one control line and multiple RNAi lines). Cells are cultured in a medium containing 1 μM β-estradiol for 3–7 days prior to imaging.

1. **Steps 1–7** of Subheading 3.4.1 are followed with some modifications. In **step 4**, 4.5 ml of the medium is poured into 1–3 wells; in **step 5**, a larger section of the agar medium is cut out; and in **step 7**, two lines are inoculated into each well.

2. To prevent the agar pad from drying out, the 6-well plate is sealed with surgical tape. In addition, 2 ml sterile water is added to each of the three empty wells. Finally, on the day of observation (3–7 days following inoculation), ~500 µl water is gently added to the wells that contain the cells. Imaging should be delayed for 1 h; imaging immediately after water addition should be avoided since the samples will move out of focus during imaging.

3. Multi-site imaging is performed with a 10× objective lens. White light can be used to illuminate the samples in between image acquisitions to activate photosynthesis; otherwise, cell growth may gradually decrease. However, illumination cannot be used if many sites are imaged at each time point.

3.6 Phenotype Screening

GFP-tubulin and histoneh2b-mRFP are good markers for several intracellular events. Through repeated viewing of time-lapse movies of microscopy images, we have identified the following types of phenotypes.

3.6.1 Mitosis

Our screening system, in which protonemal cells are imaged every 3 min for ~12 h, is particularly effective in identifying mitotic errors (Fig. 3a). During imaging, at least a few cells per imaging field enter mitosis (note that cell cycle duration of caulonemal apical cells is ~6 h). The mitotic cells are easily identifiable, since GFP-tubulin signals are strongest during incorporation into the mitotic spindle and phragmoplast. Wild-type cells have a robust spindle assembly checkpoint (SAC); thus, an error in spindle formation (improper microtubule-kinetochore attachment) can result in mitotic delay (up to several hours) [5]. Furthermore, the cell-to-cell variability in mitotic duration is extremely low (nuclear envelope breakdown to sister chromatid separation is 9.5 ± 1.7 min [SD], which corresponds to 3–4 video frames). Thus, the few minutes of delay are likely owing to SAC-accompanying spindle defects.

1. Observe GFP-tubulin and histone-RFP simultaneously on the PC monitor (we suggest a frame rate of 15 frames/s), and screen for a mitotic delay.

2. In our screen, spindle defects accompanying mitotic delay were observed following RNAi of augmin subunits, γ-tubulin and kinesin-5 (Fig. 3a) [4, 5]. By using RT-PCR or immunoblotting, we confirmed that a single RNAi construct simultaneously knocked down multiple paralogues in the case of γ-tubulin and kinesin-5.

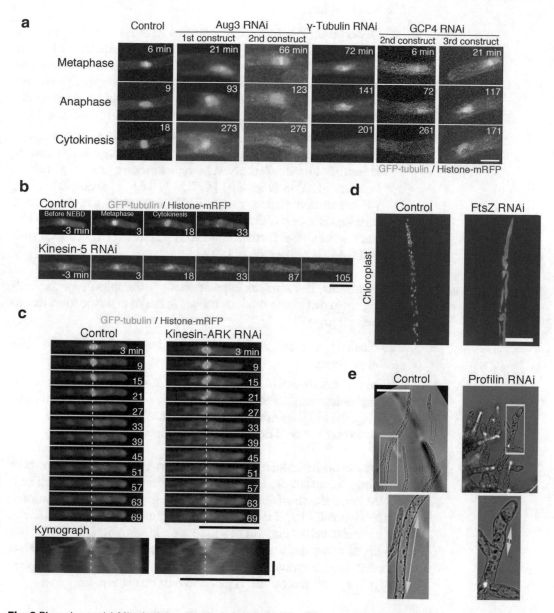

Fig. 3 Phenotypes. (**a**) Mitotic delay associated with spindle defects subsequent to augmin and γ-tubulin RNAi knockdown. Bar, 20 μm. Images originate from Fig. 3B of Nakaoka et al. [5] (Copyright American Society of Plant Biologists; www.plantcell.org). (**b**) Cytokinesis failure subsequent to kinesin-5 RNAi knockdown. Bar, 50 μm. Images originate from Fig. 5F of Miki et al. [4]. (**c**) Nuclear positioning defect subsequent to kinesin-ARK RNAi knockdown. Horizontal bars, 100 μm; vertical bar, 30 min. Images originate from Fig. 3A of Miki et al. [12] (permission of Oxford University Press and Japanese Society of Plant Physiologists). (**d**) Appearance of gigantic chloroplasts due to division failure subsequent to *FtsZ* RNAi knockdown. Bar, 50 μm. Images originate from Supplemental Fig. 3E of Nakaoka et al. [5] (Copyright American Society of Plant Biologists; www.plantcell.org). (**e**) Cell growth defect subsequent to profilin RNAi knockdown. Bar, 100 μm. Images originate from Fig. 1C of Nakaoka et al. [5] (Copyright American Society of Plant Biologists; www.plantcell.org)

3.6.2 Cytokinesis

This phenotype is also easy to identify by using the GFP-tubulin/histone-RFP line.

1. Observe GFP-tubulin and histone-RFP on the PC monitor and screen for binucleated cells in which two nuclei are located side by side in the same cell (Fig. 3b). The GFP-tubulin signal in the cytoplasm serves as an indicator of cell shape. Cytokinesis failure can stem from failure in phragmoplast formation/expansion, which is visualized by GFP-tubulin (*see* **Note 11**).

2. In our screen, cytokinesis failure accompanying phragmoplast defects was observed subsequent to RNAi of augmin, γ-tubulin, kinesin-5, kinesin-7-II (NACK-type kinesin), and microtubule bundler MAP65 (Fig. 3b) [4, 5, 11, 13]. By using RT-PCR, we confirmed that a single RNAi construct simultaneously knocked down multiple paralogues in the case of MAP65. The phenotypes were further analyzed by staining the cell wall with FM4-64 or calcofluor [11, 13].

3.6.3 Nuclear Dynamics

In apical cells, the nucleus is positioned in the middle of the cells during tip growth; the nucleus moves forward at a rate identical to that of cell growth.

1. Nuclear dynamics can be monitored by histone-RFP movement.

2. In our kinesin RNAi screen, an apical cell-specific nuclear positioning defect was identified subsequent to RNAi of kinesin-ARK (Fig. 3c) [12]. By using RT-PCR, we confirmed that a single RNAi construct knocked down multiple paralogues simultaneously.

3.6.4 Chloroplast Dynamics

Autofluorescent chloroplasts are easy to visualize by fluorescent imaging, for example, by using the Cy5 filter. We confirmed that RNAi knockdown of *FtsZ*, a well-known gene required for chloroplast division [19, 20], produced gigantic chloroplasts in the protonemal cells (Fig. 3d) [5]. In our kinesin RNAi screen, we observed other defects in chloroplast morphology and distribution in a few lines; however, we have yet to confirm whether these phenotypes are caused by the knockdown of target kinesin genes.

3.6.5 Cell Growth

Protonemal cells exhibit tip growth [21]. Genes required for tip growth have been successfully identified by using the transient RNAi method; a constitutive RNAi vector was transformed into protoplasts and cells were screened for chloronemal apical cell tip growth [8–10]. By using our inducible RNAi transgenic line system, we confirmed the results obtained for the profilin gene; RNAi knockdown significantly impaired tip growth, and therefore shorter cells were predominantly observed (Fig. 3e) [5]. However, since numerous genes are required for cell growth, off-target effects of RNAi or insertion of the RNAi vector into a locus affecting the expression of genes critical for cell growth occur more frequently.

Furthermore, we noticed that subtle differences in culture media conditions, such as the extent of culture medium dehydration, could also significantly affect cell growth.

1. Observe GFP-tubulin to assess cell growth or morphology, since GFP-tubulin is distributed throughout the cytoplasm.

2. When a phenotype related to cell growth is observed, such as slow cell growth, wavy cells, or the appearance of numerous branched cells, verify whether the culture medium is over-dehydrated.

3. If the culture medium looks normal, mark the lines as putative hits. However, a phenotype should only be associated with the target gene if it is verified by gene disruption or rescue experiments (*see* **Note 12**). Transient RNAi is also a good method for assessing cell growth phenotypes. This method can be combined with expression of an RNAi-resistant gene (rescue experiment).

4. Cell growth phenotypes are often associated with longer or shorter cell size. However, if apical cells retain tip-growing abilities, cell length varies according to cell cycle. Therefore, when cell length is quantified, the second apical cell should be measured (Fig. 3e).

3.7 Phenotype Confirmation by Using Rescue Experiments

When two non-overlapping dsRNA sequences give rise to an identical phenotype, it is quite likely that the phenotype is due to depletion of the target gene (and its paralogues). RNAi off-target effects can be completely excluded through (1) gene disruption or (2) rescue experiments. Here, we describe the procedure for rescue experiments.

1. An RNAi-insensitive gene is synthesized and inserted into the "rescue vector," which contains a constitutively active EF1α promoter and drug-resistant marker (Table 1; Fig. 4 *see* **Note 13**). The plasmids also contain *PTA1* gene sequences for integration into this nonessential locus. The gene is preferably tagged with a fluorescent marker that can be imaged separately from GFP or RFP (e.g., CFP [Cerulean]). The protein expression is confirmed by fluorescent imaging or immunoblotting.

2. Follow Subheading 3.2 and transform the plasmids into the RNAi candidate line and select by drug. The empty vector (Table 1) should be transformed as a control. Select >10 independent lines.

3. Screen for CFP (Cerulean)-expressing lines.

4. Follow Subheading 3.5 and perform time-lapse imaging.

5. Observe the phenotype; if the RNAi phenotype is the result of target gene knockdown, the CFP (Cerulean)-positive cells will not exhibit the phenotype.

Table 1
Plasmids available for inducible RNAi and ectopic gene expression

1. RNAi vector

Plasmid name	Purpose	Drug resistance in *P. patens*	Expected integration site[a]
pGG624	Inducible RNAi vector	Hygromycin	*PIG1*
pGG626	Inducible RNAi vector with partial RFP sequence	Hygromycin	*PIG1*

2. Gene over-expression vectors for RNAi-rescue experiments (Fig. 4)

Plasmid name	Purpose	Drug resistance in *P. patens*	Expected integration site[a]	Notes
pTM153	Gene over-expression vector (BSD)	Blasticidin S	*PTA1*	
pTM409	Gene over-expression vector (BSD) with mCherry	Blasticidin S	*PTA1*	mCherry codon usage is altered so that it is resistant to pGG626-based RNAi
pTM410	Gene over-expression vector (BSD) with Cerulean CFP	Blasticidin S	*PTA1*	
pTM415	mCherry over-expression vector (BSD)	Blasticidin S	*PTA1*	Used as a control. mCherry codon usage is altered so that it is resistant to pGG626-based RNAi
pTM416	Cerulean CFP over-expression vector (BSD)	Blasticidin S	*PTA1*	Used as a control
pMN601	Gene over-expression vector (NTC)	Nourseothricin (NTC)	*PTA1*	
pMN602	Gene over-expression vector (NTC) with mCherry	Nourseothricin (NTC)	*PTA1*	mCherry codon usage is altered so that it is resistant to pGG626-based RNAi
pMN603	Gene over-expression vector (NTC) with Cerulean CFP	Nourseothricin (NTC)	*PTA1*	
pMN605	mCherry over-expression vector (NTC)	Nourseothricin (NTC)	*PTA1*	Used as a control. mCherry codon usage is altered so that it is resistant to pGG626-based RNAi
pMN606	Cerulean CFP over-expression vector (NTC)	Nourseothricin (NTC)	*PTA1*	Used as a control

The plasmids are constructed on the basis of pT1OG (PHYSCOmanual). Transformation should be performed subsequent to *Pme*I digestion
[a]We have never verified whether these plasmids actually integrate at the expected site

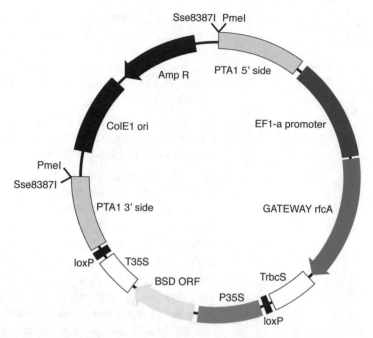

Fig. 4 Plasmid for RNAi-rescue experiments. A simplified map of gene overexpression vector pTM153. Other useful vectors are listed in Table 1. pMN601 contains a marker gene conferring resistance to nourseothricin (NTC) instead of blasticidin S (BSD). In pTM409/410 and pMN602/603, the GATEWAY *rfcA* sequence is followed by sequences that encode a fluorescent protein (mCherry or Cerulean [a CFP variant]). In pTM415/416 and pMN605/606, the GATEWAY *rfcA* sequence is replaced by mCherry or Cerulean CFP sequences

4 Notes

1. An *E. coli* strain resistant to the toxic effect of the *ccdB* sequences (e.g., the DB3.1 strain) should be used for the propagation of pGG624 and pGG626.

2. Linearization of the RNAi plasmid by *Pme*I digestion is critical for transformation. Therefore, the target sequences must not have *Pme*I cleavage sites. Furthermore, if possible, select sequences that do not contain additional cleavage sites for *Xho*I, *Kpn*I, or *Spe*I. These enzymes are useful for selecting correct plasmids following the Gateway LR reaction (Subheading 3.1.7 and Fig. 2).

3. In order to achieve co-knockdown of paralogous genes at a higher probability, multiple sequences, each 100 % identical to one of the genes, can be fused in tandem [4, 13]. However, the knockdown efficiency is not always higher using this fusion construct; a single target sequence that recognizes multiple paralogous genes sometimes induces a more complete knockdown [4].

4. In contrast, when we designed primers for kinesin RNAi screening, we avoided selecting the most homologous region that corresponds to the kinesin motor domain, since non-paralogous kinesin genes might be unnecessarily co-knocked down (note that kinesins constitute a large superfamily of 78 genes) [12].

5. It is important to ensure that the primer sets do not exactly match the paralogous genes, in particular when the regions of highest homology are selected.

6. We use the pENTR/D-TOPO vector for cloning, which should enable directional cloning. However, since the target genes are at times reversely cloned, we prefer conventional ligation by using *Not*I/*Asc*I digestion.

7. Although our RNAi screen for kinesin genes was performed with pGG626 (co-knockdown of the target protein and histone-RFP), we have recently switched to using pGG624 (knockdown of only the target protein) for the following two reasons. First, the decreased histone-RFP signals due to the use of pGG626 can hinder nuclear dynamics monitoring. Second, in our experience, inducible RNAi knockdown of a target protein is effective in at least one of the ten randomly selected transgenic lines. Therefore, RNAi screening can be conducted without the time-consuming pre-selection of candidate RNAi lines based on histone-RFP intensity.

8. The stock solution of β-estradiol (1–100 mM in DMSO) should be stored at –80 °C. Avoid repeated freezing/thawing.

9. β-Estradiol should be used only when RNAi induction is desired. RNAi efficiency gradually decreases when cells are constantly exposed to β-estradiol.

10. Importantly, the histone-RFP signal intensity is generally lower in caulonemal cells than in chloronemal cells. Therefore, transgenic lines in which the chloronema to caulonema conversion is impaired tend to have higher histone-RFP signals, even when RNAi is appropriately induced. Therefore, the histone-RFP signals should only be quantified and compared in either caulonemal or chloronemal cells.

11. Multi-nuclei can be detected without time-lapse imaging while the histone-RFP signal is quantified. However, the appearance of multinucleated cells is not necessarily because of cytokinesis failure. For example, chromosome missegregation could lead to the formation of micronuclei [4]. Time-lapse imaging can clarify the basis of multinuclear phenotype.

12. Cell growth defects are the most commonly observed phenotypes during screening. Even when two non-overlapping constructs

give rise to the identical phenotypes, we cannot conclude that the phenotype is due to the target gene without confirmation through rescue experiments (or gene disruption analysis).

13. If a UTR is targeted by RNAi, simply amplify the ORF region of the endogenous gene by PCR; the ORF sequence should not be targeted by the UTR RNAi.

Links

1. PHYSCOmanual ver. 2.0

   http://www.nibb.ac.jp/evodevo/PHYSCOmanual/00Eindex.htm

2. Phytozome—plant genome sequence database, including *P. patens*

   http://phytozome.jgi.doe.gov/pz/portal.html

Acknowledgements

We are grateful to Mitsuyasu Hasebe, Yuji Hiwatashi, Minoru Kubo, and other former and current Hasebe laboratory members for all moss reagents and valuable information regarding the techniques associated with moss culturing and imaging. We also wish to thank Akiko Tomioka and Momoko Nishina for protocol development and Moé Yamada for reading the manuscript. The moss work in our laboratory is supported by the Human Frontier Science Program, the TORAY Science Foundation, and Grants-in-Aid for Scientific Research (15H01227, 15K14540 and 26711012; MEXT, Japan).

References

1. Cove D (2005) The moss Physcomitrella patens. Annu Rev Genet 39:339–358

2. Cove D, Bezanilla M, Harries P et al (2006) Mosses as model systems for the study of metabolism and development. Annu Rev Plant Biol 57:497–520

3. Prigge MJ, Bezanilla M (2010) Evolutionary crossroads in developmental biology: Physcomitrella patens. Development 137:3535–3543

4. Miki T, Naito H, Nishina M et al (2014) Endogenous localizome identifies 43 mitotic kinesins in a plant cell. Proc Natl Acad Sci U S A 111:E1053–E1061

5. Nakaoka Y, Miki T, Fujioka R et al (2012) An inducible RNA interference system in Physcomitrella patens reveals a dominant role of augmin in phragmoplast microtubule generation. Plant Cell 24:1478–1493

6. Vidali L, Rounds CM, Hepler PK et al (2009) Lifeact-mEGFP reveals a dynamic apical F-actin network in tip growing plant cells. PLoS One 4, e5744

7. Jonsson E, Yamada M, Vale RD et al (2015) Clustering of a kinesin-14 motor enables processive retrograde microtubule-based transport in plants. Nat Plants 1, 15087.

8. Vidali L, Augustine RC, Kleinman KP et al (2007) Profilin is essential for tip growth in the moss Physcomitrella patens. Plant Cell 19:3705–3722

9. Vidali L, Burkart GM, Augustine RC et al (2010) Myosin XI is essential for tip growth in Physcomitrella patens. Plant Cell 22:1868–1882

10. van Gisbergen PA, Li M, Wu SZ et al (2012) Class II formin targeting to the cell cortex by

binding PI(3,5)P(2) is essential for polarized growth. J Cell Biol 198:235–250

11. Kosetsu K, de Keijzer J, Janson ME et al (2013) MICROTUBULE-ASSOCIATED PROTEIN65 is essential for maintenance of phragmoplast bipolarity and formation of the cell plate in Physcomitrella patens. Plant Cell 25:4479–4492

12. Miki T, Nishina M, Goshima G (2015) RNAi screening identifies the armadillo repeat-containing kinesins responsible for microtubule-dependent nuclear positioning in Physcomitrella patens. Plant Cell Physiol 56:737–749

13. Naito H, Goshima G (2015) NACK kinesin is required for metaphase chromosome alignment and cytokinesis in the moss Physcomitrella patens. Cell Struct Funct 40:31–41

14. Nakaoka Y, Kimura A, Tani T et al (2015) Cytoplasmic nucleation and atypical branching nucleation generate endoplasmic microtubules in Physcomitrella patens. Plant Cell 27:228–242

15. Yamada M, Miki T, Goshima G (2016) Imaging mitosis in the moss Physcomitrella patens. Methods Mol Biol 1413:263–282

16. Kubo M, Imai A, Nishiyama T et al (2013) System for stable beta-estradiol-inducible gene expression in the moss Physcomitrella patens. PLoS One 8, e77356

17. Zuo J, Niu QW, Chua NH (2000) Technical advance: an estrogen receptor-based transactivator XVE mediates highly inducible gene expression in transgenic plants. Plant J 24:265–273

18. Okano Y, Aono N, Hiwatashi Y et al (2009) A polycomb repressive complex 2 gene regulates apogamy and gives evolutionary insights into early land plant evolution. Proc Natl Acad Sci U S A 106:16321–16326

19. Bezanilla M, Perroud PF, Pan A et al (2005) An RNAi system in Physcomitrella patens with an internal marker for silencing allows for rapid identification of loss of function phenotypes. Plant Biol (Stuttg) 7:251–257

20. Strepp R, Scholz S, Kruse S et al (1998) Plant nuclear gene knockout reveals a role in plastid division for the homolog of the bacterial cell division protein FtsZ, an ancestral tubulin. Proc Natl Acad Sci U S A 95:4368–4373

21. Rounds CM, Bezanilla M (2013) Growth mechanisms in tip-growing plant cells. Annu Rev Plant Biol 64:243–265

22. Hiwatashi Y, Obara M, Sato Y et al (2008) Kinesins are indispensable for interdigitation of phragmoplast microtubules in the moss Physcomitrella patens. Plant Cell 20:3094–3106

Chapter 19

Data Analysis for High-Throughput RNAi Screening

David O. Azorsa, Megan A. Turnidge, and Shilpi Arora

Abstract

High-throughput RNA interference (HT-RNAi) screening is an effective technology to help identify important genes and pathways involved in a biological process. Analysis of high-throughput RNAi screening data is a critical part of this technology, and many analysis methods have been described. Here, we summarize the workflow and types of analyses commonly used in high-throughput RNAi screening.

Key words RNAi screening, Data analysis, Normalization

1 Introduction

High-throughput RNAi (HT-RNAi) screening is an efficient technique commonly used in reverse genetics and target discovery [1–7]. The ultimate goal of HT-RNAi screening is to effectively knockdown expression or silence hundreds or thousands of genes independently, in order to observe and measure any changes in a biological process caused by the knockdown of these genes. Methods for HT-RNAi screening have been mentioned in other chapters, and mainly involve the use of large commercially available libraries of either chemically synthesized short interfering RNA (siRNA) or virally delivered short hairpin RNA (shRNA) that can silence hundreds or thousands of genes. Thus, the HT-RNAi screening results in large quantities of data. Since high-throughput screening of compound libraries also produces large amounts of data, many analysis methods for HT-RNAi screening have been adapted from methods used for high-throughput compound screening. Numerous reports have described the various analysis methods used in HT-RNAi analysis [8–14]. In this chapter, we briefly describe the most commonly used methods for analysis of HT-RNAi screens.

David O. Azorsa, Shilpi Arora (eds.), *High-Throughput RNAi Screening: Methods and Protocols*, Methods in Molecular Biology, vol. 1470, DOI 10.1007/978-1-4939-6337-9_19, © Springer Science+Business Media New York 2016

2   HT-RNAi Screening Workflow

Effective data analysis for HT-RNAi screening begins with the use of a robust assay for screening. HT-RNAi screens that use siRNA libraries are predominately cell-based assays and thus involve the inherited variability associated with cell-based assays. Once an intensive assay development step has been completed, and the assay is shown to effectively detect and measure phenotypic or molecular changes in a reproducible manner, it can be expected that the HT-RNAi screen will produce robust data for analysis. The workflow of data analysis commonly used in HT-RNAi screening includes quality control, normalization, and hit selection (Fig. 1). A typical HT-RNAi screening project begins with a preliminary screen to establish the assay parameters and to confirm a high-quality assay with optimal controls. This preliminary or pilot screen is usually a smaller screen consisting of a focused set of siRNAs along with control samples. Results from the pilot screen can provide important information about the quality of the assay. Types of control siRNAs commonly used in the pilot screen include the negative and positive control siRNAs, siRNAs that result in specific phenotypic changes

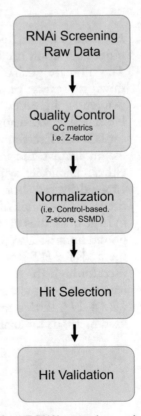

Fig. 1 Typical workflow for HT-RNAi screening analysis. The raw data from an HT-RNAi screen is assessed for quality control followed by normalization and hit selection leading to validation of the hits

for the assay readout, and siRNAs that can be used to assess transfection efficiency. The plate layout for the pilot screen should be similar to the HT-RNAi screen and contain sufficient control wells to be used in analysis. An optimal plate layout will have sufficient controls to show assay robustness and help identify inter-plate and intra-plate variations [15]. As a rule of thumb, the accuracy of the experiment increases with the number of control wells used. Other assay parameters that are assessed in a pilot screen include optimal cell density, incubation times, and readout conditions.

Depending on the goal of the HT-RNAi screen, it should be decided beforehand if assay replicates will be performed and which type of replicate should be used. Both technical and biological replicates [16] can be included in HT-RNAi screening, and the number of replicates to be performed assessed is usually determined by the question asked and the resources available. In many cases, scientists may want to discuss their individual HT-RNAi screening experiments with a biostatistician to confirm that the experiment is statistically robust and has enough replicates to generate meaningful data. Once the assay has been established, the actual HT-RNAi screen is performed using defined parameters, and the resulting raw data is collected for data analysis. Most readouts from HT-RNAi screens are measured using multimode plate readers capable of measuring absorbance, fluorescence, or luminescence. The raw data, usually txt or csv files, can be easily transferred to a spreadsheet that can be used for data formatting and several types of basic analyses. A typical plot of the raw data for a large-viability siRNA screen is shown in Fig. 2. Once the HT-RNAi data is formatted, it can be analyzed for quality control (QC) using selected metrics. Following QC, the raw data is normalized using one or more statistical methods, and statistical cutoffs are set for hit selection. If needed, further analysis is performed on the selected set of hits from the screen.

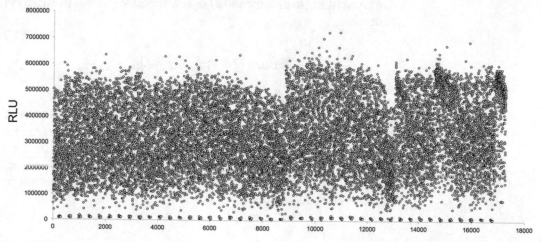

Fig. 2 Typical example of raw data for a phenotypic viability-based druggable genome siRNA library screen. RLU: relative luminescence units

3   Quality Control

Quality control (QC) is a critical part of HT-RNAi screening, and numerous reports have described the importance and challenges of QC [17, 18] and various methods of assessing QC [9, 19, 20]. Most plate-based HT-RNAi screens are performed in 96-well or 384-well plates and require a large number of plates to complete a screen of hundreds or thousands of gene targets. With such a large number of plates, QC is vital to a successful screen. Plate-to-plate variation is common in these screens, and could affect the robustness of the screen. Analysis of control wells in an HT-RNAi screen, as well as the use of QC metrics, can reveal critical information about the reliability and variability of the overall screen. Routinely used QC metrics include signal-to-noise ratio (S/N), signal-to-background ratio (S/B), and the Z-factor [19, 21]. Both S/N and S/B metrics are often used in high-throughput screening (HTS) of compounds, but they do not take into account assay variability. This variability can be significant in cell-based assays, particularly RNAi screening. The equations for S/N and S/B depend on the mean (μ) values for the negative (n) and positive (p) controls and the standard deviation (σ) of the negative control:

$$S / N = \left(\mu_p - \mu_n \right) / \sigma_n$$

$$S / B = \mu_p / \mu_n$$

The most common QC metric used to assess the robustness of each plate is the Z-factor or Z' [21]. Z-factor measures the fidelity of the assay on a per plate, per set, and per experiment basis [10, 18, 22]. Z-factor depends on four parameters including the standard deviation (σ) and mean (μ) of the negative (n) and positive (p) controls:

$$Z - factor = 1 - 3 \left(\sigma_\pi + \sigma_v \right) / \left| \mu_p - \mu_n \right|$$

Other types of analysis for assessing QC of HT-RNAi screens include using data visualization techniques such as heat maps and QC plots [9]. Both heat maps (Fig. 3) and QC plots can be used to identify trends and shifts in the HT-RNAi screen. Data that does not meet QC metrics should be removed from further analysis to improve assay reliability.

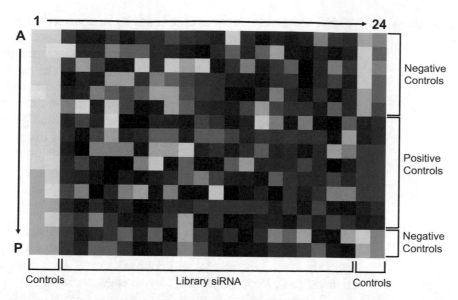

Fig. 3 Representative heat map of an assay plate used in HT-RNAi screening. The raw data from a 384-well HT-RNAi screening plate is visualized as a heat map showing relative activity of both positive and negative controls. The heat map was generated using Partek Analysis Software by Daniel H. Wai, Phoenix Children's Hospital

4   Normalization and Hit Selection

Once the HT-RNAi data has passed QC, the data is analyzed, usually beginning with a normalization step. Numerous reports of normalization and analysis methods in HT-RNAi analysis have been described [8–11, 13], and several useful Web-based analysis tools are also available [10, 23–25]. Since normalization of HT-RNAi screening data is a critical step in data analysis of HT-RNAi screens, it is often analyzed using more than one method. The two basic types of normalization are control-based and sample-based normalization [11, 18]. Control-based normalization, or percent of control (POC), is calculated by dividing the sample value (x_i) by the mean of selected control wells (μ_n) and multiplying the result by 100:

$$POC = \left(x_i \ / \ \mu_n \right) \times 100$$

This type of normalization is often favored for its straightforward calculation and ease of interpretation. It is important to use as many control values as possible to increase accuracy. Sample-based normalization, or percent of samples (POS), uses the same equation but replaces the mean of selected control wells with the mean of all samples on the plate. This method is useful when fewer potential hits are expected on a plate. The higher number of control replicates improves accuracy of the assay, but it is important to be wary of plate-to-plate variation that may cause hits to be masked and less significant data points to look more promising.

4.1   Z-Score Analysis   The Z-score or "standard score" (not to be confused with Z-factor or Z′) is based on the assumption that the data is normally distributed and that most samples will not be hits. The Z-score is generally defined as the number of standard deviations from the mean, and it is commonly used to analyze HT-RNAi screening data as it evaluates the strength of each sample compared to the other samples being analyzed [8, 11, 18]. Z-score depends on three parameters, the raw sample value (x), the standard deviation of the population (σ), and the mean (μ) of the population:

$$Z = (x - \mu) / \sigma$$

A comparison of the Z-score versus percent of control for a HT-RNAi run is shown in Fig. 4. It is common to use Z-score analysis in the primary screen, or in screens without replicates, as the Z-score assumes that each siRNA or sample will have the same variability.

A variation of the Z-score is the robust Z-score, which uses the median of the population rather than the mean, and the median absolute deviation (MAD) rather than the standard deviation [11, 26]. This method minimizes the effect of extreme outliers in the data. Similar to percent control analysis, Z-scores and robust Z-scores can be calculated on a per plate, per batch, or per experiment basis, although it is usually done on a per plate basis due to possible plate-to-plate variability. Furthermore, to eliminate bias due to the positive and negative control wells, these control values should be omitted from the Z-score

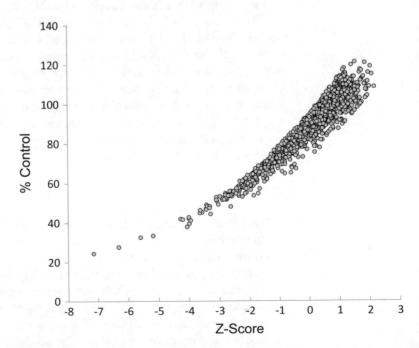

Fig. 4 Comparison of percent control and Z-score values for viability of a focused siRNA screen set

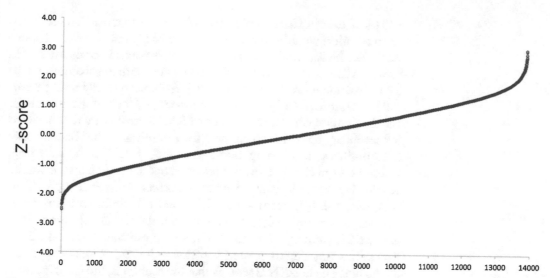

Fig. 5 Typical waterfall plot of Z-score normalized values for viability of a typical druggable genome siRNA screen

analysis. After computation of the Z-score values for a particular screen, the cutoffs or thresholds for hit selection are established. The Z-score values of RNAi screens can also be plotted as waterfall plots (Fig. 5) to more clearly depict the distribution of sample values.

4.2 Other Normalization and Analysis Methods

B-score analysis is often used to minimize or exclude positional effects that can be seen in HT-RNAi screening [8, 18]. Several groups have combined B-score analysis with subsequent Z-score analysis to use as part of their HT-RNAi analysis and hit selection [27–30]. Though mainly used in very large compound screens, B-score can be useful in analysis of HT-RNAi screening where positional effects might be an issue. Another analysis method that has more recently been applied to HT-RNAi screening is the strictly standardized mean difference (SSMD), which can be used to assess QC and hit selection [31, 32]. SSMD considers the measured sample (x), the mean (μ_n) of the negative controls, and the standard deviation (σ_n) of the negative controls. For a screen without replicates:

$$SSMD = (x - \mu_n) / (\sqrt{2}\sigma_n)$$

An advantage of using SSMD is that it can be more robust when comparing different sample size, which leads to improved comparison across different sized assays [22, 26].

4.3 Hit Selection

Hit selection can be considered the end goal in HT-RNAi screening. It is commonly done using standard statistical analytical methods including the normalization methods previously described. Several reports are available that describe the advantages and disadvantages of commonly used hit selection methods including Z-score analysis [8, 18, 22], SSMD [18, 22], t-statistics [18, 22], and clustering techniques

[33]. Hit selection for typical HT-RNAi screens that use Z-score-based normalization would require setting thresholds that are assay dependent. The hit list would consist of the samples outside of the threshold values. Many groups have used cutoff values ranging from ±1.64 to ±2.0 depending on the assay [34–36]. Another typically used threshold is a Z-score of ±1.96, which corresponds to 95% of the area under the distribution curve and a p-value of 0.5. These hits are then selected for secondary screening to confirm their significance and help identify false positives. Depending upon the type of HT-RNAi screening, researchers can choose to further categorize the hits obtained from the screen. For example, if a genome-wide screen was performed, scientists, with the help from a statistician and a bioinformatician, could perform a pathway analysis to determine if the hits are clustering into any specific pathways of interest. The group can then focus on validation of hits targeting these specific pathways instead of following up on all the hits. For HT-RNAi screens that use replicates, the use of t-statistics is useful for analysis and hit selection [18, 22, 37]. Using t-statistics allows for the comparison of several data sets, and provides p-values.

4.4 Analysis of Pooled shRNA Screening

HT-RNAi screening using pooled shRNAs can be easier to perform than plate-based siRNA screening, as it usually utilizes barcoded pooled shRNA to transduce a population of cells. This type of HT-RNAi screening involves extensive sequencing capabilities, as the hits are identified based on the analysis of barcoded shRNA. Analysis of pooled shRNA screens may use methods similar to those of siRNA screens [38], but it also involves microarray- or sequence-based analysis techniques. In many of the early genome-wide barcode-based shRNA screens, normalization often used standard microarray normalization methods such as log ratios [39]. Since next-generation sequencing is now more common than microarray-based methods, sequence-based analysis steps such as sequence alignment are integrated in the overall analysis method [40]. The resulting data, usually log ratios, can be further analyzed using many of the tools used for siRNA library screening. Another way to select hits for pooled shRNA screens is to analyze the shRNA from cells or organisms that show a phenotype of interest. In some instances, such as in dropout viability screens, hits are selected by analyzing a set of cells or organisms that remain viable or adherent. Experiments that utilize this type of analysis have identified genes essential in cell viability [40–42] and involved in synthetic lethal interactions [43]. Other types of pooled shRNA screens selected for specific phenotypes such as increased colony formation to identify genes involved in metastasis [44] or directly enriched for a specific population using immunomagnetic beads [45]. Analysis of these types of screens usually involves using standard statistical analysis. It has become a common practice to include more than one type of screening methodology in the primary and validation screens of an HT-RNAi assay. For example, if the HT-RNAi screen was performed used an siRNA platform, the validation of hits is performed utilizing specific shRNA reagents targeting these hits. Such a practice eliminates technology biases and identifies high confidence or true hits.

4.5 Analysis of Drug Sensitization HT-RNAi Screens

One popular application of HT-RNAi screening is the identification of genes that modulate drug response, particularly those that sensitize cells to a drug of interest [28, 37, 46–48]. For these types of assays, parallel sets of plates are run. These two plate sets are usually drug-treated and vehicle-treated (or untreated) sets. Analysis is focused on comparison of the drug-treated set to the vehicle (or untreated) set with the goal being to identify siRNA/shRNA that result in enhanced drug activity. Although standard normalization methods can be used, common plate-based or non-control-based normalization such as B-score, Z-score, and robust Z-score can mask differences between drug-treated and vehicle-treated (or untreated) samples [49]. Therefore, a control-based normalization is recommended, as well as having reference wells or non-drug-treated wells on all plates. Another approach requires setting up sets of plates treated with multiple concentrations of a drug to perform drug dose–response curves for each siRNA. This approach has previously been used to identify several drug-sensitizing targets [50, 51]. Analysis of these types of screens focuses on control-based normalization of the plates and calculation of dose–response curves across the differently treated sets. Hits include those siRNAs that significantly change the IC50 (half maximal response) value of the drug. Although this approach provides true chemosensitization activity, its major drawback is the big resource commitment required to perform such a screen; thus this sort of screen is more common when working with focused set libraries rather than genome-wide screens.

4.6 Other Resources

To assist researchers with HT-RNAi data analysis, several open-access data analysis packages and Web-based analysis tools have been developed [23–25]. A list of websites with tools for HT-RNAi analysis is shown in Table 1. Furthermore, websites with general information on HT-RNAi screening are described in Table 2. These websites provide a wealth of information for new and established users of HT-RNAi screening. The cellHTS2 Web application provides a user-friendly interface for RNAi screening data analysis [10, 24]. Similarly, the Web application RNAither provides complete analysis from QC, data normalization, and hit selection [23]. The Web application ScreenSifter [52] is another open-source desktop application developed to facilitate storing, statistical analysis, and rapid and intuitive biological data mining of HT-RNAi screening datasets. The application of GUItars differs from the other Web-based analysis tools by including SSMD analysis [25]. Needless to say, analysis methods for HT-RNAi screens have advanced greatly, and today there are various resources for HT-RNAi screening analysis that can facilitate HT-RNAi screening done by new and experienced investigators. HT-RNAi as a functional genomics platform has been shown to be a powerful

Table 1
Online references for HT-RNAi screening analysis

HT-RNAi analysis site	Description	Website
cellHTS2 Data Analysis Software (Bioconductor) [24]	Software for analysis of HTS data; has capabilities for B-score and other methods to normalize and score the data	https://bioconductor.org/packages/release/bioc/html/cellHTS2.html http://web-cellhts2.dkfz.de/cellHTS-java/cellHTS2/
Screensaver HTS	Application for storing RNAi screen information and facilitating data sharing between members of a lab or HTS facility	http://sourceforge.net/projects/screensaver/
Screen Sifter [52]	Desktop application for storage and analysis of RNAi data, useful for comparisons between screens	http://www.screensifter.com/
GUItars RNAi HTS Data Analysis Software [25]	Software that analyzes HT-RNAi data using the strictly standardized mean difference (SSMD) method	http://sourceforge.net/projects/guitars/
RNAither Data Analysis Software (Bioconductor) [23]	Software for analyzing HT-RNAi data; includes QC, data normalization, and different statistical test for hit selection	https://www.bioconductor.org/packages/release/bioc/html/RNAither.html
RSA RNAi Data Analysis Algorithm (GNF)	Algorithm for analyzing data using the redundant siRNA activity (RSA) method of data analysis, software available for Windows C# or Perl/Python/R language	http://carrier.gnf.org/publications/RSA/
DecoRNAi (QBRC)	Software for deconvoluting RNAi data by correcting for off-target effects; also provides corrected Z-scores	http://qbrc.swmed.edu/softwares.html
synlet (Bioconductor)	Software for synthetic lethal RNAi screening data analysis	https://bioconductor.org/packages/3.2/bioc/html/synlet.html

technique, and has laid the groundwork for the next generation of functional genomic techniques involved in gene editing.

Table 2

Online references for RNAi screening

HT-RNAi screening site	Description	Website
Cell-Based RNAi Assay Development for HTS (NIH)	In-depth walk through on setup, experimental methods, and analysis of RNAi HTS	http://www.ncbi.nlm.nih.gov/books/NBK91998/?report=reader
Minimum Information About an RNAi Experiment (MIARE)	Proposed guidelines for data reporting	http://www.miare.org
DESeq2 (Bioconductor)	Analysis package for differential gene expression based on negative binomial distribution. Can be used for HT-RNAi normalization	https://bioconductor.org/packages/release/bioc/html/DESeq2.html
NCBI probe	Searching for known siRNA sequences	http://www.ncbi.nlm.nih.gov/probe
GenomeRNAi	Database of RNAi, the genes they silence, and the corresponding phenotype in humans and fruit flies	http://www.genomernai.org/
RNAi Codex	Collection of shRNA used in RNAi screens in humans, mice, rats, fruit flies, and Arabidopsis	http://cancan.cshl.edu/cgi-bin/Codex/Codex.cgi
The RNAi Web	General guidelines for designing your own RNAi	http://www.rnaiweb.com/RNAi/siRNA_Design/

Acknowledgements

The authors would like to thank Daniel H. Wai for his valuable contribution in preparing the heat map.

References

1. Aza-Blanc P, Cooper CL, Wagner K, Batalov S, Deveraux QL, Cooke MP (2003) Identification of modulators of TRAIL-induced apoptosis via RNAi-based phenotypic screening. Mol Cell 12(3):627–637

2. Willingham AT, Deveraux QL, Hampton GM, Aza-Blanc P (2004) RNAi and HTS: exploring cancer by systematic loss-of-function. Oncogene 23(51):8392–8400. doi:10.1038/sj.onc.1208217

3. Mohr SE, Smith JA, Shamu CE, Neumuller RA, Perrimon N (2014) RNAi screening comes of age: improved techniques and complementary approaches. Nat Rev Mol Cell Biol 15(9):591–600. doi:10.1038/nrm3860

4. Iorns E, Lord CJ, Turner N, Ashworth A (2007) Utilizing RNA interference to enhance cancer drug discovery. Nat Rev Drug Discov 6(7):556–568. doi:10.1038/nrd2355

5. Falschlehner C, Steinbrink S, Erdmann G, Boutros M (2010) High-throughput RNAi screening to dissect cellular pathways: a how-to guide. Biotechnol J 5(4):368–376. doi:10.1002/biot.200900277

6. Mullenders J, Bernards R (2009) Loss-of-function genetic screens as a tool to improve the diagnosis and treatment of cancer. Oncogene 28(50):4409–4420. doi:10.1038/onc.2009.295

7. Echeverri CJ, Perrimon N (2006) High-throughput RNAi screening in cultured cells: a user's guide. Nat Rev Genet 7(5):373–384. doi:10.1038/nrg1836

8. Brideau C, Gunter B, Pikounis B, Liaw A (2003) Improved statistical methods for hit selection in high-throughput screening. J Biomol Screen 8(6):634–647. doi:10.1177/1087057103258285

9. Gunter B, Brideau C, Pikounis B, Liaw A (2003) Statistical and graphical methods for quality control determination of high-throughput screening data. J Biomol Screen 8(6):624–633. doi:10.1177/1087057103258284

10. Boutros M, Bras LP, Huber W (2006) Analysis of cell-based RNAi screens. Genome Biol 7(7):R66. doi:10.1186/gb-2006-7-7-R66

11. Malo N, Hanley JA, Cerquozzi S, Pelletier J, Nadon R (2006) Statistical practice in high-throughput screening data analysis. Nat Biotechnol 24(2):167–175. doi:10.1038/nbt1186

12. Zhang XD, Yang XC, Chung N, Gates A, Stec E, Kunapuli P, Holder DJ, Ferrer M, Espeseth AS (2006) Robust statistical methods for hit selection in RNA interference high-throughput screening experiments. Pharmacogenomics 7(3):299–309. doi:10.2217/14622416.7.3.299

13. Konig R, Chiang CY, Tu BP, Yan SF, DeJesus PD, Romero A, Bergauer T, Orth A, Krueger U, Zhou Y, Chanda SK (2007) A probability-based approach for the analysis of large-scale RNAi screens. Nat Methods 4(10):847–849. doi:10.1038/nmeth1089

14. Chung N, Zhang XD, Kreamer A, Locco L, Kuan PF, Bartz S, Linsley PS, Ferrer M, Strulovici B (2008) Median absolute deviation to improve hit selection for genome-scale RNAi screens. J Biomol Screen 13(2):149–158. doi:10.1177/1087057107312035

15. Zhang XD (2011) Optimal high-throughput screening: practical experimental design and data analysis for genome-scale RNAi research. Cambridge University Press, Cambridge

16. Vaux DL, Fidler F, Cumming G (2012) Replicates and repeats—what is the difference and is it significant? A brief discussion of statistics and experimental design. EMBO Rep 13(4):291–296. doi:10.1038/embor.2012.36

17. Boutros M, Ahringer J (2008) The art and design of genetic screens: RNA interference. Nat Rev Genet 9(7):554–566. doi:10.1038/nrg2364

18. Birmingham A, Selfors LM, Forster T, Wrobel D, Kennedy CJ, Shanks E, Santoyo-Lopez J, Dunican DJ, Long A, Kelleher D, Smith Q, Beijersbergen RL, Ghazal P, Shamu CE (2009) Statistical methods for analysis of high-throughput RNA interference screens. Nat Methods 6(8):569–575. doi:10.1038/nmeth.1351

19. Zhang XD (2007) A pair of new statistical parameters for quality control in RNA interference high-throughput screening assays. Genomics 89(4):552–561. doi:10.1016/j.ygeno.2006.12.014

20. Zhang XD (2008) Novel analytic criteria and effective plate designs for quality control in genome-scale RNAi screens. J Biomol Screen 13(5):363–377. doi:10.1177/1087057108317062

21. Zhang JH, Chung TD, Oldenburg KR (1999) A simple statistical parameter for use in evaluation and validation of high throughput screening assays. J Biomol Screen 4(2):67–73

22. Zhang XD (2011) Illustration of SSMD, z score, SSMD*, z* score, and t statistic for hit selection in RNAi high-throughput screens. J Biomol Screen 16(7):775–785. doi:10.1177/1087057111405851

23. Rieber N, Knapp B, Eils R, Kaderali L (2009) RNAither, an automated pipeline for the statistical analysis of high-throughput RNAi screens. Bioinformatics 25(5):678–679. doi:10.1093/bioinformatics/btp014

24. Pelz O, Gilsdorf M, Boutros M (2010) web cellHTS2: a web-application for the analysis of high-throughput screening data. BMC Bioinformatics 11:185. doi:10.1186/1471-2105-11-185

25. Goktug AN, Ong SS, Chen T (2012) GUItars: a GUI tool for analysis of high-throughput RNA interference screening data. PLoS One 7(11), e49386. doi:10.1371/journal.pone.0049386

26. Zhang XD, Lacson R, Yang R, Marine SD, McCampbell A, Toolan DM, Hare TR, Kajdas J, Berger JP, Holder DJ, Heyse JF, Ferrer M (2010) The use of SSMD-based false discovery and false nondiscovery rates in genome-scale RNAi screens. J Biomol Screen 15(9):1123–1131. doi:10.1177/1087057110381919

27. Tiedemann RE, Zhu YX, Schmidt J, Yin H, Shi CX, Que Q, Basu G, Azorsa D, Perkins LM, Braggio E, Fonseca R, Bergsagel PL, Mousses S, Stewart AK (2010) Kinome-wide RNAi studies in human multiple myeloma identify vulnerable kinase targets, including a lymphoid-restricted kinase, GRK6. Blood 115(8):1594–1604. doi:10.1182/blood-2009-09-243980

28. Arora S, Bisanz KM, Peralta LA, Basu GD, Choudhary A, Tibes R, Azorsa DO (2010) RNAi screening of the kinome identifies modulators of cisplatin response in ovarian cancer cells. Gynecol Oncol 118(3):220–227. doi:10.1016/j.ygyno.2010.05.006

29. Karlas A, Machuy N, Shin Y, Pleissner KP, Artarini A, Heuer D, Becker D, Khalil H, Ogilvie LA, Hess S, Maurer AP, Muller E, Wolff T, Rudel T, Meyer TF (2010) Genome-wide RNAi screen identifies human host factors crucial for influenza virus replication. Nature 463(7282):818–822. doi:10.1038/nature08760

30. Dobbelaere J, Josue F, Suijkerbuijk S, Baum B, Tapon N, Raff J (2008) A genome-wide RNAi screen to dissect centriole duplication and centrosome maturation in Drosophila. PLoS Biol 6(9), e224. doi:10.1371/journal.pbio.0060224

31. Zhang XD (2007) A new method with flexible and balanced control of false negatives and false positives for hit selection in RNA interference high-throughput screening assays. J Biomol Screen 12(5):645–655. doi:10.1177/1087057107300645

32. Zhang XD, Ferrer M, Espeseth AS, Marine SD, Stec EM, Crackower MA, Holder DJ, Heyse JF, Strulovici B (2007) The use of strictly standardized mean difference for hit selection in primary RNA interference high-throughput screening experiments. J Biomol Screen 12(4):497–509. doi:10.1177/1087057107300646

33. Gagarin A, Makarenkov V, Zentilli P (2006) Using clustering techniques to improve hit selection in high-throughput screening. J Biomol Screen 11(8):903–914. doi:10.1177/1087057106293590

34. Nickles D, Falschlehner C, Metzig M, Boutros M (2012) A genome-wide RNA interference screen identifies caspase 4 as a factor required for tumor necrosis factor alpha signaling. Mol Cell Biol 32(17):3372–3381. doi:10.1128/MCB.06739-11

35. Arora S, Gonzales IM, Hagelstrom RT, Beaudry C, Choudhary A, Sima C, Tibes R, Mousses S, Azorsa DO (2010) RNAi phenotype profiling of kinases identifies potential therapeutic targets in Ewing's sarcoma. Mol Cancer 9:218. doi:10.1186/1476-4598-9-218

36. Fisher KH, Wright VM, Taylor A, Zeidler MP, Brown S (2012) Advances in genome-wide RNAi cellular screens: a case study using the Drosophila JAK/STAT pathway. BMC Genomics 13:506. doi:10.1186/1471-2164-13-506

37. Whitehurst AW, Bodemann BO, Cardenas J, Ferguson D, Girard L, Peyton M, Minna JD, Michnoff C, Hao W, Roth MG, Xie XJ, White MA (2007) Synthetic lethal screen identification of chemosensitizer loci in cancer cells. Nature 446(7137):815–819. doi:10.1038/nature05697

38. Yu J, Putcha P, Califano A, Silva JM (2013) Pooled shRNA screenings: computational analysis. Methods Mol Biol 980:371–384. doi:10.1007/978-1-62703-287-2_22

39. Quackenbush J (2002) Microarray data normalization and transformation. Nat Genet 32 Suppl:496–501. doi:10.1038/ng1032

40. Sims D, Mendes-Pereira AM, Frankum J, Burgess D, Cerone MA, Lombardelli C, Mitsopoulos C, Hakas J, Murugaesu N, Isacke CM, Fenwick K, Assiotis I, Kozarewa I, Zvelebil M, Ashworth A, Lord CJ (2011) High-throughput RNA interference screening using pooled shRNA libraries and next generation sequencing. Genome Biol 12(10):R104. doi:10.1186/gb-2011-12-10-r104

41. Marcotte R, Brown KR, Suarez F, Sayad A, Karamboulas K, Krzyzanowski PM, Sircoulomb F, Medrano M, Fedyshyn Y, Koh JL, van Dyk D, Fedyshyn B, Luhova M, Brito GC, Vizeacoumar FJ, Vizeacoumar FS, Datti A, Kasimer D, Buzina A, Mero P, Misquitta C, Normand J, Haider M, Ketela T, Wrana JL, Rottapel R, Neel BG, Moffat J (2012) Essential gene profiles in breast, pancreatic, and ovarian cancer cells. Cancer Discov 2(2):172–189. doi:10.1158/2159-8290.CD-11-0224

42. Kimura J, Nguyen ST, Liu H, Taira N, Miki Y, Yoshida K (2008) A functional genome-wide RNAi screen identifies TAF1 as a regulator for apoptosis in response to genotoxic stress. Nucleic Acids Res 36(16):5250–5259. doi:10.1093/nar/gkn506

43. Diehl P, Tedesco D, Chenchik A (2014) Use of RNAi screens to uncover resistance mechanisms in cancer cells and identify synthetic lethal interactions. Drug Discov Today Technol 11:11–18. doi:10.1016/j.ddtec.2013.12.002

44. Gobeil S, Zhu X, Doillon CJ, Green MR (2008) A genome-wide shRNA screen identifies GAS1 as a novel melanoma metastasis suppressor gene. Genes Dev 22(21):2932–2940. doi:10.1101/gad.1714608

45. Gazin C, Wajapeyee N, Gobeil S, Virbasius CM, Green MR (2007) An elaborate pathway required for Ras-mediated epigenetic silencing. Nature 449(7165):1073–1077. doi:10.1038/nature06251

46. Turner NC, Lord CJ, Iorns E, Brough R, Swift S, Elliott R, Rayter S, Tutt AN, Ashworth A (2008) A synthetic lethal siRNA screen identi-fying genes mediating sensitivity to a PARP inhibitor. EMBO J 27(9):1368–1377. doi:10.1038/emboj.2008.61

47. Bogenberger JM, Kornblau SM, Pierceall WE, Lena R, Chow D, Shi CX, Mantei J, Ahmann G, Gonzales IM, Choudhary A, Valdez R, Camoriano J, Fauble V, Tiedemann RE, Qiu YH, Coombes KR, Cardone M, Braggio E, Yin H, Azorsa DO, Mesa RA, Stewart AK, Tibes R (2014) BCL-2 family proteins as 5-Azacytidine-sensitizing targets and determinants of response in myeloid malignancies. Leukemia 28(8):1657–1665. doi:10.1038/leu.2014.44

48. Azorsa DO, Gonzales IM, Basu GD, Choudhary A, Arora S, Bisanz KM, Kiefer JA, Henderson MC, Trent JM, Von Hoff DD, Mousses S (2009) Synthetic lethal RNAi screening identifies sensitizing targets for gemcitabine therapy in pancreatic cancer. J Transl Med 7:43. doi:10.1186/1479-5876-7-43

49. Ye F, Bauer JA, Pietenpol JA, Shyr Y (2012) Analysis of high-throughput RNAi screening data in identifying genes mediating sensitivity to chemotherapeutic drugs: statistical approaches and perspectives. BMC Genomics 13 Suppl 8:S3. doi:10.1186/1471-2164-13-S8-S3

50. Zhu YX, Tiedemann R, Shi CX, Yin H, Schmidt JE, Bruins LA, Keats JJ, Braggio E, Sereduk C, Mousses S, Stewart AK (2011) RNAi screen of the druggable genome identifies modulators of proteasome inhibitor sensitivity in myeloma including CDK5. Blood 117(14):3847–3857. doi:10.1182/blood-2010-08-304022

51. Harradine KA, Kassner M, Chow D, Aziz M, Von Hoff DD, Baker JB, Yin H, Pelham RJ (2011) Functional genomics reveals diverse cellular processes that modulate tumor cell response to oxaliplatin. Mol Cancer Res 9(2):173–182. doi:10.1158/1541-7786.MCR-10-0412

52. Kumar P, Goh G, Wongphayak S, Moreau D, Bard F (2013) ScreenSifter: analysis and visualization of RNAi screening data. BMC Bioinformatics 14:290. doi:10.1186/1471-2105-14-290

INDEX

David O. Azorsa, Shilpi Arora (eds.), *High-Throughput RNAi Screening: Methods and Protocols*, Methods in Molecular Biology,
vol. 1470, DOI 10.1007/978-1-4939-6337-9, © Springer Science+Business Media New York 2016

Printed in the United States
By Bookmasters